G. B. Bradač R. Ferszt B. E. Kendall (Eds.)

Cranial Meningiomas

Diagnosis – Biology – Therapy

With the Collaboration of
A. Riva W. Schörner J. Stevens D. G. T. Thomas
A. R. Walsh

With 150 Figures in 457 Separate Illustrations

Springer-Verlag Berlin Heidelberg New York
London Paris Tokyo Hong Kong

Professor Dr. Gianni Boris Bradač
Università di Torino
Ospedale Molinette
Via Cherasco 15
I-10126 Torino, Italy

Professor Dr. Ron Ferszt
Institut für Neuropathologie
und Psychiatrische Poliklinik
Universitätsklinikum Steglitz
Freie Universität Berlin
Hindenburgdamm 30
D-1000 Berlin 45
Federal Republic of Germany

Professor Dr. Brian E. Kendall
The National Hospital
Queens Square
London WC1N 3BG, UK

ISBN-13: 978-3-642-72583-8 e-ISBN-13: 978-3-642-72581-4
DOI: 10.1007/978-3-642-72581-4

Library of Congress Cataloging-in-Publication Data
Cranial meningiomas : diagnosis, biology, therapy / G. B. Bradač, R. Ferszt, B. Kendall (eds.) : with the collaboration of A. Riva ... [et al.]. p. cm. Includes bibliographical references.

1. Meningioma. I. Bradač, G. B. (Gianni Boris), 1939- . II. Ferszt, R. III. Kendall, Brian E. [DNLM: 1. Brain Neoplasms. 2. Meningioma-diagnosis. 3. Meningioma-therapy. WL 358 C891] RC280.M4C73 1990 616.99'281-dc20 DNLM/DLC for Library of Congress 89-26254 CIP

Softcover reprint of the hardcover 1st edition 1990

2127/3145-543210 - Printed on acid-free paper

Contents

List of Contributors

Gianni Boris Bradač, MD
Neurologist and Radiologist, Professor of Neuroradiology, Head of the Neuroradiological Department, University of Turin, Ospedale Molinette, Via Cherasco 15, 10126 Torino, Italy

Ron Ferszt, MD
Professor of Neuropathology, Consultant in Psychiatry, Universitätsklinikum Steglitz, Free University of Berlin, Hindenburgdamm 30, 1000 Berlin 45, Federal Republic of Germany

Brian E. Kendall, FRCP, FRCR
Director of Radiology, The National Hospital, Queen Square, London WC1N 3BG, UK

Antonio Riva, MD
Neurologist and Radiologist, Assistant in the Neuroradiological Department, University of Turin, Ospedale Molinette, Via Cherasco 15, 10126 Torino, Italy

Wolfgang Schörner, MD
Radiologist, Associate Professor in the Radiological Department, Klinikum Rudolf Virchow, Free University of Berlin, Spandauer Damm 130, 1000 Berlin 19, Federal Republic of Germany

John Stevens, FRCR
Consultant Radiologist, The National Hospital, Queen Square, London WC1N 3BG, UK

D. G. T. Thomas, MA, FRCP (Glas), FRCS (Edin)
Consultant and Senior Lecturer, Gough Cooper Department of Neurological Surgery, The National Hospitals, Queen Square and Maida Vale, London WC1, UK

A. R. Walsh, MA, MB, FRCS
Senior Registrar Neurosurgery, The National Hospitals, Queen Square, London WC1, UK

Introduction

Since the basic work of Cushing and Eisenhardt [67] about 50 years ago, many studies of mengiomas have been made. The aim of this further monograph is to describe the current approach to meningiomas on the basis of older, established and more recent experience in the fields of histopathology, biology, radiology and surgery.

The book contains three parts. The first part (Chaps. 1-5) deals with general diagnostic aspects. Typical histopathological features of meningiomas and the various abnormalities shown by imaging methods are discussed. Emphasis is placed on atypical findings which may cause difficulty in diagnosis and/or influence prognosis. Finally, some biological and histochemical aspects as well as possible aetiological factors of meningiomas are described.

The second, more specialized part (Chaps. 6-12) deals with the growth pattern of meningiomas arising in various locations. The value of radiological methods in demonstrating the tumours and in establishing differential diagnosis is described. Separate chapters are devoted to particular aspects of meningioma and to peritumoral oedema.

The third part (Chaps. 13 and 14) deals with the treatment of meningiomas. Surgical removal of these tumours remains the basic therapy. Adjuvant methods include the techniques of preoperative embolization, radiation and endocrine therapy.

G. B. Bradač
R. Ferszt
B. E. Kendall

1 Meningiomas: A Clinico-Pathological Synopsis

1.1 Epidemiology, Frequency, Sex and Age Predominance

Meningiomas are frequent benign growths derived from the arachnoid cells on the inner surface of the dura mater. The cells of origin of meningiomas are most abundant in arachnoid villi, and meningiomas therefore tend to arise where these structures are most frequent.

1.1.1 Frequency

It is difficult to assess precisely the incidence of meningiomas and their frequency among the primary CNS neoplasms. The annual incidence rate for primary CNS tumours has been estimated at 10–12 per 100000 standard population. In the study of Codd and Kurland [61a] meningiomas were more frequent than gliomas. This prevalence was probably due to the high incidence of asymptomatic tumours found at autopsy particularly in the elderly. In more selected surveys, meningiomas accounted for 13%–18% of primary CNS tumours [67–309a].

1.1.2 Preponderance in Women, Meningiomas in Children and Infants

There is general agreement on the preponderance of meningiomas in women, with a ratio of 2:1. This varies, depending on the meningioma type and location. In children and adolescents, meningiomas form only 1%–2% of all intracranial tumours [4, 68, 155, 192], and the sexes are equally affected. Meningiomas are very rare in children younger than 1 year old [5, 172], and prognosis is worse than that of meningiomas in general; sarcomatous changes are reported to be very frequent [155, 165].

1.1.3 Age Predominance

Clinically meningiomas present more frequently with increasing age: typically the tumours are seen in the fifth decade of life and later. However, with increasing availability of CT and MRI, more meningiomas are discovered as casual radiological findings in patients with unrelated neurological symptoms, and this may well influence the age distribution.

Table 1. Classification of meningiomas by location

Anterior cranial fossa	1. Crista galli meningioma 2. Olfactorius groove meningioma 3. Planum sphenoidale meningioma 4. Tuberculum sellae meningioma 5. Dorsum sellae meningioma 6. Orbital roof meningioma
Middle cranial fossa	1. Sphenoid wing meningioma 2. Cavernous sinus meningioma 3. Meningioma of Meckel's cave 4. Temporobasal meningioma
Tentorial meningioma	1. Medial tentorial meningioma 2. Lateral tentorial meningioma 3. Falx tentorial meningioma
Posterior cranial fossa	1. Meningioma of posterior surface of petrous bone 2. Clivus meningioma 3. Foramen magnum meningioma 4. Cerebellar convexity meningioma
Convexity meningioma	
Parasagittal – falx meningioma	
Intraventricular meningioma	1. Meningioma of lateral ventricles 2. Meningioma of the third and fourth ventricles
Primary orbital meningioma	
Ectopic meningioma	1. Meningioma of skull, paranasal, sinuses, neck etc.
Metastasizing meningiomas	

Russell and Rubinstein [236] noted that as incidental autopsy findings, meningiomas tend to become much less frequent in the very old. This corroborates our own observations of a series of patients in the 9th and 10th decade of life randomly selected from a large autopsy series, in which not a single incidental meningioma was found. It may be that this "survivor population" is resistant to these tumours or, more probably, that meningioma formation is initiated during a certain period of life which has an upper limit, and that the tumours become clinically apparent before the 9th decade is reached.

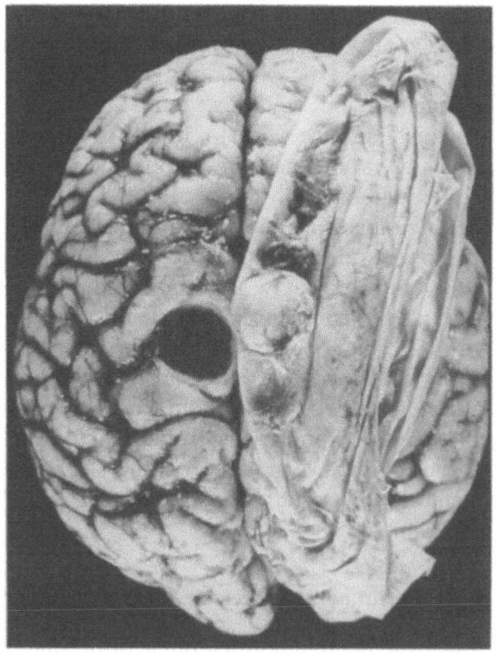

Fig. 1.1. Convexity meningioma still adhering to the dura. Note the sharply defined tumour-brain interface

1.2 Localization

With notable exceptions, meningiomas tend to grow slowly. Histological evaluation does not always reflect the biological activity of the tumour; the clinical symptoms and the outcome of treatment are often determined by location and therefore accessibility. For these reasons, it has proven useful to classify meningiomas according to their site of origin, as, for example, in Table 1.1.

1.3 Gross Pathology

1.3.1 Surface

Meningiomas tend to be round (Fig. 1.1) or, sometimes, lobulated, well-demarcated tumours, with a generally smooth surface. An important exception are en plaque meningiomas; here the tumour is a carpetlike, flat mass which may interdigitate with an underlying cerebral cortex. The latter are found more frequently on the posterior surface of the sphenoid wing, the lateral wall of the cavernous sinus, the frontobasal region and the posterior surface of petrous bone.

1.3.2 Sectioning

The cut surface usually varies in colour from yellow to white; sometimes it is mottled red (Fig. 1.2). The variation is due to lipid storage in some tumour

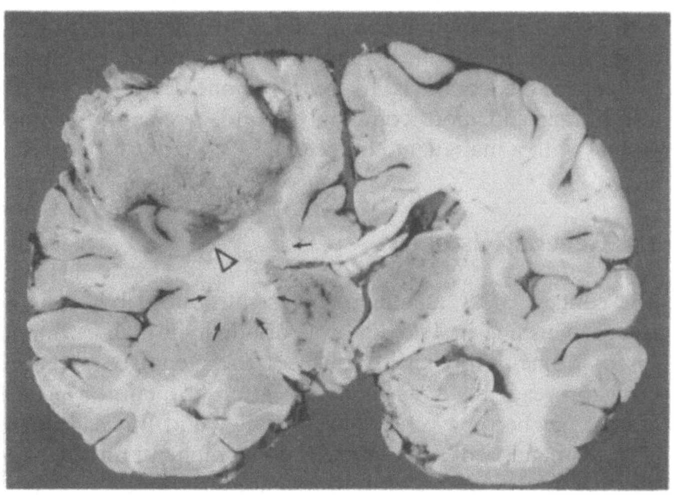

Fig. 1.2. Large convexity meningioma with dura detached. Note mottled appearance of tumour tissue. Cortex adjacent to the tumour is destroyed and partly necrotic *(arrowhead)*. The tumour is in contact with the white matter. There ist some peritumoral edema *(arrows)* with shift of the midline structures

cells, the amount of collagen formation, the degree of vascularity and the prominence of haemorrhagic changes. One type of tumour, sometimes classified as haemangiopericytoma, tends to have a red-brownish surface due to multiple microhaemorrhages of varying age; this is unusual in other types of meningiomas.

Meningiomas may necrose, undergo fatty degeneration, and form cysts. Calcification is frequent and, if disseminated, may give the tumour a gritty appearance. In some tumours, calcification progresses with age; highly calcified growths may be as hard as stone. All these features are responsible for the inhomogeneity of the tumour visible at autopsy as well as on CT and MRI. In particular, low density regions on the CT may represent cysts, necrosis, old haemorrhage or fatty degeneration [236, 237] (see also Chaps. 3, 6).

1.3.3 Peritumoral Effects

It is probable that meningiomas primarily affect the brain by simple compression. This may lead to regional thickening of the pia-arachnoid membrane, recurring microcirculatory failure, edema and, eventually, atrophy of the cortex. Cortical destruction is an important peritumoral event, as cortical tissue and the subcortical U fibres tend to prevent the spreading of edema to the white matter (see Chap. 12).

Even in patients not operated on prior to autopsy, widespread peritumoral necrosis may be found. These softenings are usually relatively fresh and related to microcirculatory failure some days or weeks prior to death.

Sometimes meningioma can infiltrate brain parenchyma, and this is frequently a sign of malignancy, though a slight degree of infiltration is compatible with a benign, slowly growing tumour. Infiltration of dura and bone with hyperostosis is typical and frequent in meningiomas. In contrast, bone destruction is rare and more commonly found in meningiomas with a malignant character.

1.4 General Histology

The concept of a "meningioma" as introduced by Harvey Cushing in 1922 [66] was originally a macroscopic one, implying a growth of the meninges. Over the years, histological classification of meningiomas has become controversial: Bailey and Bucy [12] distinguished nine types, depending upon whether fibres, blood vessels, psammoma bodies, bone formation or pigment-bearing cells were present. Cushing and Eisenhardt's [67] histological classification was even more ramified. Courville [64], Kernohan and Sayre [147], Russell and Rubinstein [236], as well as Zülch [309, 309a] gave further classifications, leading to the WHO system used by most pathologists. The current WHO classification differentiates:

- Meningiotheliomatous meningiomas (synonyms: endotheliomatous meningiomas, meningiothelial meningiomas, leptomeningiomas)
- Fibrous meningiomas (synonyms: fibromatous meningiomas, fibroblastic meningiomas, durofibroblastomas)
- Transitional or mixed meningiomas
- Psammomatous meningiomas
- Angiomatous m.
- Haemangioblastic m. } Angioblastic m.
- Haemangiopericytic m. } Angioblastic m.
- Papillary meningiomas
- Anaplastic or malignant meningiomas

To the nonhistologist even this scheme may be bewildering, and there are limits to the clinical usefulness of these detailed histological classifications. From a practical point of view, the localization of the tumour is at least as important in determining clinical symptoms, operability and, ultimately, prognosis.

The histological problem is to assess the rate of growth and recurrence from certain general parameters, such as polymorphism, rate of mitoses and necrotic tissue breakdown.

1.4.1 Meningiotheliomatous Meningiomas

Meningiotheliomatous meningiomas have a characteristic, highly cellular structure made up of compact islands of tissue separated by a three-dimensional network of collagen and reticulin fibres (Fig. 1.3). The intercellular tissue in individual islands is very sparse. The tumour cells are usually packed into sheets or strands. The cell nuclei are large, often oval and sometimes have indentations. As the cell cytoplasm is at least slightly eosinophilic, these indentations may resemble nuclear inclusions. The chromatin tends to be loosely arranged and somewhat condensed at the nuclear membrane. Small, dark pyknotic nuclei may also appear, and the number of mitoses may vary considerably; however, atypical or explosive mitoses are rare in meningiotheliomatous meningiomas. Eosinophilic inclusions in the cytoplasm of meningioma cells also occur in about 1 in 20 tumours. These inclusions

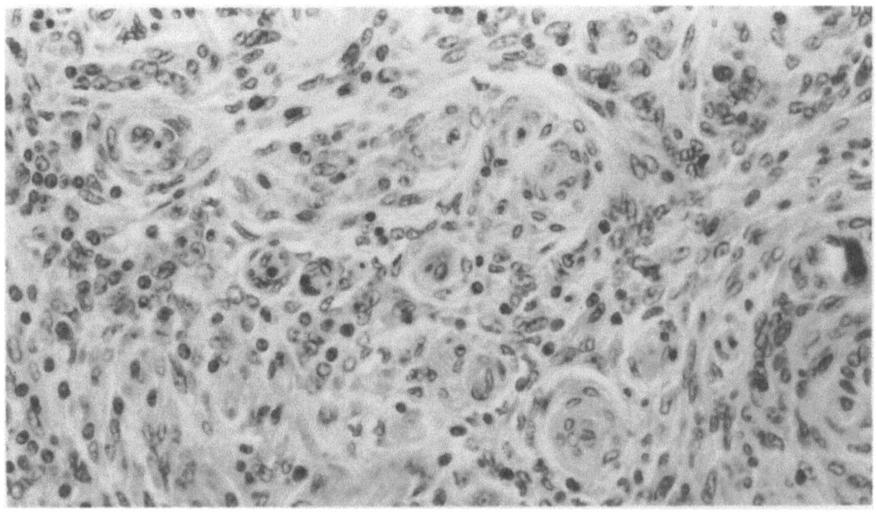

Fig. 1.3. Meningiotheliomatous meningioma. Highly cellular tumour with typical whorl-like concentrical arrangement of tumour cells (H. E. stain, ×160)

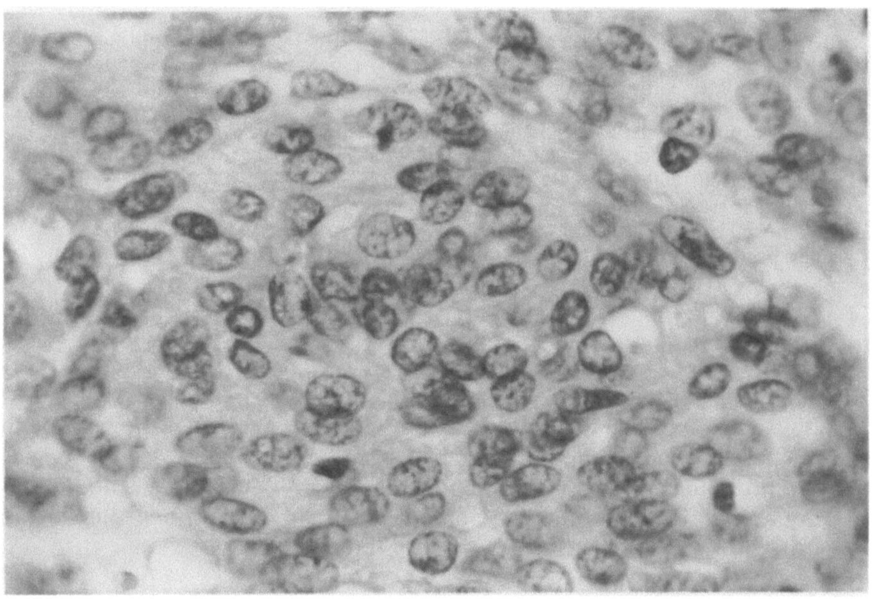

Fig. 1.4. Typical foamy nuclei of meningiotheliomatous meningioma. Note that the cytoplasms form a pale homogeneous background with ill-defined cell borders (H. E. stain, ×100)

are made up of a PAS-positive glycoprotein formed by the tumour cells.

The cytoplasmic borders of the tumour cells may often elude light microscopy (Fig. 1.4). Under the electron microscope (Fig. 1.5), cytoplasmic indentations with junctional complexes between tumour cells are quite frequent. Within the islands, the cells tend to assume a whorl-like arrangement (Fig. 1.6a). The centre of the whorl may become hyalinized. With the deposition of mineral salts in these hyalinized central areas of a whorl, sandlike or psammoma bodies are formed (Fig. 1.6b–c). Kubota et al. [157] did an excellent electron microscopic study of the fine structure of psammoma bodies around blood vessels in meningioma. It seems that meningiocytic cells invest the outer aspect of the blood vessels, which are constituted by multilayered basal lamina, collagen fibres, microfibrils and pericytes. The perivascular space may contain remnants of degenerated cells. X-ray microanalysis gives evidence for the presence of both calcium and phosphorous in psammoma bodies. Psammoma body formation in the meningiocytic whorls then represents degeneration of centrally localized mesenchymal cells, producing cell debris which calcifies and, subsequently, the mineralization process may extend to neighbouring connective tissue fibres.

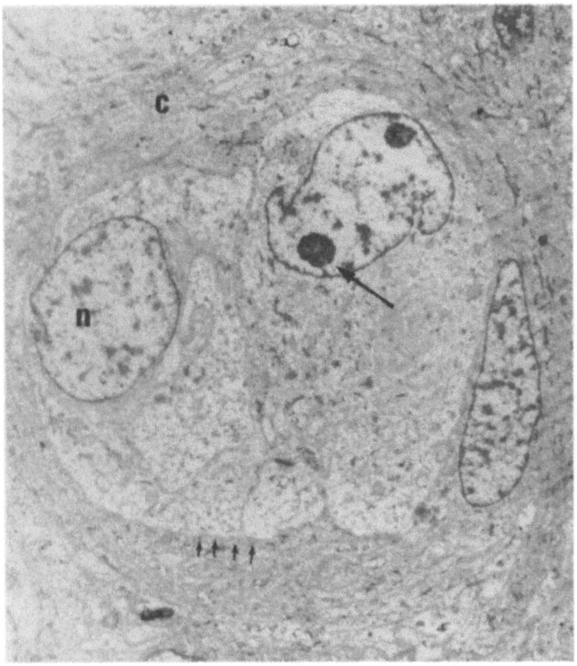

Fig. 1.5. Two tumour cells in meningiotheliomatous meningioma. Nucleus(n). Note slight nuclear indentations and prominent nucleoli *(long arrow)*. At the ultrastructural level the cell borders are clearly visible *(short arrows)*. Both tumour cells are embedded in a dense feltwork of collagen fibres *(c)* (Original magnification, ×6600)

1.4.2 Fibrous Meningiomas

Fibrous meningiomas differ from the meningiotheliomatous type and histologically tend to resemble fibroma (Fig. 1.7). The tumour cells are spindle shaped and lie loosely next to one another, tending to produce pallisadelike structures. Some degree of whorls and psammoma bodies is also present. The tumour cells are embedded in an extensive network of collagen fibres; these tend to form hyalinelike masses, which may calcify. As a rule, fibromatous meningiomas are less vascular and quite often less cellular than the meningiotheliomatous type. Oedema is less frequent and extensive around this type of tumour.

1.4.3 Transitional Meningiomas

Those meningiomas incorporating features of both the meningiotheliomatous and fibromatous types are transitional. They tend to form whorls of banana-shaped cells compactly layered, forming onionlike structures. The centres of these structures may undergo necrobiosis, and psammoma bodies may be formed.

1.4.4 Psammomatous Meningiomas

Psammomatous meningiomas form abundant psammoma bodies. They occur most often on the dorsal aspect of the thoracic spinal cord and on the skull base.

1.4.5 Vascularization

Vascularization varies considerably from one tumour to another and, also, in different regions within a single tumour. In many tumours the periphery is somewhat more vascular than the central part and often the base of the tumour, which transmits feeding vessels, is very vascular.
Meningiomas do not have a barrier between the lumen of their blood vessels and the tumour paren-

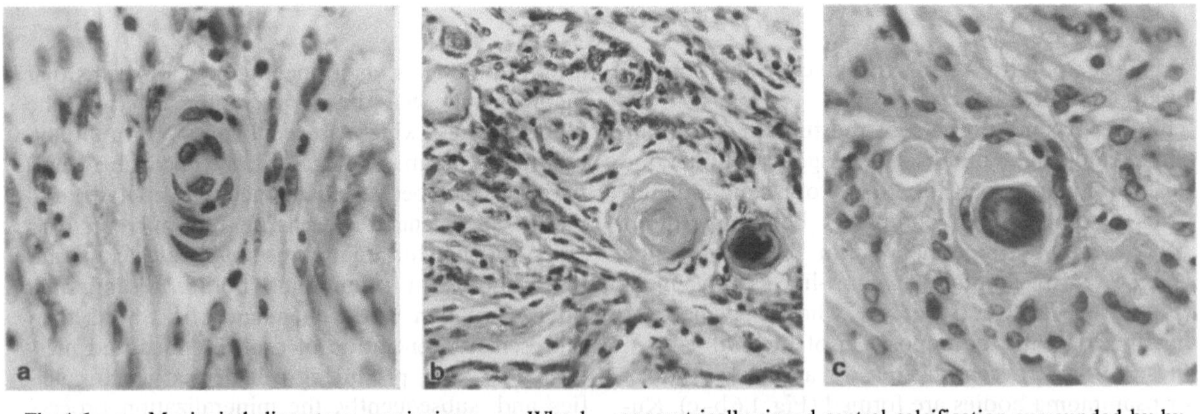

Fig. 1.6a–c. Meningiotheliomatous meningioma. **a** Whorl structure (H. E. stain, ×1000). **b** Various types of psammoma bodies (H. E. stain, ×160). **c** Psammoma body with typical concentrically ringed central calcification surrounded by hyalinized tumour cells (H. E. stain, ×1000)

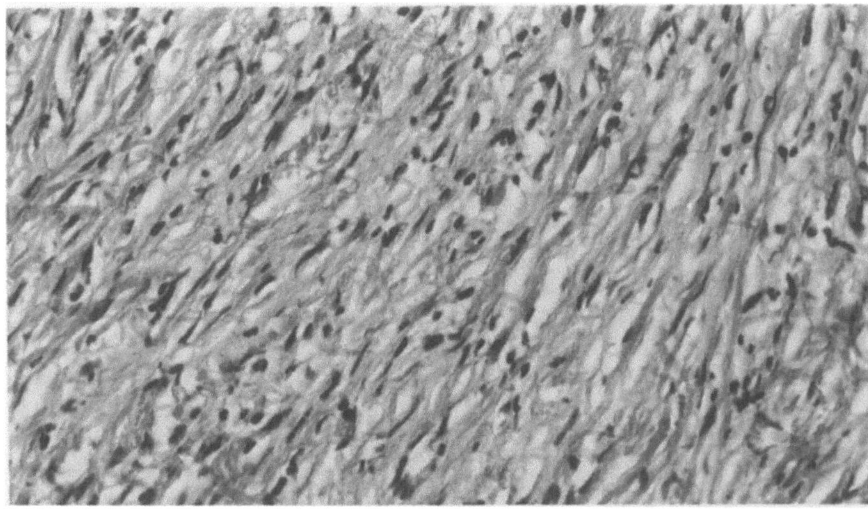

Fig. 1.7. Fibromatous meningioma. Note typical elongated cytoplasms and slitlike nuclei (H. E. stain, ×160)

chyma. A detailed ultrastructural study of these vessels has been made by Long [171] who showed that the lack of such a barrier is due to three factors:

1. Widely open endothelial junctions
2. Marked pinocytotic vesicles in endothelial cytoplasms
3. Fenestrated endothelial cells

Contrast medium can easily pass through the open junctions from vessels into the extracellular space and contribute to the enhancement of the tumour visible on CT (Fig. 1.8a-b).

1.4.6 Highly Vascular Meningiomas

The classification of highly vascular meningiomas is controversial. While most of these meningiomas are clearly derived from arachnoidal cells, some may actually be of vascular origin. Haemangiopericytomas or haemangiopericytic meningiomas (Fig. 1.9) do not differ from haemangiopericytomas elsewhere in the body. In the central nervous system they are compact, solid growths, as a rule attached to the meninges. In contrast to the other meningiomas already mentioned, haemangiopericytomas are more frequent in men and occur at a younger age, often diagnosed in the fourth decade of life. The typical histology is a mass of packed cells with oval or elongated nuclei forming polycystic structures around a multitude of capillaries, giving the impression of an irregularly shaped sponge. Reticulin staining shows fine fibres surrounding either single cells or small islands of tumour cells.

Mitoses, sometimes atypical, are a frequent finding. As a rule there is no infiltration of the surrounding tissue, but they may metastasize. Numerous deposits of iron document their tendency to haemorrhage, which is not common in other types of meningioma. Microhaemorrhages may not be clinically apparent, but profuse bleeding may lead to acute neurological symptoms. Surgical excision may be hampered by haemorrhage; this aspect, and the fact that they belong to the group of malignant meningiomas explain the high frequency of recurrence of these tumours [131, 146].

Nakamura et al. [205] analysed seven intracranial haemangiopericytomas morphologically. Their results suggest that this kind of tumour is a poorly specialized mesenchyma-related growth of the meninges. In vitro, at least some of the cells possess a potential for aggressive growth and some for differentiation into smooth muscle cells.

Peña [219], in an electron microscopic study, found that the tumour cells in haemangiopericytoma did not seem to have the capability of forming junctional complexes, such as desmosomes and gap or other tight junctions present in other types of meningiomas. This may account for the biological differences between the haemangiopericytoma cell and those of other types of meningioma.

However, Holden et al. [120], using immunohistochemical techniques, showed a posistive response for vimentin and partially for keratin in normal arachnoid cells and in meningiomas, including those of haemangiopericytic type. Soft-tissue haemangiopericytomas and normal pericytes were negative for both vimentin and keratin. They concluded that meningeal haemangiopericytoma is a variant of meningioma and not of pericytic origin.

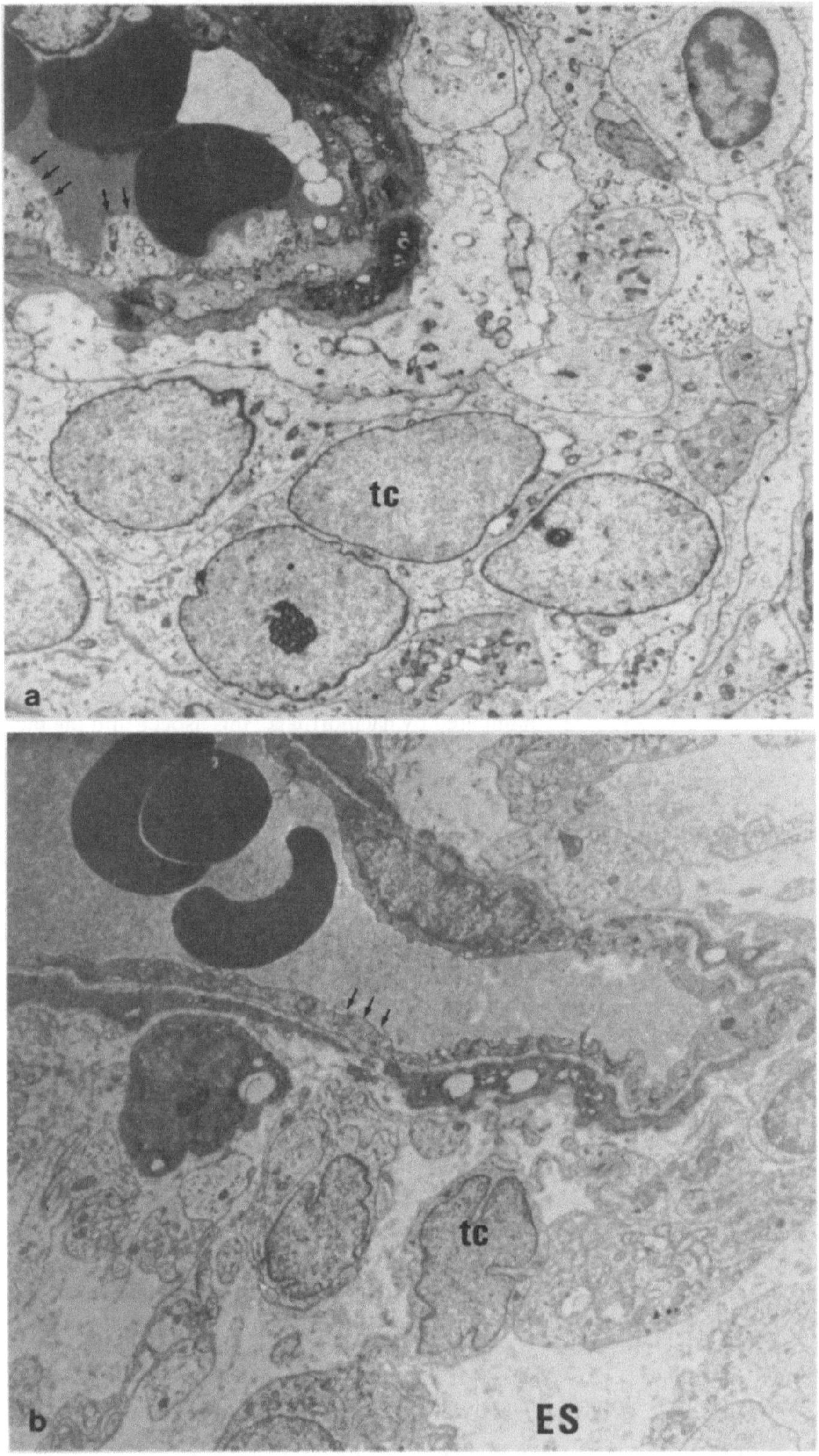

Fig. 1.8 a, b. Venule in meningiotheliomatous meningioma. Erythrocytes are visible in the vessel lumen. Endothelial cells *(arrows)* are swollen and contain pinocytotic vesicles. A compact layer of tumour cells *(tc)* surrounds the vessel (Original magnification, ×4000), courtesy of Prof. I. Cervos-Navarro). **b** Venule in meningiotheliomatous meningioma. Note necrotic endothelial cells *(arrows)*. Tumour cells *(tc)* are loosely arranged in the perivascular extracellular space *(ES)*

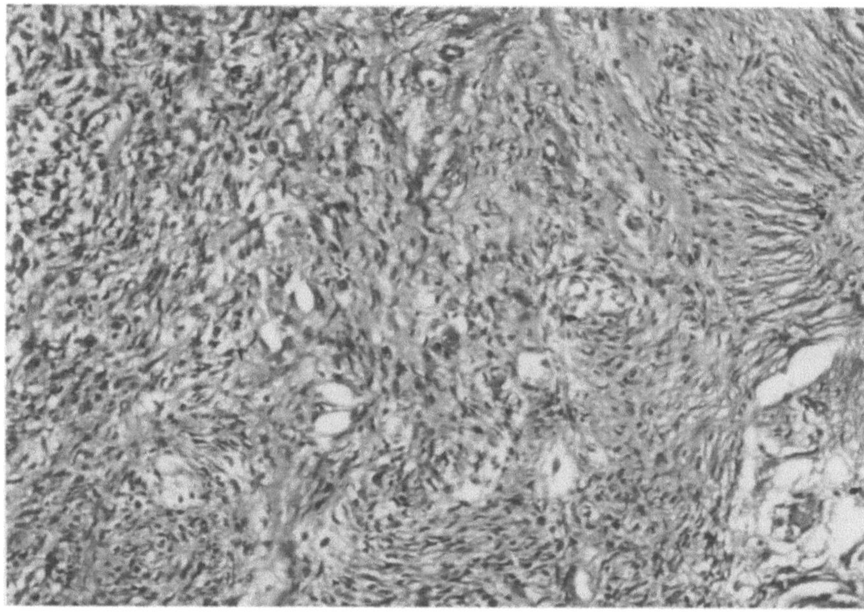

Fig. 1.9. Haemangiopericytoma. Highly cellular tumour with many slitlike small vessels (H. E. stain, ×160)

Finally, examples are documented [145] in which the tumours have morphological features of both of an haemangiopericytoma and an endotheliomatous meningioma. Similar considerations can be made for the haemangioblastic meningiomas. Indeed there are cases where features of an haemangioblastic meningioma are associated with patterns of a capillary haemangioblastoma.

1.4.7 Atypical Features

1.4.7.1 Cystic Meningiomas

Meningioma cysts deserve particular attention since they may cause misinterpretation of diagnostic studies. The frequency of cystlike structures associated with meningiomas varies between 4% and 10% of all the tumours [61, 216, 237].

It is interesting to note that the predominance of women noted in meningiomas in general is reversed in cystic meningiomas, where men are clearly overrepresented. Cystic meningiomas are also comparatively frequent in children [5, 137, 155].

According to Nauta et al. [206] and Worthington et al. [298] five types of cysts can be distinguished:

1. A cyst located centrally and completely surrounded by solid tumour mass.
2. A cyst eccentrically located, but still within the tumour mass.
3. A cyst eccentrically located at the periphery of the tumour with its wall made up of fibrous tissue and nests of tumour cells.
4. A cyst outside the tumour with a capsule of gliotic tissue. According to Worthington et al. [298] this is the most frequently found lesion.
5. A cyst caused by local distension of the subarachnoid space due to disturbance of CSF drainage caused by the tumour.

Although all five types of cystlike structures are associated with meningiomas, only tumours containing cavities of the first three types may be termed cystic meningiomas.

Intratumoral cysts may be caused by degeneration of tumour cells or secretion of fluid by tumour cells, or may be the result of absorption of a haemorrhage into the tumour. Peritumoral cystlike structures evolve in the course of necrosis and gliotic scarring [68, 206, 298]. In some cases cystlike hypodensities in CT can arise from distended extracellular spaces in oedematous brain tissue near the tumour [264]. Finally, loculation of cerebrospinal fluid adjacent to the tumour is also possible.

1.4.7.2 Lipomatous Changes

Kepes [145] described two forms of fatty transformation. One is apparent in the so-called lipoblastic meningiomas, characterized by an accumulation of fat droplets in the cytoplasm of tumour cells. These droplets may become confluent and completely fill the cell body. In the same tumour, varying degrees of fatty degeneration of the meningiothelial cells are observed. Another type of fatty change is seen in the so-called xanthomatous meningiomas in which the lipid material is limited to tiny vacuoles within the cytoplasm. The inhomogeneous feature in CT of these meningiomas can make the differential diagnosis from other lesions difficult (Fig. 11.2).

1.4.7.3 Other Changes

Meningiomas may form bone. The formation of bone in a meningioma is not necessarily related to the intensity of hyperostosis in bone adjacent to the tumour. Cartilage is rare in meningiomas, chondromas and osteochondromas, and chondrosarcomas should be ruled out as well.

Myxomatous changes are also very rare. If they are extensive, differential diagnosis from myxoma of the meninges should be made.

In unoperated and otherwise unmanipulated meningiomas, plasma and lymphocellular infiltrates are also uncommon. This contrasts strikingly to other intracranial tumours, both gliomas and neurinomas. It might be taken to indicate a negligible cellular immunological response of the organism to the tumour.

1.4.8 Papillary Meningiomas - Malignant Meningiomas

While many of the meningiomas with a malignant clinical course, as made manifest by multiple recurrences in spite of apparently total extirpation and postoperative irradiation, are of the haemangiopericytic type, other types of meningioma also may behave in a similar fashion; these are:

1. Papillary meningiomas: as the name suggests, these tumours have a papillary structure and typically show multiple mitoses.
2. Anaplastic or malignant meningiomas: in a stricter sense these are intermediate in position between the classical benign growth classified as Grade I according to WHO, and the meningiosarcomas. Malignant meningiomas have an age curve corresponding to that of benign meningiomas.

Jääskeläinen et al. [126] found malignant meningiomas in 12% of the men and only 4% of the women. The frequency of meningiomas considered malignant on histological grounds varies according to the authors: 1.4% in the series of Jellinger and Slovik [131], 11.1% in that of McCarty and Taylor [190], 5.7% in the material of Jääskeläinen et al. [126].

There are some histological features, such as high cellularity, great number of mitoses, necrosis and invasion of the brain tissue, which may be regarded as potential signs of malignancy [65, 131, 146, 258].

Note: Meningeal Meningiomatosis (Primary meningeal Sarcomatosis). This is a very rare tumoural form characterized by a diffuse involvement of the leptomeninges, without a presence of a circumscribed mass. The tumour can infiltrate the adjacent sulci and brain and histologically corresponds frequently to a sarcoma [236, 309].

1.5 Recurrence

The important aspect of any classification of meningiomas is its value in the assessment of postoperative prognosis in a given patient; the tumours of haemangiopericytic, papillary or anaplastic type tend to be malignant, but, also, meningiomas classified as benign from general histological criteria may recur in up to 27% of patients [191]. There is general agreement that the most important factor determining recurrence is incomplete removal of tumour [2, 14, 32, 191, 200], but recurrence in cases with macroscopically complete extirpation of the tumour, its dural attachment and adjacent bone is documented. Adegbite et al. [2] in review of 114 surgically treated meningiomas over a period of 24 years found recurrence in 22 (19.3%). The grade of initial surgery (total removal or not) was the most important factor for recurrence. The recurrence rate was 18% and 52% 5 years after surgery evaluated respectively as Grade II-IV according to Sympson (see also Chap. 14, Sect. 14.4.1). However, after total removal of the tumour (Grade I) there was still a recurrence rate of 14%. Similar results have been reported more recently by Mirimanoff et al. [200]. The recurrence rate at 5 years was 37% for meningiomas partially resected and 7% for lesions totally removed.

Recently, tumour cell aggregates, in the form of microscopic nodules on the inner surface of the dura mater at a distance of 1-3 cm from the site of attachment of meningiomas, have been demonstrated [30, 31]. This finding corroborates the theory of regional multicentric origin. Resection of a wide area of dura around the tumour should improve surgical results.

Some histological criteria which may influence the prognosis of meningiomas have already been described in Sect. 1.4.8. Recently, a review of the relevance of histopathological data for meningioma prognosis was given by Kepes [146]. He found haemangiopericytomatous patterns, papillary formations, high cellularity, either focal or diffuse, as well as invasion of the brain to correlate with the potentially aggressive behaviour, whereas a large number

of mitoses, prominent nucleoli and cell necroses at least suggest a guarded prognosis. As Kepes [146] must also admit, however, some meningiomas with no detectable histological features of malignancy at all may nevertheless recur and even metastasize. On the other hand, meningiomas with atypical and polymorphic histological character may take a benign clinical course [79, 126].
In a further attempt to attack this dilemma, Iwaki et al. [125] have studied the cell kinetics of meningiomas by means of a bromodesoxyuridine BRDU-uptake examination. BRDU is a thymidine analogue which is incorporated into nuclear DNA. It was given intravenously to 40 patients with meningioma shortly before operation and studied in the nuclei of cells in the resected tumour. The labelling indices of tumour cells of benign meningiomas were usually less than 1%, while in tumours in which a rapid recurrence occurred, the index was much higher, and a high labelling index is considered to be a reliable sign of the risk of recurrence.
Di Chiro et al. [70] investigated glucose metabolism in meningiomas using positron emission tomography (PET). They described a relatively higher rate of glucose metabolism in tumours with rapid recurrence after surgery. High glucose metabolism correlates well with high cellularity and with an increased mitotic rate. Finally, several angiographic and CT findings have been described as possible signs of malignancy. These are discussed in Chaps. 3 and 5.

1.6 Metastasizing Meningiomas

Metastasizing meningiomas are rare: they are estimated to constitute about 0.1% of all meningiomas [261]. This is quite surprising considering the frequency with which the dural sinuses are invaded, and tumour tissue is bordering the cerebrospinal fluid.
In recent reviews [146, 261] less than one third of the metastasizing meningiomas were of the haemangiopericytic and other malignant types, the rest were presumably "benign" meningiomas.
About two thirds of the extracranial metastases are to lung, followed by liver, pleura, lymph nodes, bone and kidneys [135, 198, 261, 280, 288, 299]; the central nervous system is rarely involved [174]. Histologically, the metastases are usually similar, if not identical, to the primary lesion.
Dissemination is usually haematogenous. This accounts for the high incidence of pulmonary seedings: spreading through the cerebrospinal fluid is rare, but does occur (Fig. 1.10) [125, 153, 174].
In relation to metastases, the location and the size of the meningiomas seems to be irrelevant. Surgical intervention has been considered a potentiating factor in the spread of metastases through both blood and CSF, but the evidence is unconvincing [133, 135, 198].

1.7 Multiple Meningiomas

This entity was first described by Cushing and Eisenhardt [67]. Prior to the introduction of CT, the in vivo diagnosis of multiple meningiomas was comparatively infrequent. In vivo visualization gives a frequency of about 8%–9% of all meningiomas, which is remarkably high [176, 255]. It is quite possible that the frequency of multiple meningiomas diagnosed with CT (Figs. 1.11, 1.12) will increase further and might even approach the figure of 16% of all meningiomas, as reported in a study of 100 intracranial meningiomas found incidentally

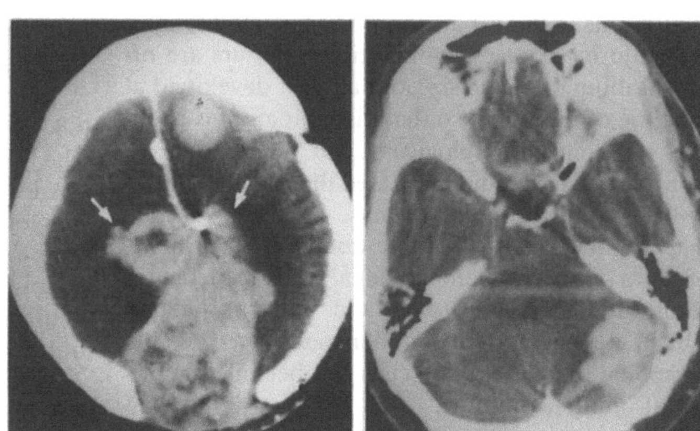

Fig. 1.10. Recurrent and metastasizing haemangiopericytic meningioma. After contrast medium CT shows an evident enhancement of the recurrent tumour in the parasagittal area. There are rounded and finger-like extensions of the tumour at its periphery. In addition, two other lesions not recognizable in previous CT images are visible in the frontal region and in the posterior fossa

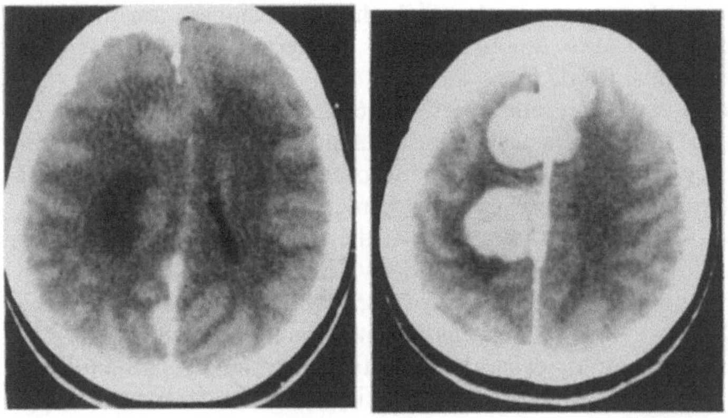

Fig. 1.11. Multiples meningiomas

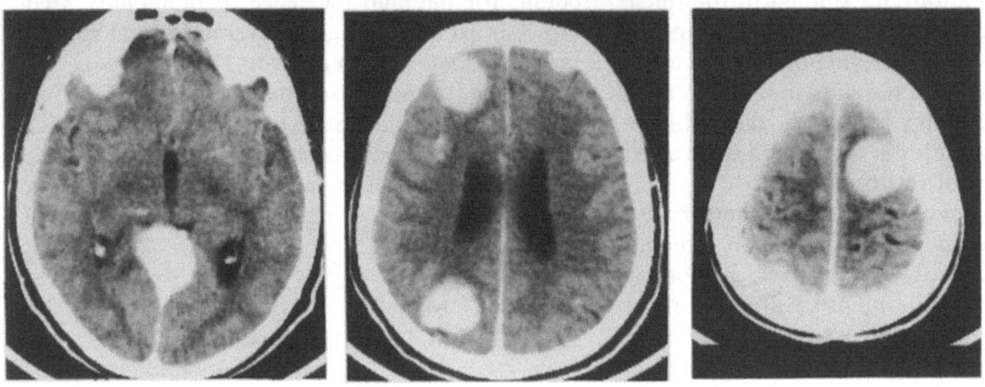

Fig. 1.12. Multiples meningiomas

at necropsy [297]. The predominance of women seems to be greater in multiple meningiomas than in meningiomas in general: in Sheehy and Crockard's study [255], all of the 10 reported patients were women.

Multiple meningiomas may be associated with neurofibromatosis, and some authors [97, 176] suggest that all cases of multiple meningiomas are a variant of that disease. Multiple meningiomas could also be the result of secondary dissemination of meningioma cells in the subarachnoid space. However, in the majority of cases, the multiple tumours are often of about the same size and all well developed at the time of diagnosis, so that dissemination is probably not a major aetiological factor.

Borovich et al. [31] demonstrated the regional multicentric origin of meningiomas. It seems feasible that in patients with multiple tumours, many areas of dura carrying meningothelial cells capable of forming tumours are present and, under influences which are not currently understood, but possibly hormonal in nature, these cells can become the origin of multiple tumours.

1.8 Experimental and Biological Aspects

1.8.1 Aetiological Factors

1.8.1.1 Trauma

The possibility that head trauma may predipose to meningioma formation is controversial; while single case studies seem to indicate a predisposition, more extensive statistical material is not available to prove any significant association between head injury and brain tumour. The same holds true for tuberculosis and irradiation [27, 203, 235, 260].

1.8.1.2 Viruses

The infectious Inoue-Melnick virus (IMV) was present in and isolated from six to seven human meningioma-derived cell cultures, but was not isolated from six other brain tumour cell cultures as reported by Inoue et al. [124]. Sera of 145 consecutive neurosurgical patients were tested for an IMV-neutralizing antibody. Of 26 patients with meningioma, 22 were positive for IMV antibody, of the remaining 119 patients, only 16 were positive. According to the authors mentioned above, continuous production of infectious IMV may be elicited in some meningioma cell cultures. Over 90% of these cultured cells we found to have IMV-associated cytoplasmic antigens. The role of this virus for the promotion or initiation of the disease process remains unclear; even the possibility of a serological test for meningiomas certainly warrants further research.

1.8.2 Histochemical Aspects

Yamashima [301] reported meningiothelial clusters with formation of numerous rosettes observed in the canine subarachnoid space after a single injection of adrenaline. Ultrastructurally, these cell packages were knitted together by numerous functional devices, desmosomelike junctions as well as interdigitations strongly reminiscent of meningiomas.

Chen et al. [57] saw extensive intracellular mucoid changes within tumour cells together with deposits of polyvinyl pyrrolodine (PVP) granules. Both of the patients had received intravenous PVP as a plasma expander. Recipients of PVP are known to develop PVP storage within mesenchymal cells and also exhibit mucoid changes; the findings indicate that the behavioural characteristics of meningioma cells are typical of other mesenchymal cell elements.

Immunohistochemical techniques have been increasingly used in investigating meningiomas, and these will probably be very useful to characterize these tumours in the near future. Collagen-type and noncollagenous glycoproteins such as fibronectin (FN) and laminin (LN) normal components of the extracellular matrix have been demonstrated in certain meningiomas [21, 59, 154, 240]. Other authors [113, 120] have identified in meningiomas vimentin and cytokeratin, two intermediate filament proteins of the cytoskeleton. Schwechheimer et al. [249] showed the association of vimentin with desmosome junctions in all types of meningiomas and in arachnoid cells. This suggests that meningiomas are derived from the arachnoid layer. Rutka et al. [239] have shown that both leptomeningeal cells and meningiomas in vitro can synthesize and secrete several glycoproteins found in the normal extracellular matrix. This similarity supports the notion that meningiomas are indeed derived from arachnoid cells.

In a more recent study on 50 meningiomas, Hitchcock and Morris [117] found FN, vimentin and to a lesser extent cytokeratin in all types of tumours. In addition, other proteins such as Neuron Specific Enolase (NSE) and S100 were demonstrated to varying degrees. The latter might play a role in determining malignancy and recurrence in meningiomas.

1.8.3 Meningiomas Associated with Other Neoplasms

Meningiomas are most frequently associated with glioma [196, 236], but also other lesions such as adenoma, teratoma and melanoma of the choroid plexus have been reported [7, 44, 160]. The association of meningiomas with other primary intracranial tumours may be partly coincidental. However, sometimes meningiomas and other tumours are found in one area, which might lead one to speculate on a common aetiology. The immediate neighbourhood of a meningioma and a glioma can have considerable practical consequences: one of our patients, a 56-year-old woman, presented with focal neurological symptoms which were related to a convexity meningioma visualized in CT. A peritumoral hypodensity was interpreted as oedema, and the meningioma was excised. Some 7 months later, the patient presented with a progressive focal syndrome; the hypodensity underlying the first site of the operation had enlarged. The patient was reoperated, the biopsy diagnosis was astrocytoma, grade II.

1.8.4 Endocrine Effects

Reubi et al. [227] report a high incidence of somatostatin receptors in human meningiomas. This agrees with our own experience and could be of therapeutic interest. The inhibitory effect of somatostatin on meningioma tumour growth has been demonstrated on the proliferation of meningioma cells in vitro [158]. However, one should note that in our series [85], a number of malignant glial tumours also provide some evidence of somatostatin receptors.

Furthermore, the possibility of endocrine influence of meningiomas in vivo is supported by unquestionably higher incidence in women by reports of tumour exacerbation during pregnancy [23] and the frequent association of meningioma with breast and genital cancer in women [15, 128, 247]. Finally, oestrogen and progesterone receptors have been noted in both breast cancer and meningioma. In contrast to breast cancer in which oestrogen receptor positivity is more common, meningiomas are more frequently characterized by a positivity for progesterone. This has been demonstrated in several studies [25, 63, 177, 188, 246, 278, 291, 306].

Markwalder et al. [185] used the anti-oestrogenic agent tamoxifen in the treatment of six patients with meningioma. The 2-year study did not show a positive response to therapy. Also, the use in clinical setting of medroxy progesterone acetate (MPA) which has anti-oestrogenic properties failed to demonstrate positive results [127, 186] (see also Chap. 14).

Jay et al. [130] attempted to assess the effects of estradiol, progesterone and the anti-oestrogen tamoxifen on the growth of meningioma cells in culture. The authors achieved an inhibition of estradiol-induced growth stimulation either by progesterone or tamoxifen in the majority of their cultures, but it remains to be clarified whether these effects are mediated by a hormone receptor or caused by alterations in cell metabolism independent of specific hormone binding. This in vitro technique apparently can be used to study the hormones which biologically effect human meningiomas. More recently the hormone receptor status and the hormone sensitivity have been investigated by Grunberg et al. [105] on specimens of meningioma obtained from 17 patients. This study has confirmed that positivity for progesterone receptor is more common than that for oestrogen receptor. In 40% of the cases with progesterone receptor positivity, growth suppression of meningioma specimens could be achieved with pharmacological levels of progesterone. In tumours such as meningiomas in which progesterone receptors seem to predominate, modulation of progesterone levels with either progestin agonists or antagonists may be a possible therapeutic approach. The inhibitory effect of the antiprogesterone agent RU38486 on meningioma in vitro has been demonstrated by Olson et al. [212].

Finally, androgen receptors [213] have also been reported. Whether endocrine therapy of meningiomas will one day present a realistic alternative to surgery remains to be seen.

2 The Skull X-Ray

2.1 General Observations

The plain skull x-ray has proven more valuable in the diagnosis of meningioma than of any other intracranial neoplasm. A positive diagnosis of meningioma may be made in 30%-50% of patients [274], whereas CT is abnormal in 98.8% [223]. En plaque meningiomas which can be difficult to demonstrate with computed tomography (CT) can now be recognized reliably with magnetic resonance imaging (MRI). Bone changes associated with meningiomas are well demonstrated by high definition CT and often even with MRI. For these reasons the plain skull x-ray has lost most of its importance. However, particularly in nonspecialized centres many patients have plain x-rays as the first diagnostic step and so it remains useful to define briefly the typical radiological signs which can be suggestive of intracranial meningioma. These should lead to more precise investigation with CT or MRI.

2.2 Specific Features

The plain film abnormalities in meningiomas may be grouped into direct and indirect signs. The direct signs are, in descending order of importance, hyperostosis, hypervascularity and tumoral calcification.

2.2.1 Hyperostosis

2.2.1.1 Incidence and Pathogenesis

The incidence of hyperostosis reported radiologically varies, depending upon the localization of the meningioma. It is generally far higher than the 4.5% quoted by Cushing and Eisenhardt in 1938 [67] and endorsed by many pathologists since [236]. Radiologically, incidences of between 23% and 44% are reported overall [149] and for meningiomas involving the sphenoid wings over 90% [28]. The incidence may be higher with endotheliomatous than fibrous lesions [236].

Hyperostosis has been associated with aggregates of tumour cells in the medullary spaces of bone, and it has been suggested that new bone formation is closely linked with the activity of meningioma cells. Biopsy specimens of hyperostotic bone shown radiologically have revealed invasion by tumour cells in some cases, but [28] in others only minimal numbers of meningothelial cells have been identified. Therefore, the extent and severity of radiological hyperostosis bear no relation to the extent of bone invasion, or even its presence, since some of the textural changes and thickening are known to occur in response to local hypervascularity alone [76, 236, 274].

A localized hyperostosis of the inner table often occurs at the site of the vascular pedicle in the base of a meningioma, usually assuming the form of a nipplelike enostosis. This is thought to be caused by detachment of dura from the underlying bone which stimulates subperiosteal bone formation. The bone trabeculae beneath this hyperostosis are usually thin and sparse, the intervening spaces being occupied by large blood vessels, and tumour cells are absent [236].

2.2.1.2 Appearance

The inner table, diploë and outer table all may be involved. The inner table is most frequently affected. Histologically this usually takes the form of multiple lamellae of compact bone parallel to the table, which assumes a denser and thickened appearance on radiographs. Hyperostosis involving only the inner table is most frequent in convexity meningiomas (Fig. 2.1).

Involvement of the diploë may give rise to a poorly circumscribed spongy type of hyperostosis in which the endosteal surfaces become indistinct, especially that of the inner table. Often, however, the spongy appearance of the diploë is lost.

The outer table also is particularly affected where the bone is thin, as in parts of the sphenoid wing [274] (Fig. 2.2; see also Fig. 7.9). In some cases, per-

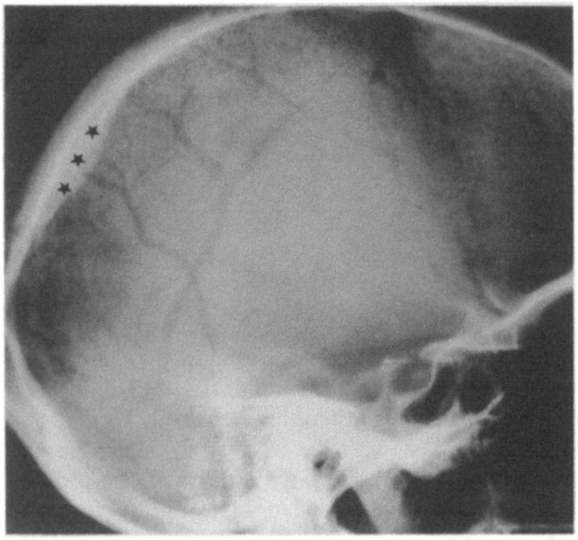

Fig. 2.1. Hyperostosis in convexity meningiomas involving only the inner table *(stars)*

pendicular trabeculae from the outer table are laid down resulting in spicule formation. This pattern typically occurs in convexity and parasagittal meningiomas invading through the vault and into the scalp.

Hyperostosis is usually maximal beneath the centre of the tumour, and tomography may reveal a small exostosis at the site of entry of dural vessels.

2.2.2 Hypervascularity

Enlarged vessels causing enlargement of the vascular grooves, intradiploic channels and nutrient foramina in the skull are a more common finding than hyperostosis in convexity meningiomas. Subtle changes are more easily interpreted in retrospect or when the level of suspicion is heightened due to clinical or other radiological features. The least ambiguous changes are seen in the arterial grooves for the middle meningeal artery on the inner table of the vault because their appearance in normal subjects is more constant than other vascular markings. Suggestive features are increase in size of the grooves, failure to taper distally, tortuosity - especially of confined segments - and visibility of usually invisible branches such as those taking course anterosuperiorly from the anterior division. Although parasagittal lesions may receive dural supply from both sides, significant changes tend to be predominantly unilateral so that comparison with the more normal side is useful. A tendency for more than one arterial groove to converge towards a single region of the vault is sometimes a helpful feature. One large foramen spinosum occurring in isolation is not helpful because of the wide range of normal variation [76, 274].

At the site of tumour attachment, multiple small round lucencies in the inner and outer tables and in the diploë may be present, giving the bone a stippled appearance. The lucencies are usually produced by transcalvarial nutrient vessels derived

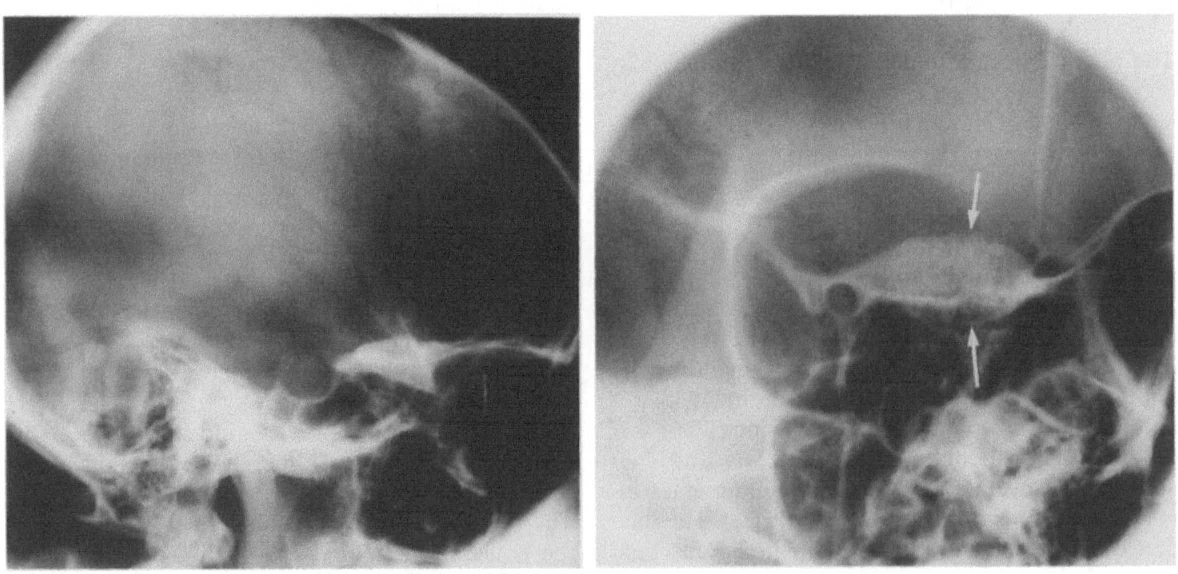

Fig. 2.2. Hyperostosis involving the three layers in medial sphenoid wing meningioma *(arrows)*

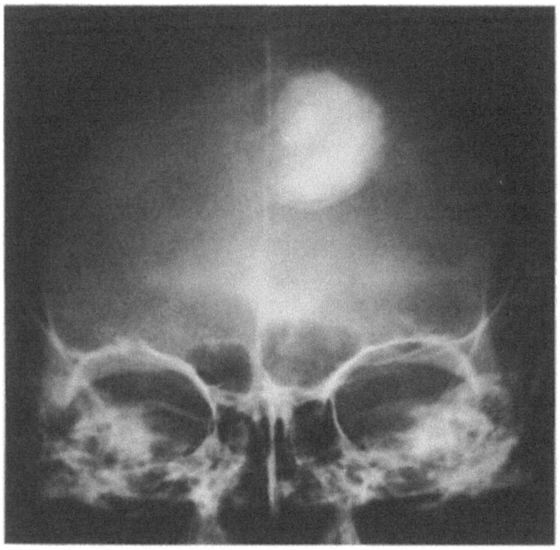

Fig. 2.3. Almost completely calcified falx meningioma

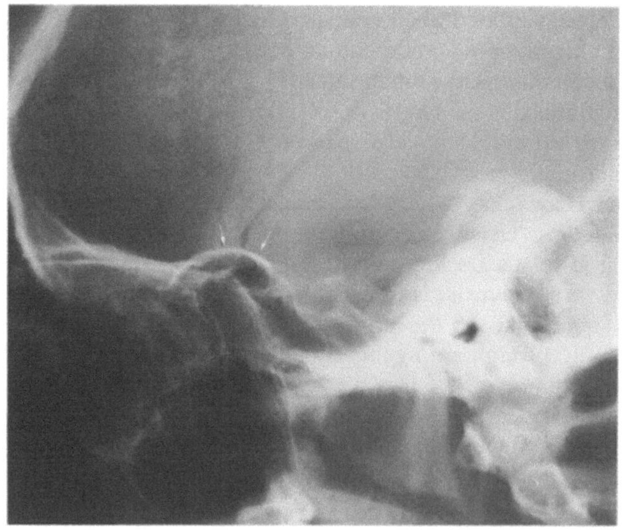

Fig. 2.4. Enlargement *(arrows)* of sphenoid sinus *(blistering)* in tuberculum sellae meningioma extending to the planum sphenoidale

from scalp arteries, and their presence suggests osseous invasion [76, 274].

2.2.3 Calcification

Calcification in the matrix of a meningioma is usually associated with psammoma bodies and generally produces an amorphous, cloudlike appearance on plain x-rays. Less commonly, curvilinear calcification forms in the surface layers of the tumour, and in about 2% of patients dense ossification develops in deeper parts (Fig. 2.3). Most authorities agree that calcification is visible on plain x-rays in less than 10% of patients [76, 274], and usually indicates that the tumour matrix is firm or hard.

Dural ossification may also be seen appearing as plaques or bands; it has been reported in just over 70% of patients with meningioma en plaque, though usually requiring tomography or high definition CT for its demonstration [149] (Fig. 8.3). In this special situation meningioma often spreads subdurally, and osseous metaplasia develops in the dura where it is separated from the underlying and usually hyperostotic calvaria. Extensive ossification seen in the petroclinoid and interclinoid ligaments and the dura of the dorsum sellae with some meningiomas of the sellar region presumably has an analogous origin.

2.2.4 Indirect Signs

Remote and therefore indirect signs of intracranial meningioma on plain skull x-rays are mainly those of raised intracranial pressure. Since 90% of meningiomas occur in adults, sutural diastasis and accentuated convolutional markings are not usually present. However, over half the patients show demineralization of the sella turcica, usually without enlargement. Far less common is erosion of the tip of the dorsum sellae and thinning and depression of the floor of the anterior cranial fossa [76, 274].

2.2.5 Bone Erosion and Blistering

Bone erosion is seen in less than 2% of meningiomas. Erosion can be due to cortical pressure from the tumour mass or bone destruction in the form of osteolytic invasion.

Some meningothelial meningiomas evoke a partly osteoclastic response from invaded bone. More often there is a mixed osteoblastic and osteoclastic response so that destruction and sclerosis coexist. The incidence of purely lytic bone lesions is greater in sarcomatous meningiomas and some forms of malignant meningiomas such as haemangiopericytomas and papillary tumours.

Pressure erosion is usually seen in the body of the sphenoid from parasellar tumours, in the dorsum sellae from suprasellar tumours, and in the walls of foramina, most often but still rarely, of the internal auditory and optic canals.

A closely related phenomenon which is confined to meningiomas of tuberculum sellae and planum sphenoidale is the phenomenon of "blistering" or pneumosinus dilatans [77, 274]. The roof of the posterior ethmoid air cells, planum sphenoidale and chiasmatic groove, each or all, may develop an upward convexity which can be very striking indeed (Fig. 2.4). Usually the normal planum and chiasmatic sulcus are flat or concave, and a pronounced upward convexity is unusual, though not necessarily abnormal. In the appropriate clinical setting it should prompt a diligent search for another sign, in particular evidence of a spongy type of hyperostosis which is nearly always associated when the appearance is due to meningioma. The blistering is thought to be due to softening of the sinus wall where it is invaded by tumour, and air pressure in the sinus causes remoulding of the sinus wall.

2.3 Differential Diagnosis

Hyperostosis is an important sign of meningioma on plain skull x-rays. However, the commonest hyperostosis to be found in the vault is hyperostosis frontalis interna, occurring in about 15% of women over the age of 40 and rarely in men. This involves the inner table and characteristically spares a median strip around the superior sagittal sinus; in hyperostosis from bifrontal meningioma there is no midline sparing.

Fibrous dysplasia can be difficult to distinguish from hyperostosis due to meningioma. Fibrous dysplasia usually presents with symptoms in childhood or adolescence when differential diagnosis is less of a problem. It commonly affects the anterior part of the skull base along the orbital roof and sphenoidal ridge and in this site causes thickening, sclerosis and foraminal stenosis. It may be progressive although this is unusual after bone growth has ceased. The textural change tends to be homogeneous, like ground glass rather than spongy as in many meningiomas; the surface of the hyperostosis is smooth in fibrous dysplasia, whereas it is usually irregular in meningiomas [48, 150]. Some forms of fibrous dysplasia affect the vault, and these may show mixed sclerosis and cystic change. The bone also may show evidence of hypervascularity with stippling and enlargement of vascular grooves, though virtually never specifically of middle meningeal arterial channels, and being a lesion mainly of the diploë, the inner table is normally not involved.

Osteoma usually arises from the outer table and rarely from the inner table [150, 293]. It does not extend into diploë nor grow across suture lines as meningiomas frequently do. Paget's disease alters the diploë and preferentially thickens the outer table; involvement of the base in continuity with the convexity is also common in Paget's disease. Sclerotic metastases can present serious difficulties, but again, these are usually lesions of the diploë and often are multiple or diffuse. A variety of metabolic and congenital bone disorders can result in sclerosis of all or part of the skull.

2.4 Meningiomas in Unusual Locations

Plain skull x-rays are usually normal in intraventricular meningioma. However, demineralization of the dorsum sellae due to raised intracranial pressure may be seen and occasionally, calcification in the tumour [143]. The mass may displace physiological calcification in the choroid plexus, to which such lesions are often closely related. Meningiomas arising in the paranasal sinuses cause clouding of the sinuses, sometimes with erosion and hyperostosis. The rare meningiomas apparently arising in the diploë and/or outer table of the skull cause hyperostosis occasionally associated with areas of osteolysis. Parapharyngeal tumours are usually partly calcified on CT, but most often are invisible on plain skull x-rays. Primary meningiomas of the petrous bone often cause bone destruction, centered on or near an opaque or partially opaque tympanic cleft.

3 Computed Tomography

3.1 General Efficacy

Even in the early years of computed tomography (CT) only about 2% of all intracranial meningiomas were not detected by CT, and they were not recognized as meningiomas in only 4%-7% of cases [61, 207, 223, 237]. Missed lesions are usually located in the posterior fossa and floor of the anterior and middle cranial fossae, and are usually low and flat; misdiagnoses usually result when lesions display atypical features. The sensitivity of CT is similar for all types of supratentorial neoplasm, but specificity is better for meningioma, diagnostic errors being made about twice as often with other types of neoplasms [13]. The commonest error has been to misdiagnose a meningioma for a malignant lesion, usually lymphoma, metastasis and glioblastoma.

The appearances of meningiomas in different regions will be detailed in other chapters, together with the relation of CT to other tests and the differential diagnosis. Only general principles will be indicated in this section.

3.2 Typical Features

3.2.1 Site

Meningiomas are usually superficial with a broad base contacting a dural surface. However, some meningiomas have no dural attachment, being attached to tela choroidea and choroid plexuses.

3.2.2 Margin and Shape

Meningiomas are usually circumscribed. They are usually either globular or flat and plaquelike in shape. The cerebral surface is smoothly convex or undulating, although in some tumours small fingerlike projections extend into the cortex (Figs. 3.1, 9.9); the dural surface, on the other hand, conforms to the shape of that surface and is usually flat. The margin of the dural attachment usually forms an obtuse angle with the dural surface, which in some cases actually tapers along that surface for a variable distance beyond the main bulk of the mass. This latter finding in particular is more sensitively shown by magnetic resonance imaging (MRI; Figs. 6.1, 10.1). Choroidal meningiomas are globular in shape and only slightly lobulated, or not at all.

3.2.3 Attenuation

Most meningiomas attenuate x-rays a little more than normal grey matter, but 11%-19% are isodense or slightly hypodense [207, 264]. In 14% HU values of over 100 have been recorded in parts of the lesion [264]. There is an inconsistent relation between attenuation value and tumour consistency at surgery, the denser lesions are usually, though not always firmer [142].

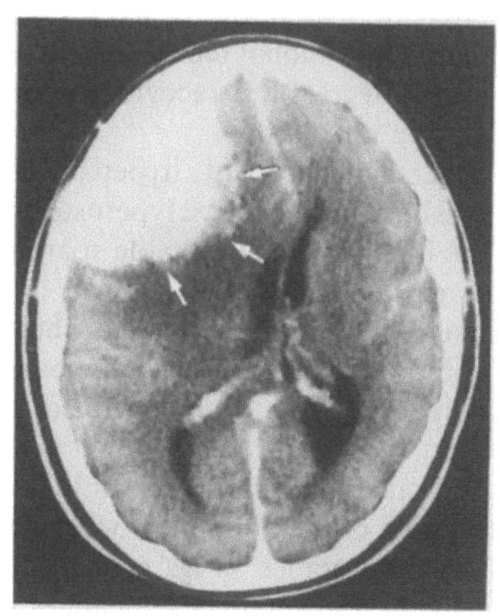

Fig. 3.1. Endotheliomatous meningioma. The tumour shows a rich contrast enhancement. The borders of the tumour are irregular with fringes of tumour extending into the cortex *(arrow)*. No signs of malignancy histologically

3.2.4 Calcification

Calcification may appear as nodular foci of varying size. Calcified meningiomas occur especially in the posterior fossa where a prevalence as high as 53% has been recorded [207]. Calcification also is relatively more frequent in frontobasal and sphenoid wing tumours. Totally calcified meningiomas may occur (Figs. 9.12, 12.5). Apparently calcification is rare in malignant types of meningioma [126, 208].

3.2.5 Contrast Enhancement

Enhancement after intravenous contrast administration probably occurs in all meningiomas and is detectable in about 97% [61, 223]. Characteristically it is diffuse and homogeneous. Peak enhancement is achieved within a few minutes of the contrast injection; subsequent decline parallels renal excretion, but enhancement remains several times greater than that of surrounding vascular structures, sometimes for several hours. The degree of enhancement is not closely linked with vascularity shown by angiography or encountered at operation. The important factor for contrast enhancement is the tumoral microvasculature, characterized by high capillary permeability permitting the passage of contrast medium into the tumoral interstitium [37, 93, 94, 264].

3.2.6 Effect on Adjacent Structures

Hyperostosis is a characteristic feature of meningiomas involving bone beneath the dural attachment. High definition CT is significantly more sensitive than conventional techniques at detecting it, though minor degrees are recognizable only down the operating microscope.

Several patterns of hyperostosis may be distinguished on CT [150]. Hyperostosis may involve only the inner or the outer table sparing the diploë, or all three layers may be involved in which the diploë may or may not be distinguishable as a less dense component; occasionally hyperostosis seems to involve only the diploë. Mixed patterns are common.

With meningioma of the vault, inward and outward bulging of the bone may occur resulting in a biconvex appearance (Figs. 6.10, 6.11); the surface is usually irregular. These changes may be associated with globoid tumours (Figs. 13.1, 8.2), but are more typical of en plaque meningiomas (Figs. 8.3, 8.4, 8.12, 8.15, 8.16). The en plaque portion of the tumour is generally evident on CT as a thin strip next to the hyperostotic bone, enhancing after contrast medium, though it is not invariably detectable (Figs. 6.10, 8.4).

MRI is inferior to CT in demonstrating hyperostosis, but is useful in distinguishing hyperostosis from tumour, which is sometimes difficult on CT (Figs. 7.5, 7.9), and, particularly when Gd-DTPA is given, in demonstrating the en plaque portion of a meningioma (Figs. 8.4, 7.9). Finally "blistering" (Chap. 2) may be demonstrated better with MRI using sagittal planes (Figs. 7.5, 7.8, 7.9 d).

Low attenuation is visible in the cerebral parenchyma surrounding meningiomas in 50%–70% of patients [37, 207, 264]. This is usually due to peritumoral oedema and will be discussed in Chap. 12. It is worth noting that about 17% of small lesions have shown typical oedema [37, 264] and in these it may be the oedema which draws attention to the presence of the meningioma.

3.2.7 Differential Diagnosis

In some cases hyperostosis needs to be differentiated from other diseases involving bone, usually fibrous dysplasia and osteoma. The diagnosis of meningioma is clear when a soft tissue tumour can be demonstrated adjacent to the hyperostosis. As a rule the surface of hyperostosis induced by meningioma is irregular, whereas it is smooth in fibrous dysplasia [48, 150] and involvement of the inner table is rare in fibrous dysplasia [150, 163]. Osteoma involves the outer table, or sometimes the inner table, usually sparing the diploë [150, 293]; its surface is smooth and it does not extend across suture lines as meningiomas frequently do.

Extra-axial soft tissue masses such as neurinomas and aneurysms are uncommonly as homogeneous on CT as meningiomas. The lack of a broad dural attachment, and formation of an acute rather than obtuse angle at the tumour-dural margin are typical of neurinomas and aneurysms. Aneurysms are most often confused with meningioma in the region of the skull base; neurinomas more often cause erosion of parts of the skull base. Some types of intra-axial tumour may be both homogeneous and slightly hyperdense, and when superficial may exhibit a broad, flattened area of contact with a dural surface; in particular this has been seen with medulloblastoma, haemangioblastoma, glioma, primary cerebral lymphoma [223] and in a few other circumscribed superficial lesions (Figs. 3.2, 3.3, 3.4, 6.13).

Occasionally metastases, especially those to the dura, are impossible to differentiate from meningiomas.

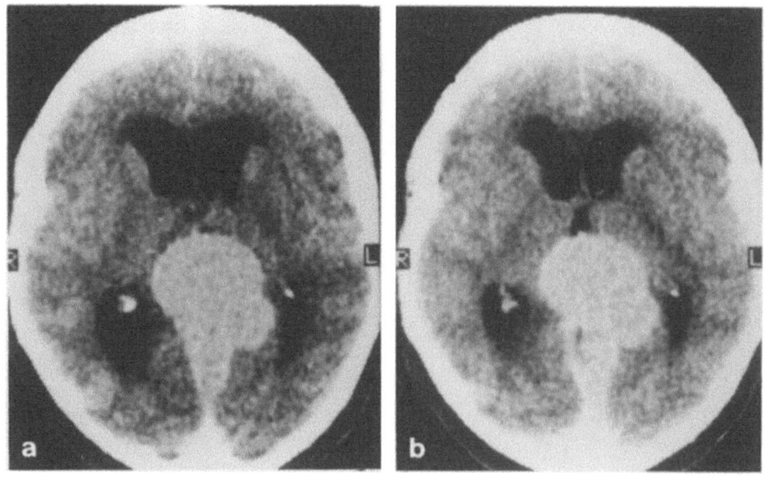

Fig. 3.2 a, b. Medulloblastoma in contact with tentorium and falx, simulating meningioma. CT without (**a**) and with (**b**) contrast medium. Compare with Fig. 9.9

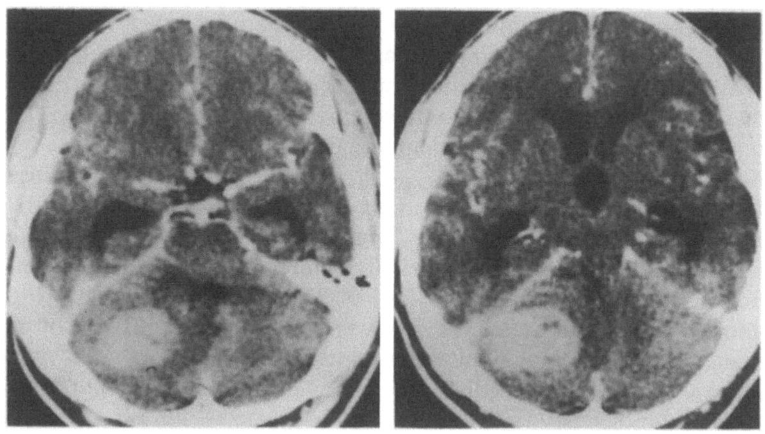

Fig. 3.3. Medulloblastoma of the left cerebellar hemisphere in an 25 year-old man misdiagnosed as meningioma. The tumour displays a rich and homogeneous contrast enhancement. It seems to be partially in contact with the tentorium

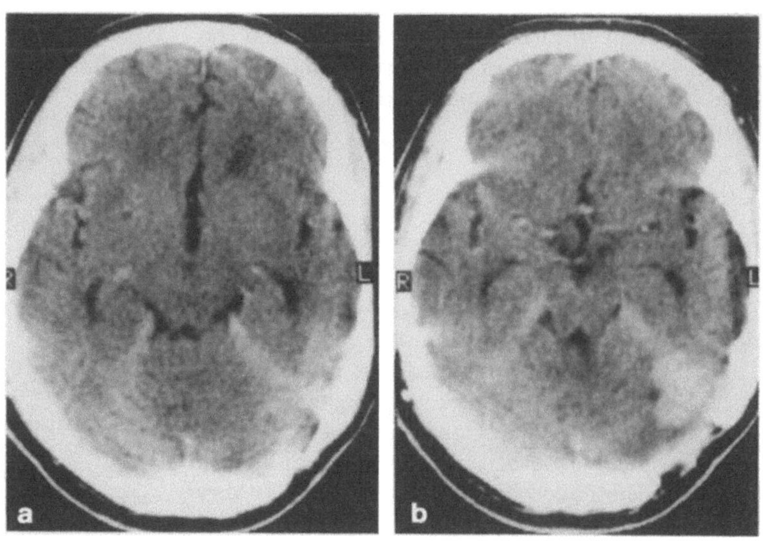

Fig. 3.4 a, b. Recurrent Haemangioblastoma in the left cerebellum. Examination without (**a**) and with (**b**) contrast medium. The tumour had a dural attachment. The picture can simulate a meningioma. Compare with Fig. 9.14

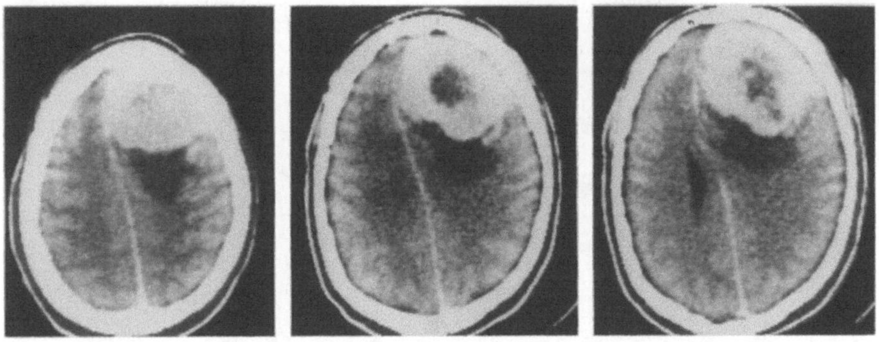

Fig. 3.5. Endotheliomatous meningioma of the convexity with degenerative changes in the central part of it

3.3 Atypical Features

3.3.1 Heterogeneity

Between 11% and 15% of meningiomas are of heterogeneous consistency. In about 45% of these the greater part of the lesion is of relatively low density [223, 237, 264]. This is a common cause of misdiagnosis. The low density regions which represent either necrosis, dense fibrosis, old haemorrhage and/or cysts generally are not enhanced after intravenous contrast medium.

Xanthomatous change, characterized by accumulations of viable lipid-laden cells, may be encountered in some large meningothelial meningiomas, not infrequently in angioblastic lesions. The attenuation of such regions on CT is lower than white matter, but rarely actually in the fat range, and after intravenous contrast medium they are enhanced similarly to the rest of the lesion (Fig. 11.2).

At operation most meningiomas containing hypodense areas are soft and necrotic or cystic, but some have been hard and fibrous [142] (Figs. 3.5, 5.4, 6.8, 6.9, 11.1, 11.2, 13.4).

Finally, recent intratumoral haemorrhage may be responsible for partial or sometimes almost complete hyperdensity of the tumour on CT, but this is distinctly uncommon.

3.3.2 Surface Irregularity

Only 10 of 160 supratentorial meningiomas reviewed by Stevens et al. [264] were associated with fingerlike extensions into the underlying brain, and none were significantly unusual histologically. However, it has been suggested that such appearances are a common feature of malignant meningiomas (Fig. 1.10) [208]. Confusion with an intra-axial mass can arise because this may result in a poorly circumscribed cerebral surface on CT. Very occasionally this surface is indistinct even in lesions with a relatively smooth surface, and more subtle signs such as inward displacement of cortex and compression or buckling of the white matter become important in establishing the extrinsic nature of the lesion. Some meningiomas have a small dural attachment, and some are pedunculated, so that the marginal tumour-dural angle becomes acute rather than obtuse.

3.3.3 Unusual Effects on Adjacent Structures

Some meningiomas excite little sclerosis, but mainly bone destruction. It is seen with some benign (Fig. 3.6) meningothelial tumours, but is a feature of meningeal haemangiopericytoma, malignant meningioma (Fig. 10.5) and meningeal sarcoma [207, 253] and of meningiomas arising in some extracranial sites.

In about 20% of supratentorial meningiomas [264,

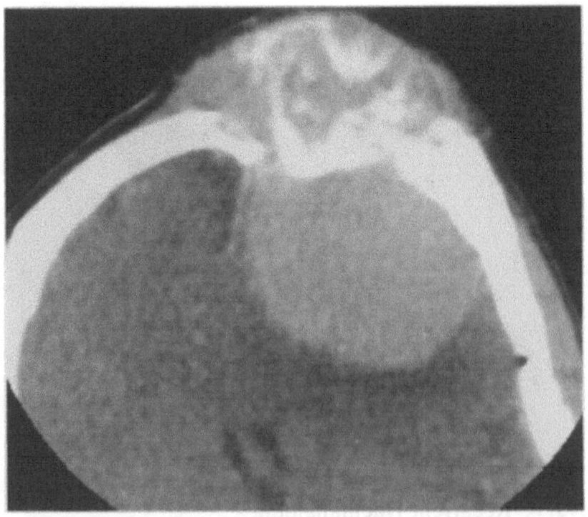

Fig. 3.6. Meningioma of the frontal convexity extending intra- and extracranially. There is an evident osteolysis associated with osteoclastic areas. The histologic examination revealed an endotheliomatous tumour without any signs of malignancy

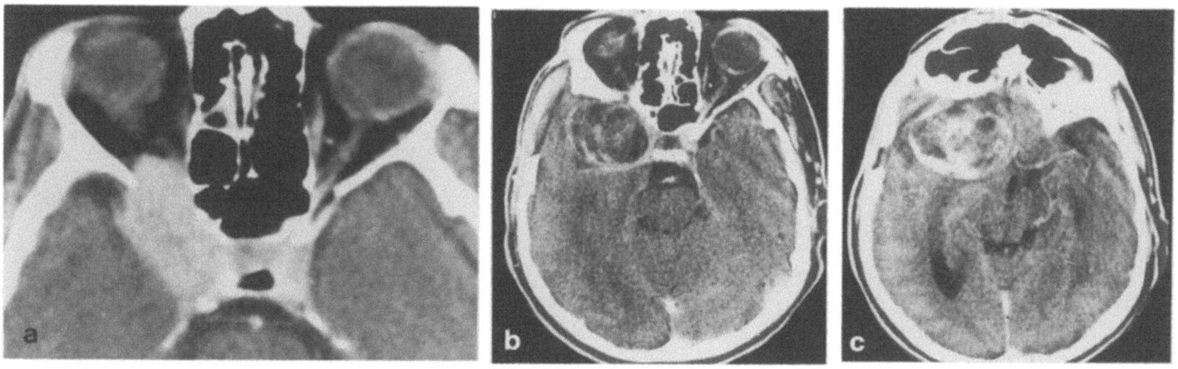

Fig. 3.7a–c. Malignant degeneration of an endotheliomatous cavernous sinus meningioma. **a** CT with contrast medium. Cavernous sinus meningioma, histologically classified as typical "benign" endotheliomatous tumour. **b, c** CT with contrast medium. Examination 8 months after partial surgical removal. There is recurrence with a tumour displaying atypical features

265] a round, circumscribed region of low density may be visible in the adjacent brain, suggestive of a cyst. However, in only 50% of these are cysts actually found at operation, and in the others only markedly oedematous brain. Cysts are either unilocular glial-lined intracerebral structures or complex arachnoid cysts invaginated into brain substance. In some meningiomas the low density region surrounding the tumour corresponds to localized cortical atrophy [256, 264].

Very occasionally, meningiomas are associated with intracranial haemorrhage. Russell et al. [237] have identified 31 reported cases, of which only 3 were associated with angioblastic meningiomas. Haemorrhages were subdural, subarachnoid and intracerebral and adjacent to the cerebral surface of the tumour [26, 129, 237]. Their aetiology is unclear.

3.4 Criteria for Malignancy

In meningiomas with inhomogeneous appearance due to large intratumoral low-density areas, irregular borders, particularly with parts of tumour growing far from the globoid mass and inhomogeneous enhancement, the possibility of a malignant character of the lesion should be taken into consideration [71, 208]. In a recent review on atypical and anaplastic meningiomas [126] these CT findings were present in 74% of the cases. However, these are not definite criteria of malignancy since the same appearance may be recognizable in lesions which are benign. Moreover, malignant meningiomas can appear identical with typical benign lesions (Figs. 3.7, 5.3).

4 Magnetic Resonance Imaging

4.1 General Aspects

While conventional x-ray methods, including computed tomography (CT), visualize varying degrees of x-ray absorption in different tissues, magnetic resonance imaging (MRI) is based on a completely different principle. There are some excellent reviews explaining the physical aspects of this technique [224] to which we refer. Very briefly we can say here that nuclei containing an unpaired number of protons rotate on their own axis (Spin) and in doing so produce a discrete magnetic field. By means of static and electromagnetic fields we can temporarily influence these nuclei and their reactions can be measured and finally transformed to images with the help of a computer. These depend on the quantity of nuclei influenced in a given area, on their motion and on the biological properties of the tissue examined, expressed by T1 and T2 relaxation times. In the clinical setting MRI uses the nuclei of hydrogen, which are in a very high concentration in the human body and possess a strong magnetic moment.

4.2 Technical Aspects and Material

A total of 77 patients with histologically confirmed intracranial meningiomas, the majority of them investigated at the University of Turin, have been considered. In the following pages we will describe the aspects of these tumours recognizable on MRI as well as the advantages and disadvantages of this method based on our experiences and on those of others reported in the most recent literature.
Most of the images demonstrated in this monograph have been obtained with a superconducting whole-body-scanner (ESATOM-ANSALDO) operating at 0.5 Tesla.
Routinely spin-echo (SE) sequences with different repetition times (TR) and echo delay time (TE) were applied. Proton-density, T1, T2-weighted images were routinely used. More rarely the examinations involved the inversion recovery technique.

4.3 MRI Features of Meningiomas

4.3.1 Aspects of the Tumour Mass

Commonly the degree of contrast of meningiomas related to the normal parenchyma is less than that of glioma [39, 49, 262, 281, 307]. Zimmerman et al. [307] report isointensity of the meningiomas to the adjacent brain in 62.5% of the tumours examined on T1-weighted images and in 51% on the T2-weighted images. In a previous study [39] we found isointense meningiomas on all sequences in about 40% of the patients (Figs. 4.1, 4.2, 4.3, 8.5). Using multiecho techniques, prolonging TE up to 240 msec there are in general no significant changes in the signal intensity, although occasionally a slightly increase or decrease of the signal is recognizable (Figs. 4.4–4.5). A slightly greater contrast between tumour and cerebral parenchyma can be achieved with high field MRI [262]. Meningiomas often appear slightly inhomogeneous due to their different tissue components. 84% of the cases of Spagnoli et al. [262] and 70% of the cases of Bradac et al. [39] were inhomogeneous, though gross inhomogeneity is less frequent. This can be due to nodular and/or linear areas characterized by a void signal on all sequences used. This finding can be due to calcifications and in general there is a good correlation between large calcifications visible on CT and corresponding black areas on MRI. In other cases a mottled appearance of the meningioma is due to intratumoral vessels; the absence of calcifications in CT further strengthens the assumption of a highly vascularized tumour (Figs. 9.9, 7.11). In a minority of patients (5% in our experience) large areas of low signal intensity visible on all the sequences used are recognizable in absence of calcifications and large vessels.

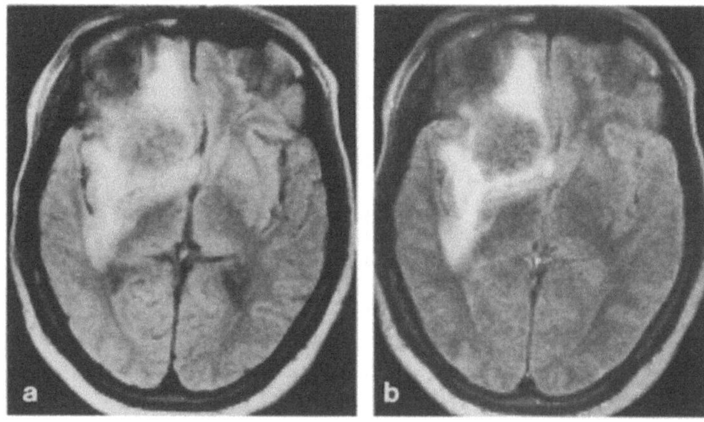

Fig. 4.1 a, b. This middle-sized sphenoid wing meningioma appears to have a signal of intensity quite similar to that of normal parenchyma on **a** the proton density-weighted (SE 1600/30) as well as **b** on the T2-weighted (SE 1600/70) scans. The tumour is recognizable by the evident oedema

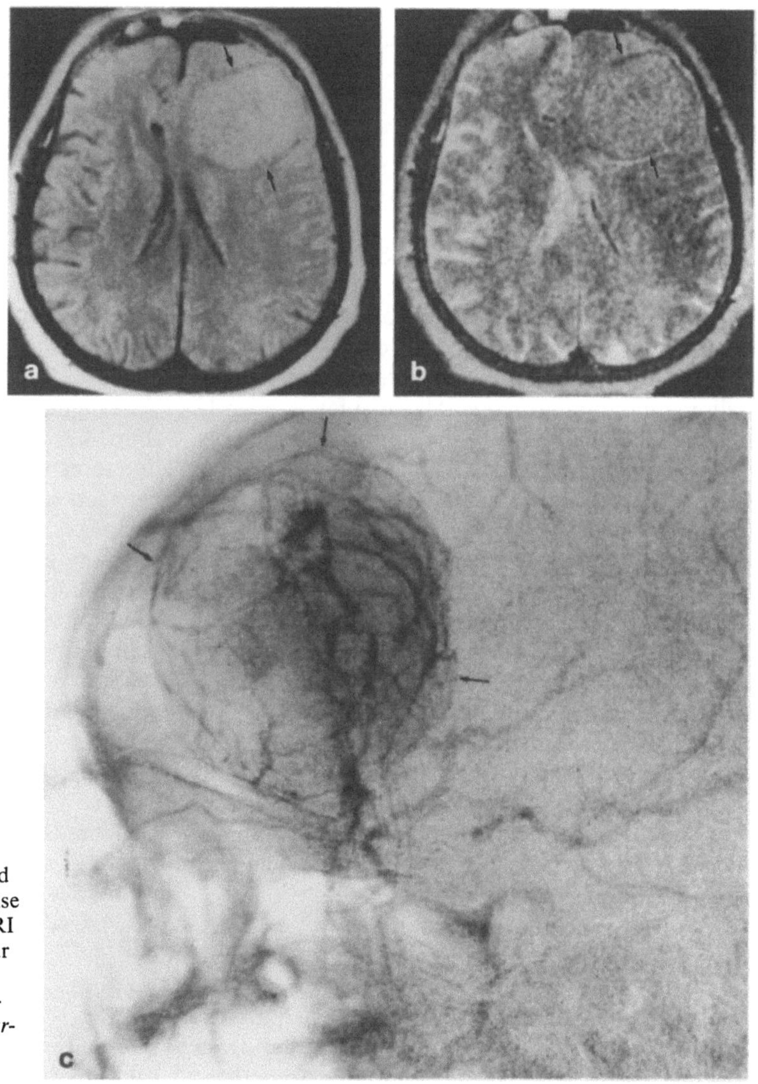

Fig. 4.2 a–c. Frontal convexity meningioma. **a** MRI (SE 1600/30) Proton density-weighted scan. The tumour appears slightly hyperintense to the surrounding brain parenchyma. **b** MRI (SE 1600/100) T2-weighted scan. The tumour is now isointense to the brain parenchyma. There is no oedema. The meningioma is surrounded on both sequences by a black rim *(arrows)*. **c** On the angiogram venous channels surrounding the tumours are visible

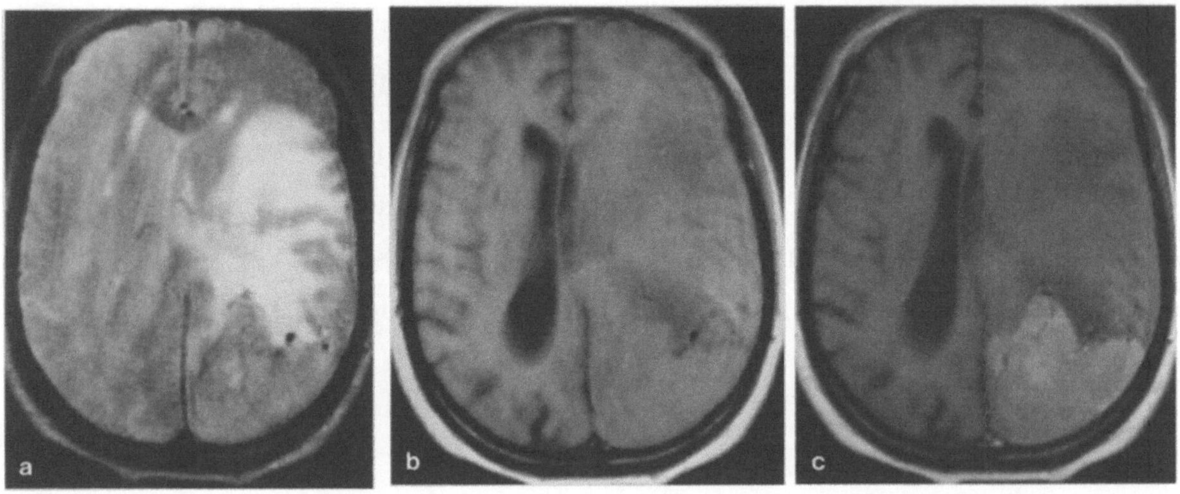

Fig. 4.3a–c. Occipital convexity meningioma. **a** MRI (SE 1600/30). There are some movement artefacts. The tumour appears isointense to the normal brain parenchyma. On the periphery of the meningioma there are some enlarged tumoral vessels. A large peritumoral oedema is present. **b** MRI (SE 500/50). Also on this T1-weighted scan the tumour appears isointense. **c** MRI (SE 500/50). Tumoral enhancement after Gd-DTPA

This finding is probably due to the presence of numerous psammoma bodies (Figs. 4.4, 4.10). Cystic parts of the tumour appear as areas of decreased signal intensity on T1 and/or proton density-weighted images and of increased signal intensity on T2-weighted scans (Figs. 4.5, 4.14).

In an attempt to find out some features specific for the different subtypes of meningiomas, Hiyama et al. [118] report that on T2-weighted images, endotheliomatous tumours generally display a slightly higher signal than those of the fibrous type. Highly vascularized meningiomas appear frequently characterized by a high signal, and the presence of psammomatous bodies is associated with areas of low signal on all the sequences used. A precise biophysical explanation of these phenomena is lacking. The higher signal intensity of endotheliomatous compared with fibrous meningiomas is probably due to the greater tissue-water content in the former, depending on their richness in large, round cells within sparse intercellular matter. The high intensity signal in highly vascularized tumours could be correlated with the richness of vessels with a very slow flow. The presence of numerous psammoma bodies probably explains the hypointensity areas in this type of meningioma.

4.3.2 Tumour Margins

In about 50%–60% of the patients [39, 307] a complete or partial rim separating the tumour from cerebral parenchyma is recognizable. Sometimes this finding is clearly due to major cerebral arteries surrounding the tumour [39] (Figs. 7.5, 7.11). Also, tumoral arteries or large venous channels located on the periphery of the tumour can partially explain this picture (Figs. 4.2, 4.9, 4.10, 4.11, 9.6). In these patients the rim is characterized by a void signal on all the sequences used. In several other patients, however, its signal intensity changes and so it appears hypointense on T1-weighted while on T2-weighted images it becomes hyperintense (Figs. 4.7, 4.8). This has been interpreted [39, 262] as due to cerebrospinal fluid (CSF), probably trapped between surface of the tumour and cerebral parenchyma.

In many cases CSF and vessels are probably present simultaneously and so the image on MRI is a result of both factors (Fig. 4.9). Finally, is worth remembering that the rim is frequent in meningiomas but it is not specific of these, since it can be found occasionally in other extraaxial lesions also.

4.3.3 Peritumoral Oedema

Oedema is well recognizable on T2-weighted scans where it is characterized by a high signal intensity, well discernable from the tumour itself (Figs. 4.1, 4.3, 4.4, 4.7, 4.8, 4.9, 4.10, 4.13).

4.3.4 Bone Changes

Normally the inner and outer tables are seen as linear hypointensities, while the diploë is character-

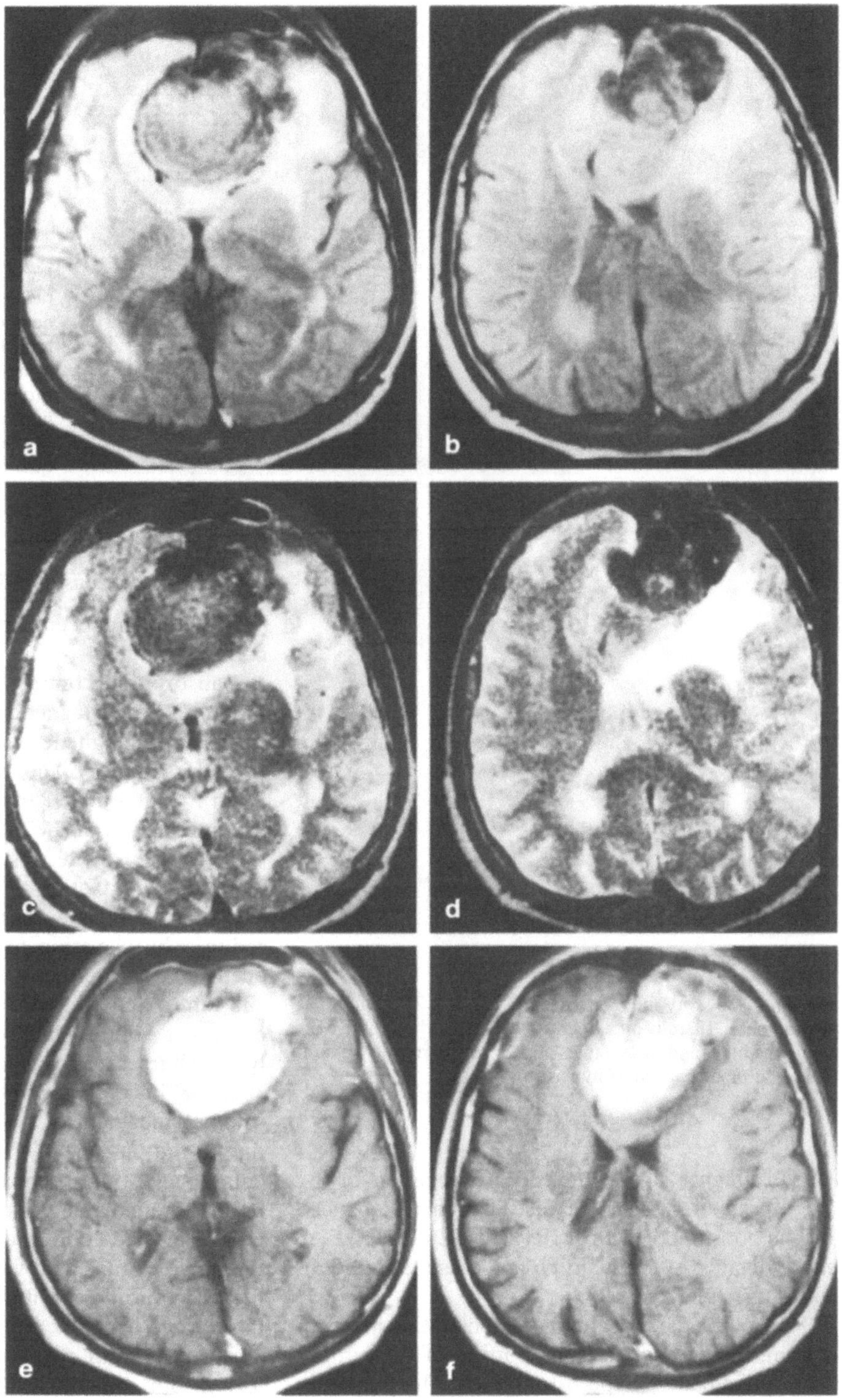

Fig. 4.4 a–f. Frontobasal meningioma appearing not calcified on CT with atypical MRI aspect. **a, b** (SE 1600/30). There are portions of the tumour with different signal intensity (iso-hypohyperintensity). There is a black rim and a peritumoral oedema. **c, d** (SE 1600/100). The hypointense areas inside the meningioma are even more evident. The black rim on the periphery of the tumoral mass probably corresponding to vessels shows no changes. **e, f** (500/50) After injection of Gd-DTPA. There is an evident enhancement even if it is slightly inhomogeneous

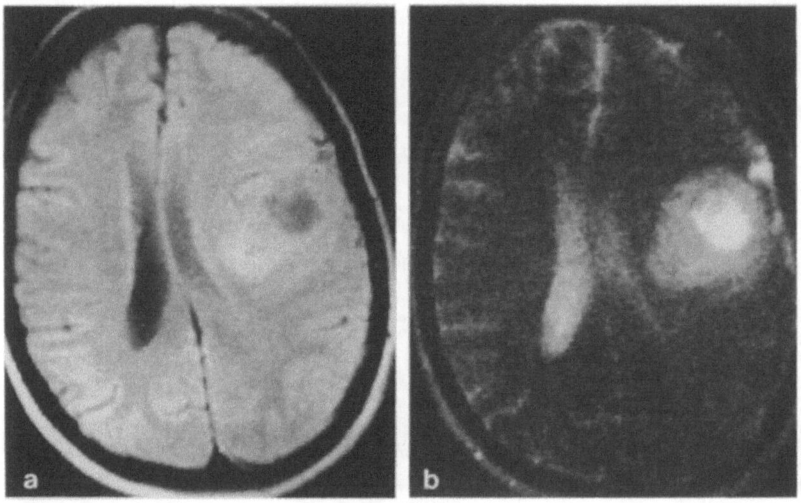

Fig. 4.5 a, b. Meningioma of the parietal convexity with cystic component. (SE 1600) with **a** short and **b** long TE. There is an increase of the signal intensity in the tumoral mass prolonging the TE. The cystic portion of the tumour shows a signal similar to that of CSF in the two sequences used

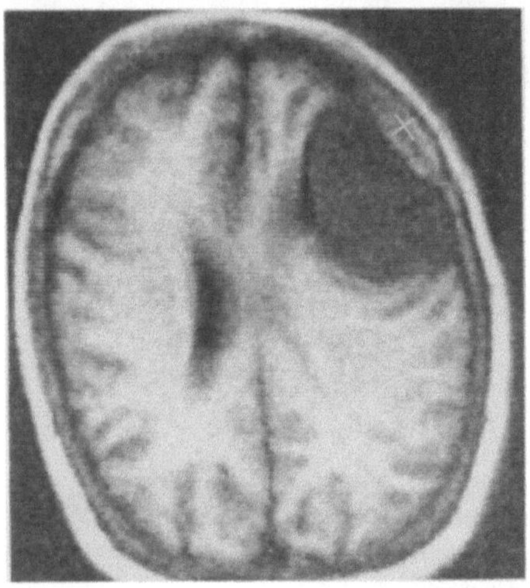

Fig. 4.6. Convexity meningioma. MRI (I. R.). The tumour is hypointense. There is an evident thickness of the diploë (+), while the inner and outer tables appear nearly normal. Example of "diploë" pattern of hyperostosis

ized by higher signal intensity. Changes involving these structures as in the case of hyperostosis can be demonstrated with MRI (Fig. 4.6). However, more detailed studies can be made using high definition CT (see Chap. 3).
MRI is particularly useful in demonstrating and separating the parenchymatous portion of the tumour from the adjacent hyperostotic area. The dilatation of the sphenoid sinus (blistering) frequently associated with hyperostosis in tuberculum sellae and sphenoid plane meningiomas is also easily demonstrated (Figs. 7.5, 7.8, 7.9).

4.4 Contrast Medium

4.4.1 General Considerations

While the enhancement obtained with iodinated contrast medium is due to its elevated grade of x-ray absorption, contrast medium for MRI acts by modifying the magnetic environment of hydrogen nuclei. Paramagnetic substances, like gadolinium, have this property. The magnetic moment of gadolinium is much higher than that of hydrogen nuclei. The interaction of the paramagnetic substance with the hydrogen nuclei results in a shortening of the T1 and T2 relaxation times of the tissue.
The relative toxicity of gadolinium can be markedly reduced by chelation to diethylenetriamine pentaacetic acid to produce gadolinium-DTPA. With this substance Schering AG (Berlin) has developed a contrast medium which when injected intravenously is well tolerated, as clinical studies [22, 40, 41, 53, 102, 248] have demonstrated.
The enhancement of normal organs of the body is due to the passage of Gd-DTPA into the extravascular space; but no enhancement occurs in normal brain parenchyma because the contrast does not cross normal blood-brain barrier (BBB). Usually, the only enhancement visible intracranially is in the plexus choroideus, pituitary gland and infundibulum. Some irregular enhancement is also recognizable on the dura of the convexity, the falx, the tentorium and on the walls of sinuses. Arteries and venous channels are not enhanced with the exception of the cavernous sinus, which always shows an increased signal intensity after Gd-DTPA due to the slow blood flow. The signal intensity is also increased in the mucosa of the nasopharynx and paranasal sinuses.

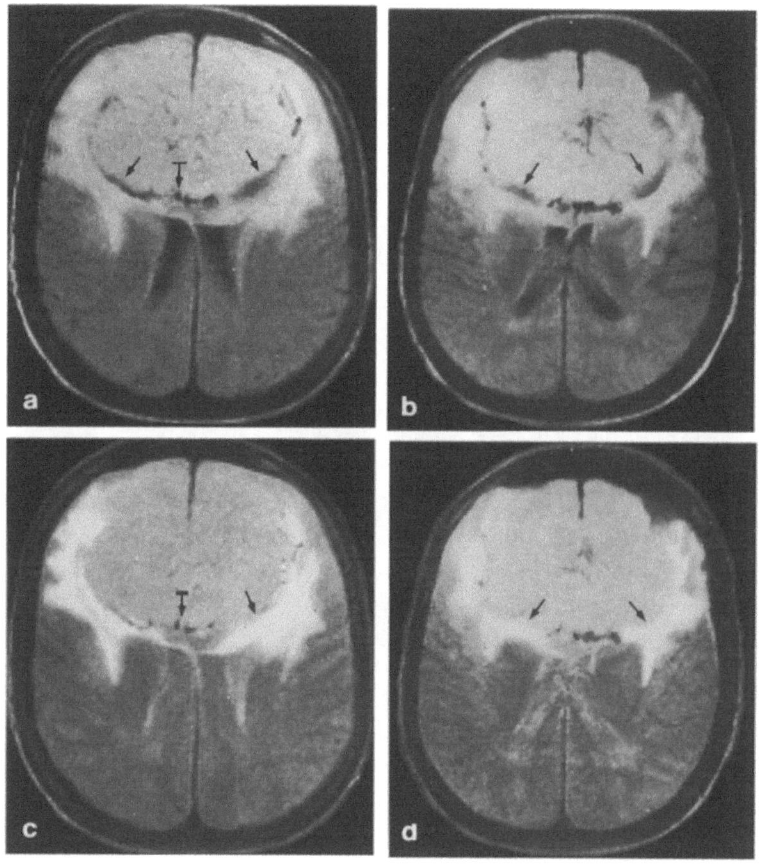

Fig. 4.7 a–d. Very large frontobasal meningioma. **a, b** (SE 1600/30), **c, d** (SE 1600/70). The tumour is hyperintense on the two sequences used. There is evident peritumoral oedema. Branches of anterior cerebral arteries (⊢→) are well visible. They appear dark on the proton-density (**a, b**) and on the T2-weighted (**c, d**) scans. On the periphery of the tumour there is a thick rim which turns from dark to bright in the T2-weighted scan (→). This phenomenon is due probably to incarcerated CSF surrounding the tumour

4.4.2 Contrast Enhancement in Tumours

It is well accepted [93, 94] that enhancement of iodinated contrast medium in cerebral tumours is due mainly to an alteration of the BBB, allowing a diffusion of contrast medium into tumoral tissues. In brain tumours examined both with CT and MRI, the enhancement following iodinated contrast medium and Gd-DTPA correlates well, suggesting that the mechanism of enhancement is similar. With regards to the specific problem of meningiomas, histological studies [18, 37, 82, 171] with electron microscopy have clearly shown features of intratumoral vessels which allow passage of molecules of contrast medium into the tumoral parenchyma.
Once penetrated into the meningioma, Gd-DTPA leads to changes of the T1-T2 relaxation times. On plain T1-weighted scans, tumoral tissue with long T1 values is characterized by decrease of signal intensity and so tumour appears dark. After application of Gd-DTPA, the passage of this paramagnetic substance into tumoral tissue leads to shortening of T1. Therefore, there will be an increase of signal intensity and the tumour will appear bright.

As described previously, meningiomas are frequently characterized by a poor signal intensity and so enhancement with Gd-DTPA clearly improves their demonstration and definition [22, 39–41, 49]. Enhancement is frequently inhomogeneous and this is sometimes very pronounced due to large cysts, calcifications, psammoma bodies or intratumoral vessels (Figs. 4.4, 4.14, 7.11, 9.9). Very often, however, the inhomogeneous enhancement is subtle, and due probably to variation in histological pattern within the tumour mass (Figs. 4.3, 4.12, 4.13, 4.15). Quite frequently there is also strong enhancement forming a rim at the periphery of the tumour [22].
The enhanced tumour gives a sharper image with well-defined borders. Furthermore, it is relevant that only the injection of Gd-DTPA allows the diagnosis of some meningiomas en plaque [39] (Fig. 8.4) and the demonstration of additional parts of other tumours (Figs. 6.1, 7.9, 8.14–8.16, 10.1), not detected on plain MRI sequences.

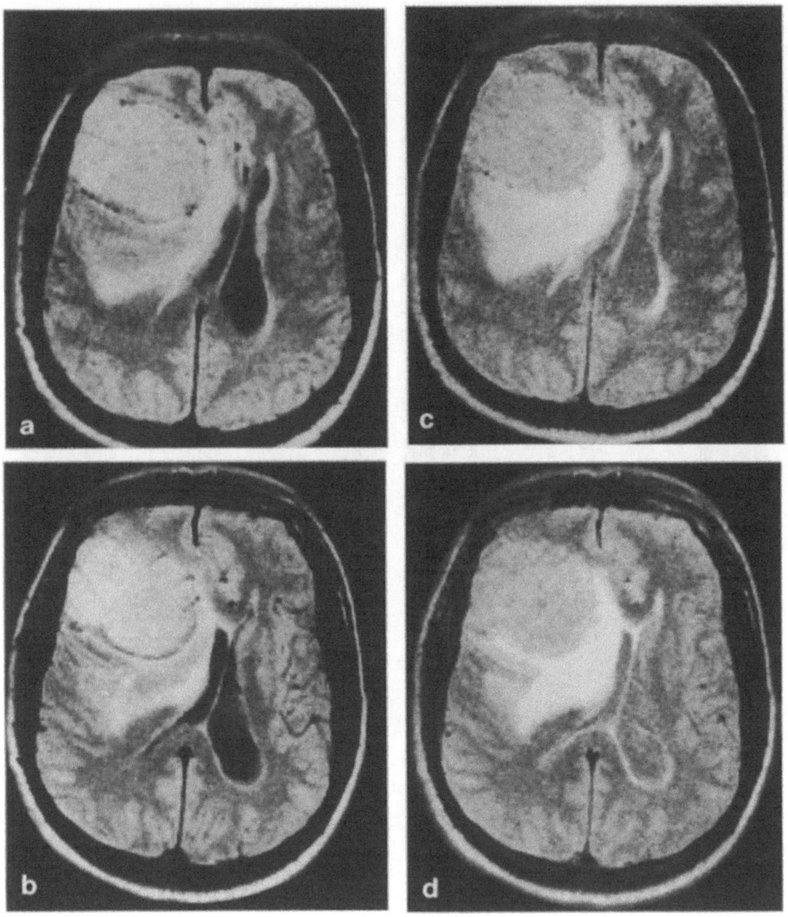

Fig. 4.8 a–d. Large meningioma of the frontal convexity. **a, b** Proton density-weighted and **c, d** T2-weighted sequences. The tumour appears slightly hyperintense on the two sequences used. There is evident peritumoral oedema. On the periphery of the tumour there are several nodular foci, corresponding to surrounding arteries, which appear dark in the two sequences. The tumour is surrounded partially by a rim which turns from dark to bright. This phenomenon could be due to CSF

4.5 Topographic Localization

4.5.1 Topographic Analysis

MRI allows visualizing tumours in multiple planes, providing topographic analysis superior to CT. The relationship between tumour and brain tissue as well as distortion and/or compression of these structures are well demonstrated.

4.5.2 Brain Vasculature

MRI gives considerable information on brain vasculature and its relationship to a tumour. In MRI, arteries display a void signal. This is due to the fact that stimulated protons which are responsible for the signal on MRI follow the blood flow, and so when the signal is recorded, they are no longer present in the plane studied, but they are substituted by nonstimulated protons which do not deliver signals. This allows easy separation of parenchyma and vessels. Tumoral encasement of arteries is frequently easy to recognize, while often impossible on CT in which arteries only become clearly visible after injection of contrast medium: contrast enhancement of the tumour usually masks vessels (Figs. 8.9, 8.10, 8.13–8.16, 10.7).

4.5.3 Sinus Infiltration

Infiltration of sinuses may also be well demonstrated (Figs. 4.13–4.14, 6.12, 8.13–8.16, 9.9, 9.11). Sometimes, however, this diagnosis is difficult, because there are areas inside venous sinus where an increase of signal intensity on proton density- and T2-weighted scans is frequently present as a normal finding. This phenomenon, due to a local slowing of venous circulation, can be misinterpreted as a sign of tumoral infiltration in cases of parasagittal and parasellar meningioma. The application of contrast medium can be useful, but it is also a potential source of errors. It may be very difficult to differen-

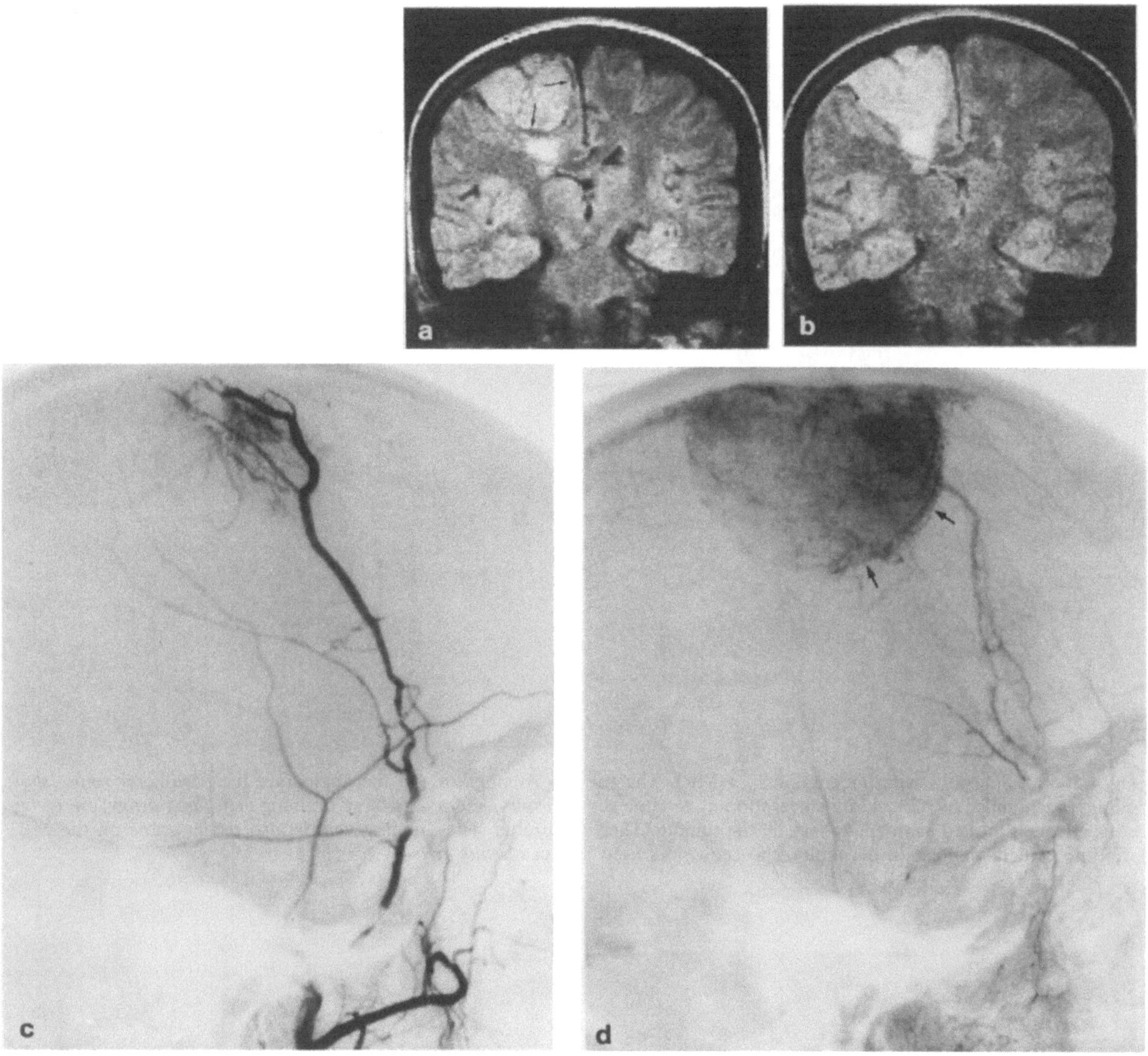

Fig. 4.9 a–d. Parasagittal meningioma. MRI. The meningioma is surrounded on the sequence in **a** (SE 1600/30) by a black rim *(arrows)* which displays on the sequence in **b** (SE 1600/70) a signal of slightly increased intensity. There is a peritumoral oedema only on one sector of the surface of the meningioma. The sagittal sinus is not infiltrated. **c, d** Angiogram of the external carotid artery. On the periphery of the tumour large venous channels *(arrows)* are recognizable

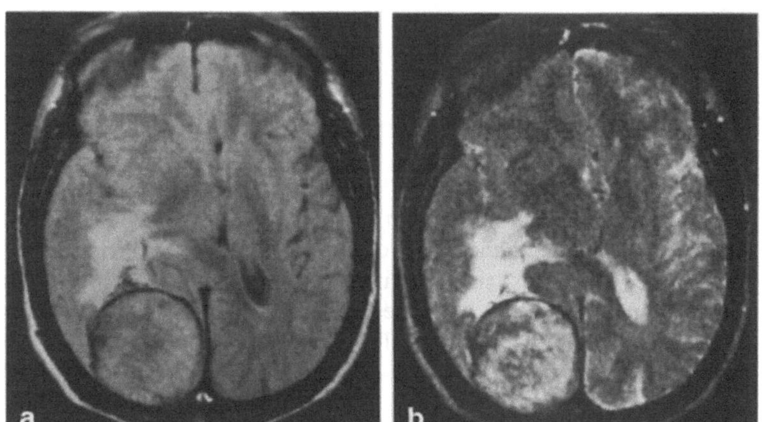

Fig. 4.10 a, b. Parasagittal meningioma. MRI. The black rim, probably due to vessels surrounding the meningioma, shows no changes in the **a** proton density and **b** T2-weighted sequences used. The tumour shows inhomogeneity with black area probably corresponding to psammoma bodies. There ist evident oedema which is better visible on **b**

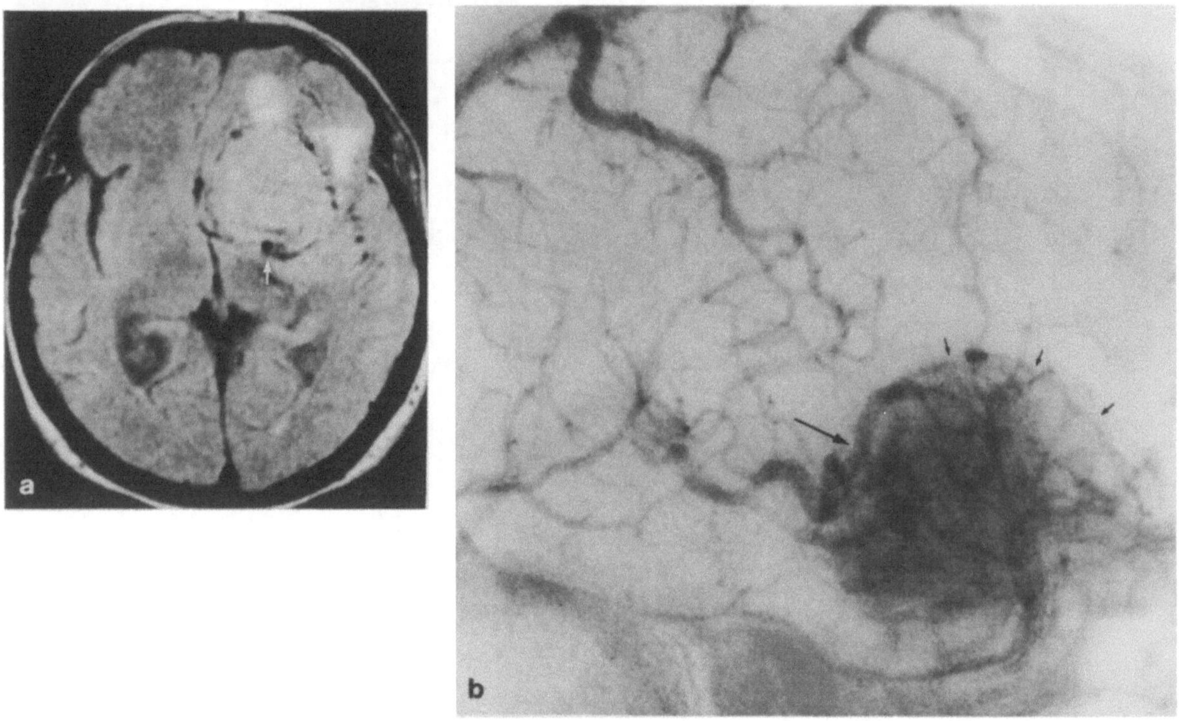

Fig. 4.11 a, b. Sphenoid wing meningioma. **a** MRI. The tumour is surrounded by a black rim corresponding to large venous channels located at the periphery oh the tumour. There were no evident changes in the multi-echo sequences used. **b** Angiogram. On the angiogram the peripheral veins *(short arrows)* and a very large draining vein *(long arrow)* are recognizable. The draining vein is also recognizable on the MRI scan *(white arrow)*

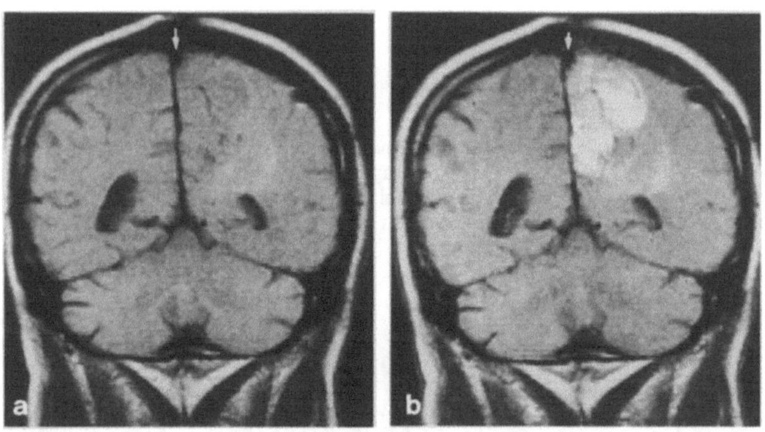

Fig. 4.12 a, b. Parasagittal meningioma. Examination **a** without and **b** with Gd-DTPA. The tumour, which appears isointense to the parenchyma on the T1-weighted scan, shows clear enhancement after contrast medium. The sinus *(arrow)* appears normal

tiate a partial tumoral infiltration of the sagittal sinus from normal enhancement of dura and falx. When the cavernous sinus is involved, the enhanced tumour together with the outward bulging of the lateral wall of the sinus will be helpful in establishing the diagnosis [38].

4.6 Conclusions

CT still remains a valuable method to be used first in the diagnosis of meningiomas. It is more sensitive in detecting these tumours since the contrast between them and brain parenchyma is quite frequently poor on MRI. Furthermore, intratumoral calcifications and bone changes are well recognized

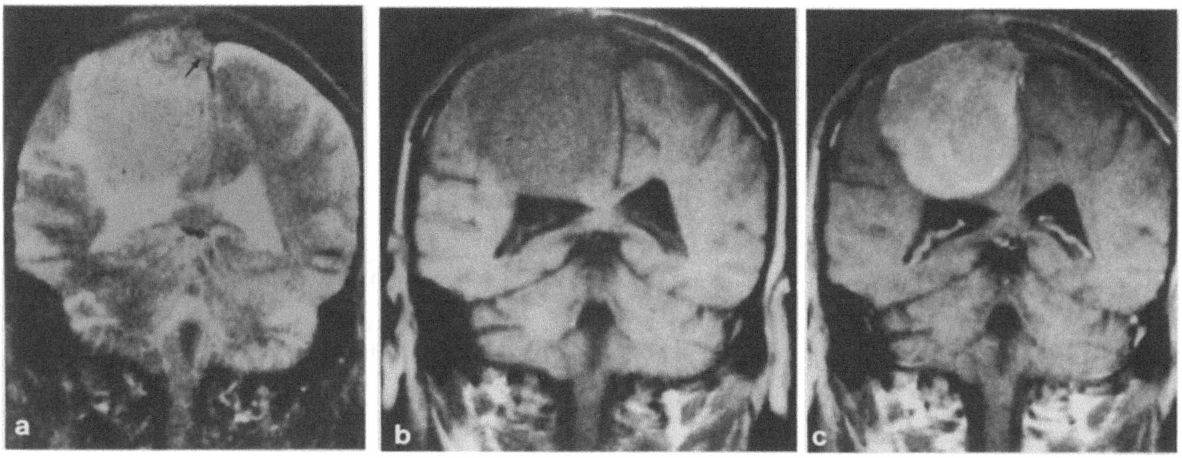

Fig. 4.13a–c. Parasagittal meningioma with sinus infiltration. **a** SE 2000/120). On this T2-weighted scan the tumour is slightly hyperintense. There is infiltration of the sinus which does not display its typical void signal *(arrow)*. Mild peritumoral oedema is present. **b** (SE 500/50). The tumour appears hypointense on T1-weighted scan. **c** (SE 500/50). Tumoral enhancement after Gd-DTPA also involving the sinus. Note the slight inhomogeneity of the enhancement

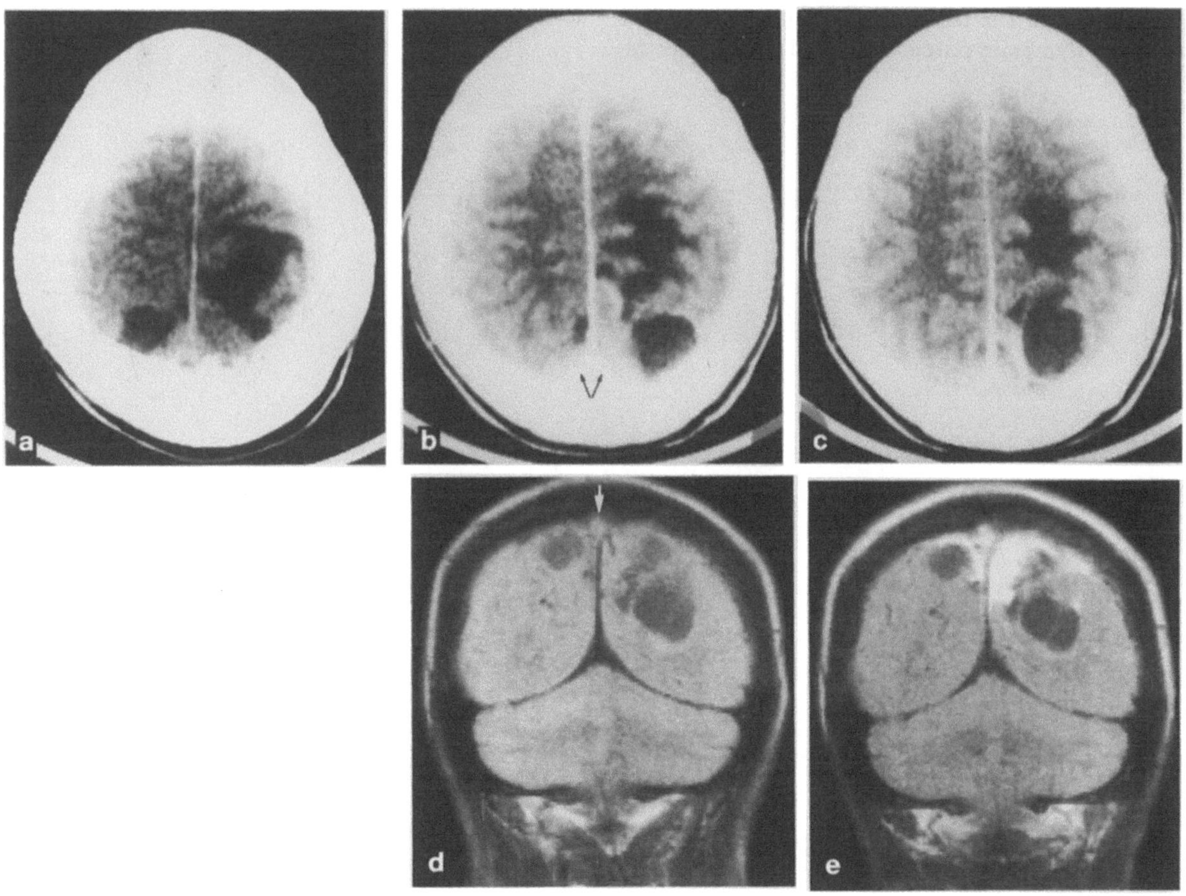

Fig. 4.14a–e. Atypical parasagittal meningioma with bilateral extent and sinus infiltration. **a–c** CT. A solid *(double arrow)* and a cystic part of the tumour are well recognizable. There is some peritumoral oedema. **d, e** MRI. Coronal planes (**d**) before and (**e**) after Gd-DTPA. The superior sagittal sinus *(arrow)* displays a signal of intensity similar to that of the solid part of the tumour. This can be interpreted as a sign of sinus infiltration, which was confirmed angiographically. After Gd-DTPA the solid part of the tumour shows evident enhancement. The dural attachment is well demonstrated

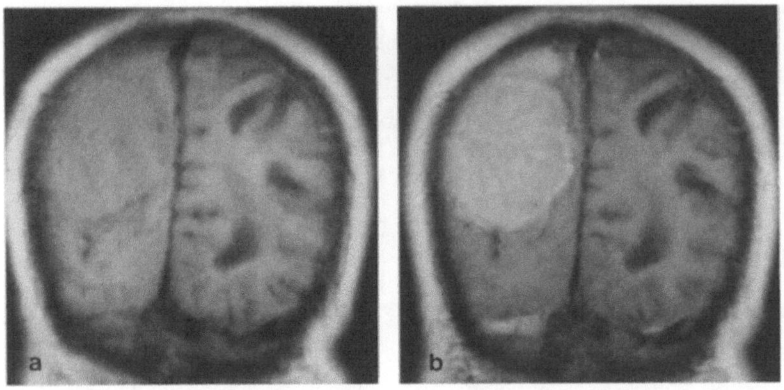

Fig. 4.15a, b. Convexity meningioma. MRI, Coronal planes. The tumour appears isointense with the surrounding parenchyma on this T1-weighted scan. There is an evident enhancement after injection of Gd-DPTA

on CT. MRI, with its facilities of multiplanar study, is superior in delineating the tumour in its complete extension and in showing the relationship to surrounding cerebral parenchyma and vessels. Encased arteries as well as sinus infiltration can be demonstrated. The presence of a rim separating the tumour from brain parenchyma and the demonstration of a dural contact is particularly useful in the diagnosis of atypical meningiomas. Finally, small tumours near the skull base and in the posterial fossa and particularly en plaque lesions which can be missed on CT are generally visible on MRI, especially if Gd-DTPA is used.

5 Angiography

The mass effects of meningiomas depend on their individual location and will be considered by region in the appropriate *chapters*.

5.1 Angiographic Features

The following angiographic patterns are frequent in intracranial meningiomas:

1. Vascular supply from meningeal branches, which are often hypertrophied, arising from the internal, and/or external carotid and/or vertebral arteries
2. A radial pattern of tumour vascularization in the arterial phase
3. Tumour blush which persists late in the venous phase
4. Delayed filling of veins draining the tumour

These findings are not always present, and they are not specific for meningiomas. In principle, a meningeal supply can occur in any tumour adherent to the dura mater.

Meningiomas can also cause 'early filling of veins' draining the tumour, which was once considered typical of glioblastoma or metastasis. Wickbom [292] first described its occurrence in a few meningiomas and considered it suggestive of malignancy. It has been noted in many series with varying frequency (5% El-Banhawy and Walter [78]; 14% Stattin [263]; 19% Leeds and Taveras [164]; 37.5% Kieffer et al. [148]). Early filling of tumoral draining veins occurred in about 15% of our cases and, in accordance with previous reports [148, 276], these meningiomas were of angiomatous or endotheliomatous type; none had signs of malignancy. It can be safely concluded that 'early filling of tumoral veins' is frequent in meningiomas and not of prognostic significance (Figs. 5.1, 5.2).

5.2 Angiographic Vascularization and Histological Type of Meningioma

On angiograms, fibrous meningiomas tend to appear poorly vascularized and endotheliomatous meningiomas richly vascularized. Angiomatous, an-

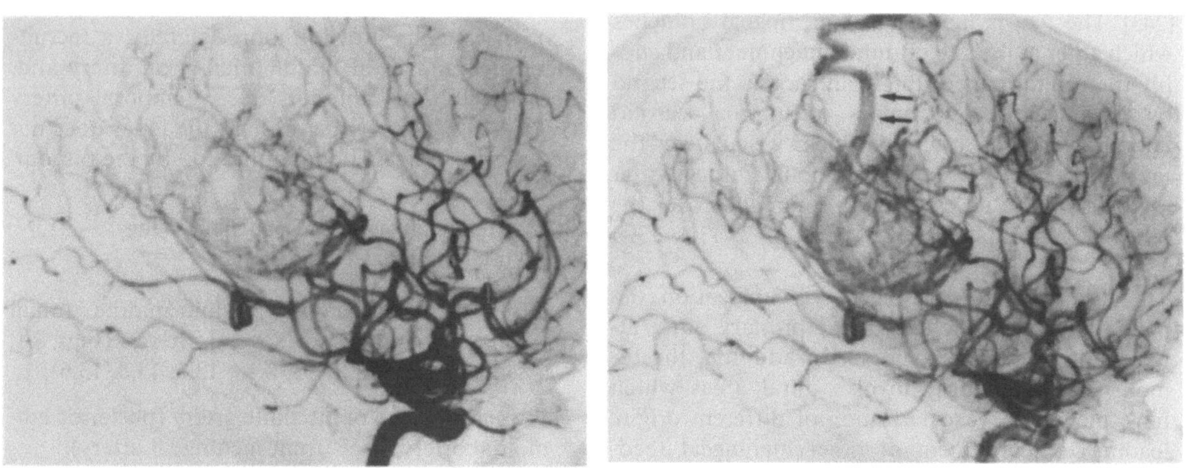

Fig. 5.1. Convexity endotheliomatous meningioma. Early filling of draining vein *(arrows)*

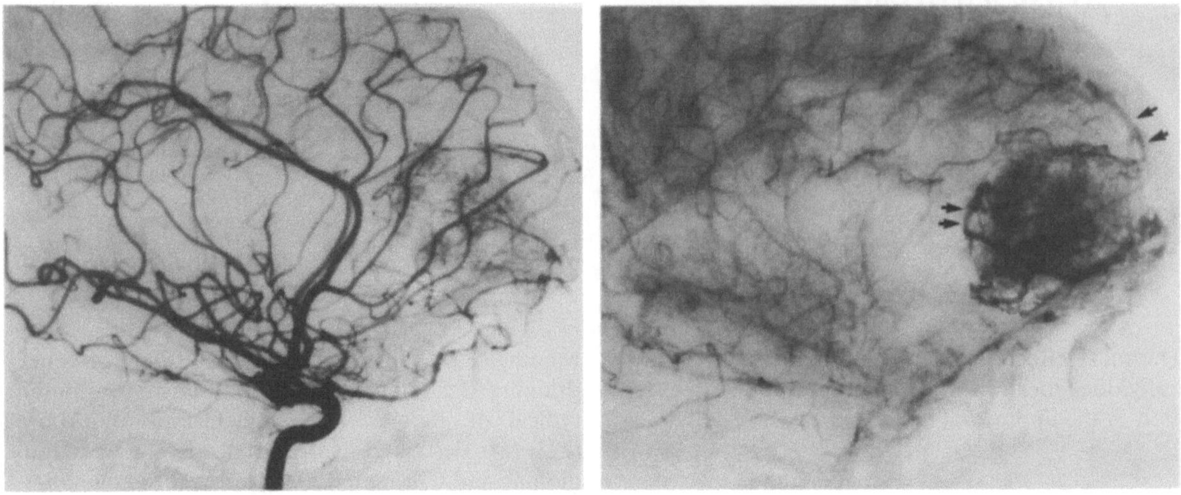

Fig. 5.2. Frontobasal endotheliomatous meningioma. Early filling of draining veins *(arrows)*

gioblastic meningiomas and most meningiosarcomas are characterized by a very rich vascularization [253, 300]. In general, however, angiography alone does not allow a definite diagnosis of histological type (Figs. 5.1-5.4, 8.1, 8.18, 13.1-13.8).

The degree of vascularization in the angiogram does not relate to the frequency of microvessels reported by the histologist. This explains the frequent discrepancy between the density of 'angiographic' vascularization and the degree of enhancement visible in CT and MRI, the latter being linked mainly to permeability of the tumour microvasculature, which lacks a barrier for contrast medium.

5.3 Meningeal Vascularization

Meningiomas have two groups of supplying arteries [243]. The first is made up of meningeal branches which enter at the site of dural attachment and supply the central part of the meningioma, the second by leptomeningeal branches of internal carotid and/or vertebral arteries which vascularize the more peripheral part of the tumour. One vascular sector can have an evident predominance over the other (Figs. 5.3, 5.4, 6.1, 8.1, 8.18, 13.2, 13.3, 13.5, 13.8).

The origin of the meningeal vascularization depends largely on the site of the primary dural attachment of the meningioma. In addition, the tumour can secondarily involve dural areas which have meningeal vascularization of different origin, leading to recruitment of other meningeal feeders.

Vascularization of dura of the skull base and vault is from multiple branches of external and internal carotid and the vertebral arteries, which richly anastomose. There are many anatomical variations; in particular, any artery can be hypoplastic or absent, and its vascular territory is taken over by neighbouring arteries. Nevertheless, basic patterns of vascularization in the different regions are recognized.

Excellent works on meningeal vascularization already exist [73, 161]. The more important practical aspects are summarized here.

5.3.1 Meningiomas of Frontal Cranial Fossa (Frontobasal Meningiomas)

Tumours located on the midline can be sùpplied by meningeal branches of posterior and anterior ethmoidal branches of the ophthalmic artery (Figs. 7.3, 7.5). In tumours growing more laterally, a recruitment of branches of middle meningeal artery and, occasionally, of anterior deep temporal artery (Figs. 7.10, 7.11) may be present; the latter does not necessarily indicate bone infiltration by the tumour.

5.3.2 Meningiomas of the Sphenoid Wing and Middle Cranial Fossa

Tumours of the sphenoid wing and middle cranial fossa may be supplied by several arteries (Figs. 8.1, 8.2, 8.4, 8.5, 8.7, 8.12, 8.13, 8.18, 13.3, 13.5, 13.6):

- Branches of the ophthalmic artery (posterior ethmoidal artery - recurrent meningeal artery).
- Meningeal branches of the internal maxillary artery.

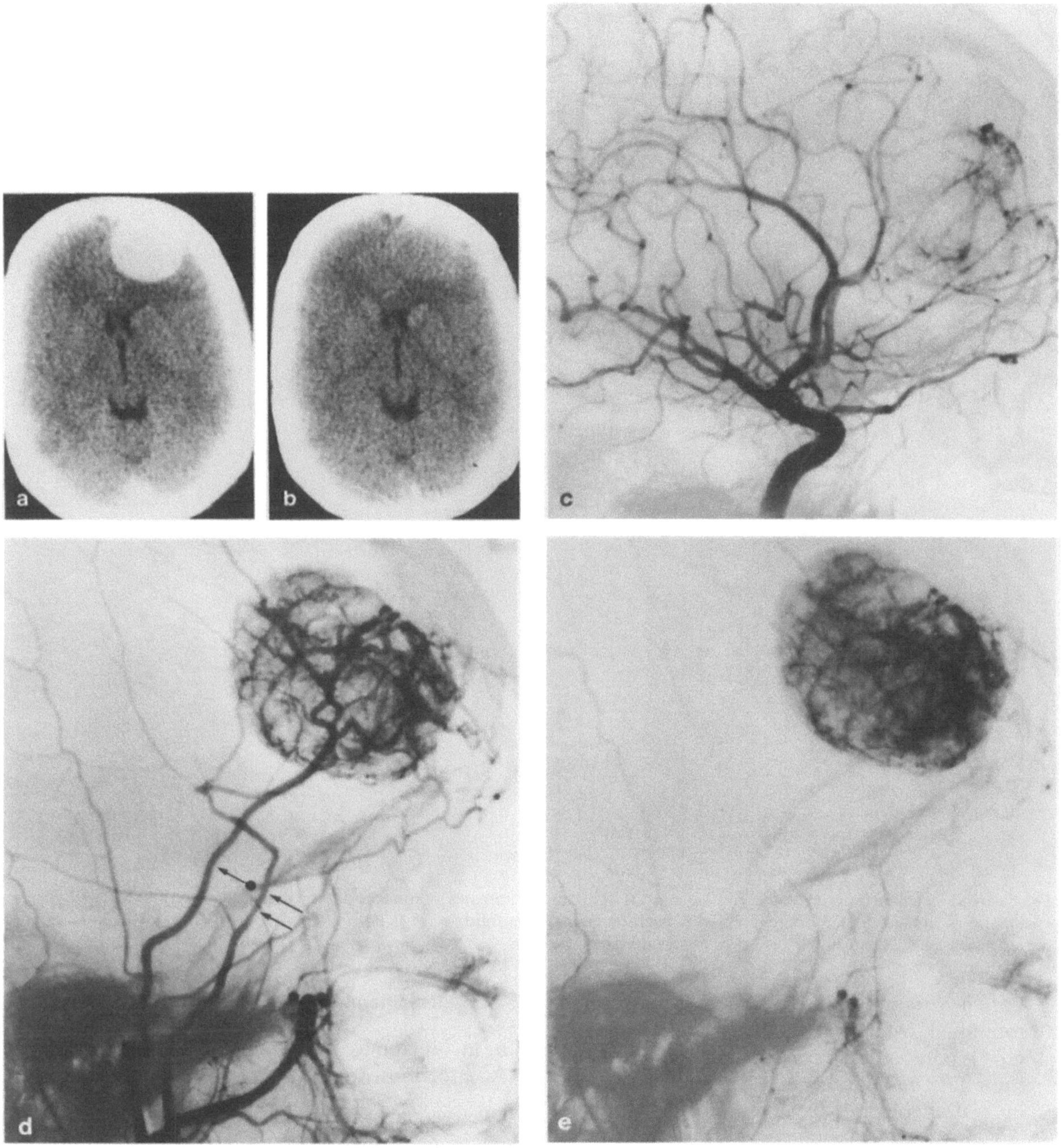

Fig. 5.3a–e. Haemangiopericytic meningioma. **a, b** CT. Examination with and without contrast medium. Sharply defined tumour with surrounding oedema. **c–e** Angiogram. Richly vascularized tumour supplied by branches of anterior cerebral artery and particularly by the frontal branch of the superficial temporal *(arrow with circle)* and middle meningeal *(double arrow)* arteries

- Middle meningeal artery (MMA). This artery is frequently involved in the supply of these meningiomas, as well as meningiomas located elsewhere. It usually enters the middle cranial fossa through the foramen spinosum; variants originating from the ophthalmic artery (Figs. 5.5, 5.6) enter through the superior orbital fissure and those from the carotid artery (ICA) (Fig. 5.7) may pass through the middle ear (stapedial) or arise within the cranium from the C_4 segment.
- Accessory meningeal artery, entering the skull through the foramen ovale.

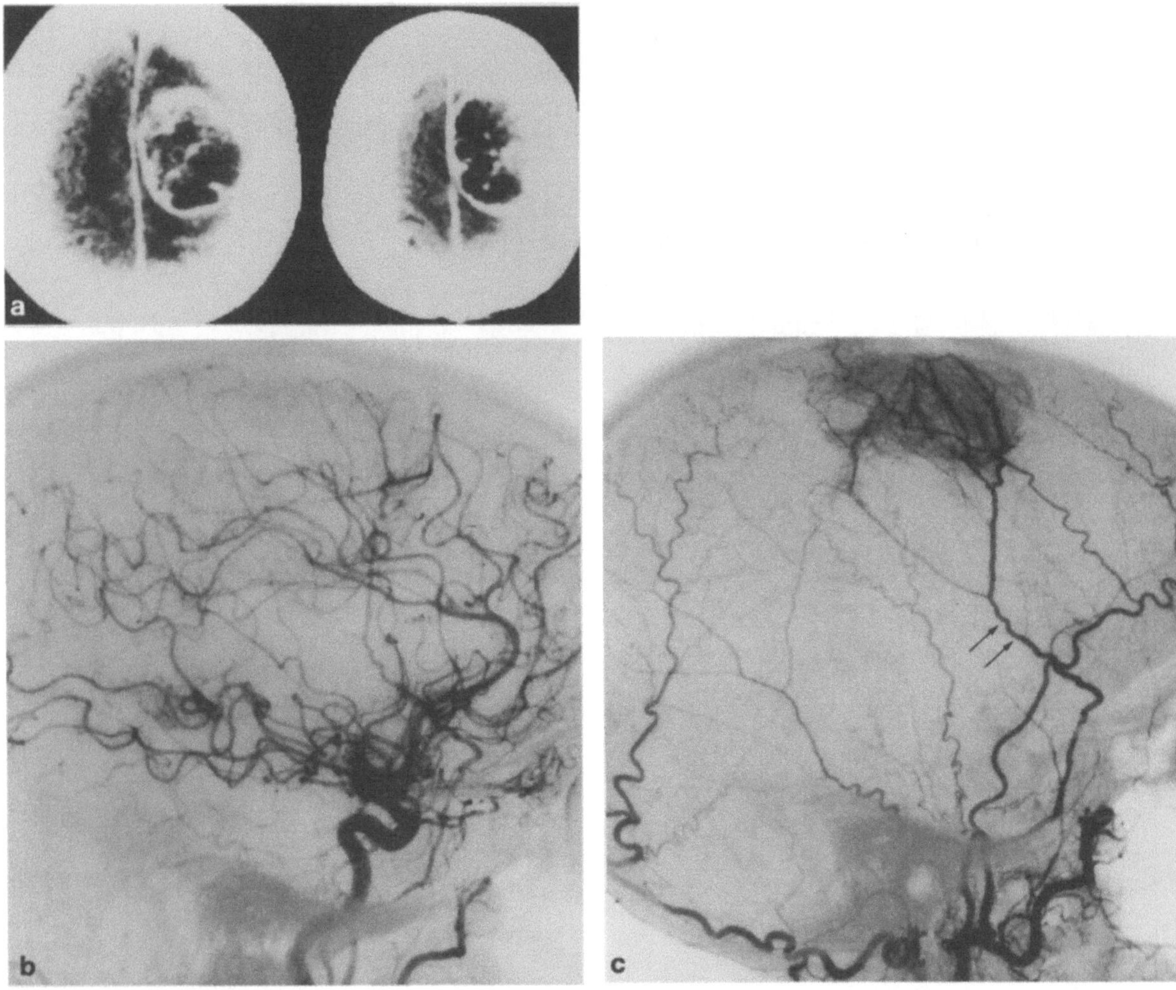

Fig. 5.4 a–c. Haemangiopericytic meningioma. **a** CT. The tumour shows enhancement. There are large necrotic areas. **b, c** Angiogram. The tumour is richly vascularized by branches of middle meningeal artery *(arrows)*. The internal carotid sector is not involved

Foramen rotundum artery, entering via foramen rotundum. Anastomoses between branches of C_4–C_5 portion of the carotid siphon and foramen rotundum, middle meningeal and accessory meningeal arteries can occur.

- Anterior deep temporal artery (DTA) which, particularly, supplies meningiomas with intraorbital extension. It enters the orbit via the inferior fissure or through the malar bone.
- The petromastoid artery gives a meningeal supply via the stylomastoid foramen. It may originate from the posterior auricular or occipital arteries and can supply meningiomas located more dorsally in the middle cranial fossa.
- Meningeal branches of C_5 and C_4 portion of carotid siphon.

5.3.3 Meningiomas of Posterior Cranial Fossa

In meningiomas of cerebellar fossa (Figs. 10.12, 13.8), the most frequent arteries involved are:

- Petrosquamosal branch of MMA.
- Meningeal-mastoid branch of occipital artery entering the skull through the mastoid emissary foramen.
- Posterior meningeal artery (PMA). This is a branch of vertebral or occipital arteries. PMA, after having circumvented the foramen magnum, runs near the midline along the insertion of the falx cerebelli, and anastomoses dorsally with the artery of the falx cerebri. Its territory can be taken over by the meningeal branch of the hypoglossal branch of the ascending pharyngeal artery. The latter is further from the midline and is

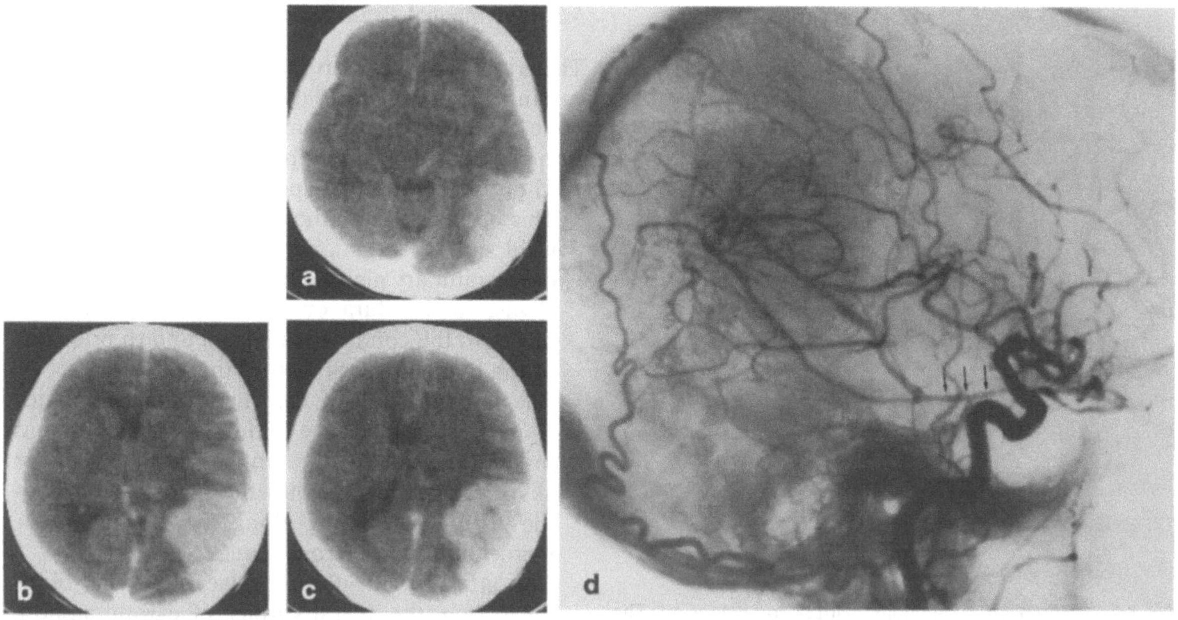

Fig. 5.5 a–d. Temporo-occipital endotheliomatous convexity meningioma. **a–c** CT. After contrast medium. The tumour shows slightly irregular borders. Peritumoral oedema is present. **d** Angiogram. The MMA *(arrows)* supplies the tumour areas from the ophthalmic artery

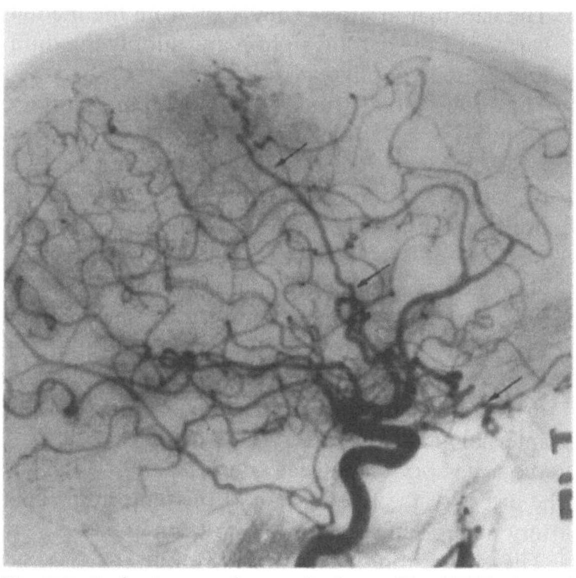

Fig. 5.6. Parietal convexity meningioma. The MMA *(arrow)* supplying the tumour arises from the ophthalmic artery

therefore projected somewhat lower than the former on the lateral angiogram.

Meningiomas of clivus and pontocerebellar angle (Figs. 10.3, 10.10) may be supplied by several arteries:

- Meningeal branches of C_5 and C_4 portion of carotid siphon.
- Petrosquamosal branch of MMA.
- Meningeal-mastoid branch of occipital artery.
- Meningeal branches of the posterior branch of the ascending pharyngeal artery (APA), namely:
  D1, the jugular branch, which enters the cranial cavity through the jugular foramen. It supplies nerves IX, X, XI and partially nerve XII
  D2, the hypoglossal branch, which is more medially located and passes through the hypoglossal foramen. This artery frequently gives off an important branch to the cerebellar fossa reciprocating with the supply from the vertebral and/or occipital arteries. The hypoglossal artery may give a branch anastomosing with a meningeal branch of vertebral artery through the odontoid arch system [161].
  D3, the artery of foramen lacerum (see Sect. 5.3.6).

Meningiomas of the foramen magnum are rare. These tumours can be supplied by branches of APA, occipital and vertebral arteries.

5.3.4 Convexity, Parasagittal, Falx Meningiomas

Dura of the convexity is mainly supplied by branches of the MMA which is frequently involved

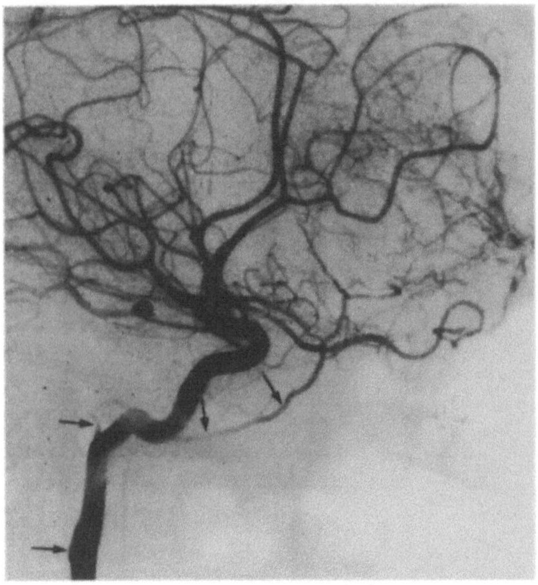

Fig. 5.7. Frontobasal meningioma with lateral extension. The tumour is richly vascularized by meningeal branches arising from anterior ethmoidal artery (ophthalmic artery). The MMA *(arrows)*, also partially involved, originates from the ICA

in the vascularization of meningiomas of this region. Meningeal branches of the occipital and posterior auricular arteries supply blood to the occipital convexity dura. Branches of superficial temporal artery can also be involved, particularly if the meningioma has invaded the bone (Figs. 5.3, 5.5–5.6, 6.1, 6.2, 6.3, 13.1, 13.2).

Peripheral branches of both MMA form a vascular arcade which extends along the junction of the lateral wall of superior sagittal sinus and the dura of the convexity. This arcade anastomoses anteriorly with the anterior falx artery arising from the anterior ethmoidal artery and posteriorly with the PMA. The arcade supplies parasagittal meningiomas (Figs. 5.4, 13.4), and from it arteries supply the falx and meningiomas arising from it (Fig. 6.6).

5.3.5 Tentorial Meningiomas

The vascular supply of tentorial meningiomas depends on their location and their extension supra- or infratentorially. There is almost always some supply from the cavernous branches of C_5–C_4 portion of carotid siphon. MMA, APA, occipital and vertebral arteries may also contribute (Figs. 9.2, 9.4, 9.6, 9.7, 9.10).

5.3.6 Meningeal Branches of the Carotid Siphon

These include several arteries which can supply into varying degrees tentorial, parasellar, clivus and pontocerebellar meningiomas.

Branches arising from C_5 portion:

- The posteroinferior hypophyseal artery (PIHA). This originates from the medial surface of the carotid siphon and supplies: (1) the posterior lobe of the pituitary gland, (2) the medial artery of the clivus, to the dura on the clivus, with anastomoses to the contralateral vessel and to branches of the hypoglossal branch of the APA.
- The lateral artery of the clivus. This originates from the lateral surface of the carotid siphon and branches: (1) to the dura on the lateral part of the clivus, anastomosing with the jugular branch of the APA, (2) running along the attachment of tentorium to the petrous bone.
- The artery of the foramen lacerum. This originates from the lateral surface of carotid siphon, runs dorsally to the foramen lacerum and anastomoses with branches of APA and MMA.
- An artery to the trigeminal ganglion and surrounding dura.

Branches arising from C_4 portion:

- The capsular arteries. They arise from the medial surface of the carotid siphon and supply the dura lining the hypophyseal fossa.
- The inferolateral trunk (ILT), also called artery of inferior cavernous sinus. This is a relatively large artery arising from the inferolateral surface of carotid siphon. It gives off several small branches supplying the dura of the cavernous sinus and of Meckel's cave, the third, fourth and sixth nerves and the trigeminal ganglion. An anterior branch may anastomose with the ophthalmic artery after crossing the superior orbital fissure. A lateral branch may anastomose with the artery of the foramen rotundum, a branch of the internal maxillary artery, and with branches of the accessory meningeal artery.

The artery of the free margin of the tentorium. This artery may originate from:

- The C_5 portion of the carotid siphon
- The middle/accessory meningeal arteries
- The ophthalmic artery

5.3.7 Intraventricular Meningiomas

The primary supply to intraventricular meningiomas is from choroidal arteries. Adhesion to brain substance induces supply from parenchymal vessels.

5.3.8 Ectopic Meningiomas

Depending on location, various branches of the external carotid artery may be involved in the supply of ectopic meningiomas. Sometimes the vascularity is abundant and the differential diagnosis from other richly vascular tumours, particularly chemodectomas, may be impossible (Fig. 11.9).

5.4 Changes in the Venous Circulation

Infiltration of sinuses is relatively frequent in meningiomas located in certain regions:

- Parasagittal meningiomas may infiltrate the superior sagittal sinus (Figs. 6.4, 6.5).
- Laterally located tentorial meningiomas may infiltrate the transverse sinuses (Figs. 9.13, 9.14).
- Falcotentorial meningiomas may infiltrate the straight sinus and/or the Galenic vein (Fig. 9.12).
- Meningiomas of the cerebellopontine angle can infiltrate the superior and/or inferior petrous sinuses (Fig. 10.3).
- Meningiomas laterally in the cerebellopontine angle or cerebellar convexity may infiltrate the sigmoid sinus.
- Infiltration of cavernous and/or sphenoparietal sinus may occur in parasellar and in sphenoid wing meningiomas. Involvement may be evident from segmental stenosis or occlusion of a sinus and/or diversion of venous drainage (see Chap. 8).

5.5 Indications for Angiography

In general, meningiomas are diagnosed by CT and/or MRI. Angiography is performed to obtain complementary information which may be useful for treatment.
A high degree of vascularization, possible encasement and sinus infiltration may be diagnosed or, at least, suspected after CT and, particularly, MRI examination, but precise demonstration is best achieved by angiography. In certain situations, detailed knowledge of the venous anatomy may be crucial in deciding operability in an individual case (see Chaps. 6, 8, 9, 10).
Studying the external carotid artery can add confirmatory evidence in the diagnosis of atypical meningiomas (see Chap. 11, Sect. 11.1). In tumours richly supplied by the external carotid artery preoperative embolization may facilitate surgery.

6 Convexity, Parasagittal, and Falx Meningiomas

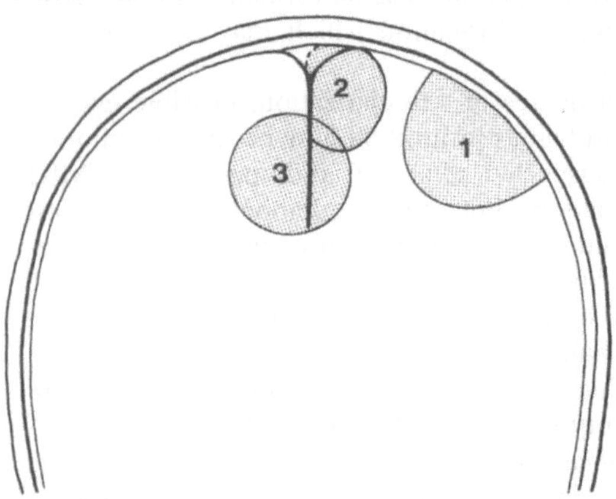

1 Convexity meningiomas
2 Parasagittal meningiomas
3 Falx meningiomas

6.1 Incidence and Localization

6.1.1 Convexity and Parasagittal Tumours

Tumours of the convexity and those located in the parasagittal area are the most frequent of the intracranial meningiomas. Together they account for about 40% of all meningiomas, and about 50% of them occur in women [128].

Convexity meningiomas are attached to the dura of the convexity and are most prevalent in the parietal and frontal regions. Tumours in the temporal and occipital areas are relatively rare.

Parasagittal meningiomas are located at the point where the dura of the convexity continues in the dura forming the lateral wall of the superior sagittal sinus. They are generally located along the middle third of the sinus: meningiomas located along the anterior third are less frequent and along the posterior portion are relatively rare. The sinus itself is often infiltrated by the tumour.

6.1.2 Falx Meningiomas

Falx meningiomas are relatively uncommon, constituting about 5% of all intracranial meningiomas, with a high frequency in women (ca. 90% of patients according to Jacobs et al. [128]). They are generally attached to the anterior and middle portion of the falx, growing bilaterally in about a third of patients.

Convexity, parasagittal and falx meningiomas are frequently very large when diagnosed. Tumours more than 7 cm in diameter occur, sometimes causing considerable atrophy of the surrounding brain. Epileptic seizures and/or a slowly progressive psychosyndrome are the most frequently presenting symptoms.

6.2 Computed Tomography and Magnetic Resonance Imaging

Using computed tomography (CT) and/or magnetic resonance imaging (MRI), the diagnosis of these meningiomas and the amount of compression of brain parenchyma poses no great difficulty. Occasionally growing with their long axis parallel to the vault (Figs. 6.1, 13.1), the tumours appear as roughly rounded, well-circumscribed masses (Figs. 6.2–6.7), commonly showing a broad surface of contact with the meninges of the convexity and/or falx.

Fig. 6.1 a–f. Frontoparietal convexity endotheliomatous meningioma. **a, b** MRI (SE 500/50). Study after Gd-DTPA. The tumour displays an evident enhancement. There is a small cyst *(black area→)* in the peripheral portion of the meningioma close to the cerebral parenchyma. Note the thickened dura extending far from the globoid mass due to a flat portion of the tumour *(arrow from circle)*. **c** Angiogram. There is no pathological vascularization on the angiogram of the internal carotid artery (ICA). **d, e** Very large middle meningeal artery *(arrows)* supplying the tumour. **f** Angiogram after embolization showing occlusion of the middle meningeal artery *(arrow)*

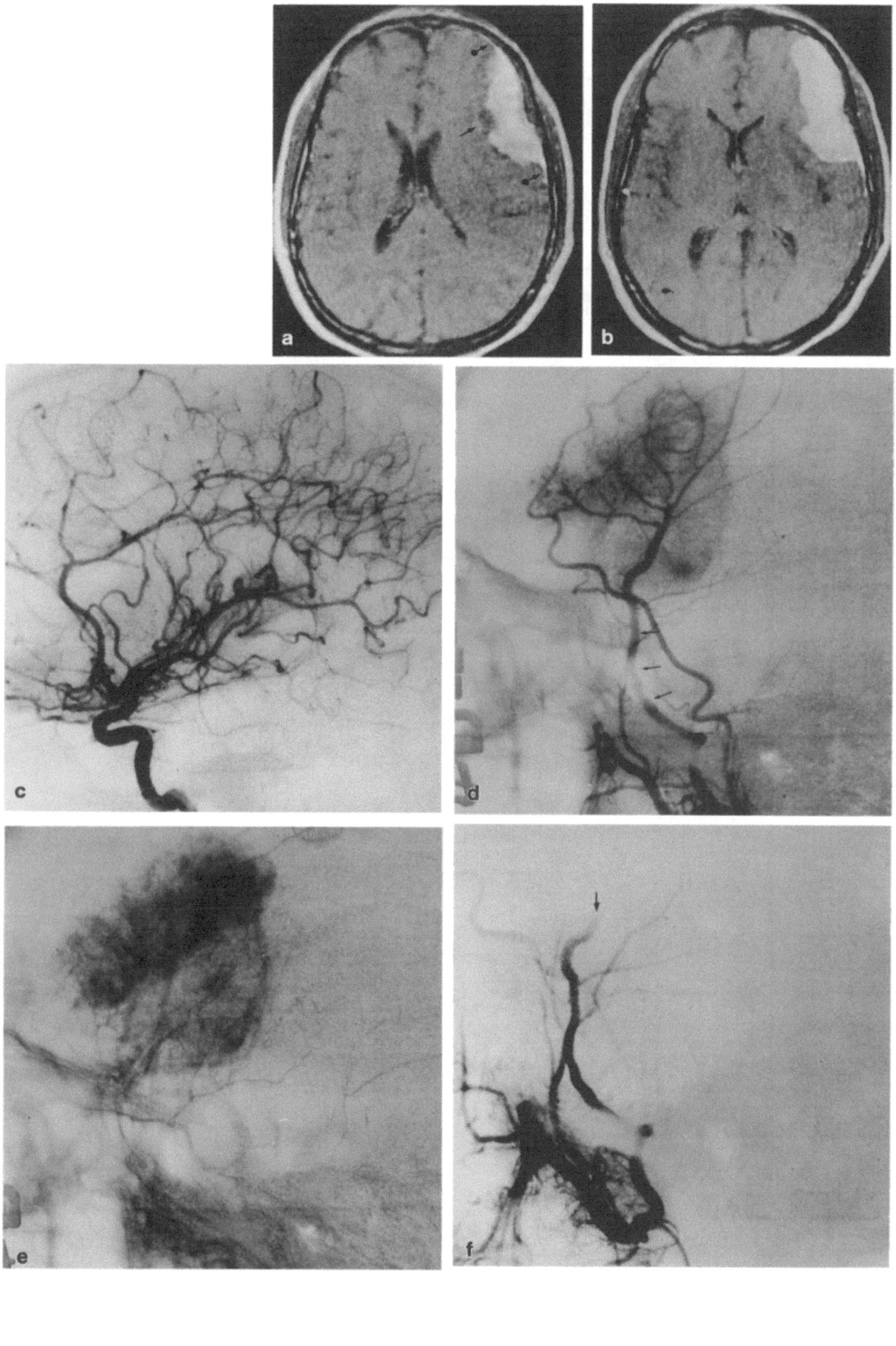
a
b
c
d
e
f

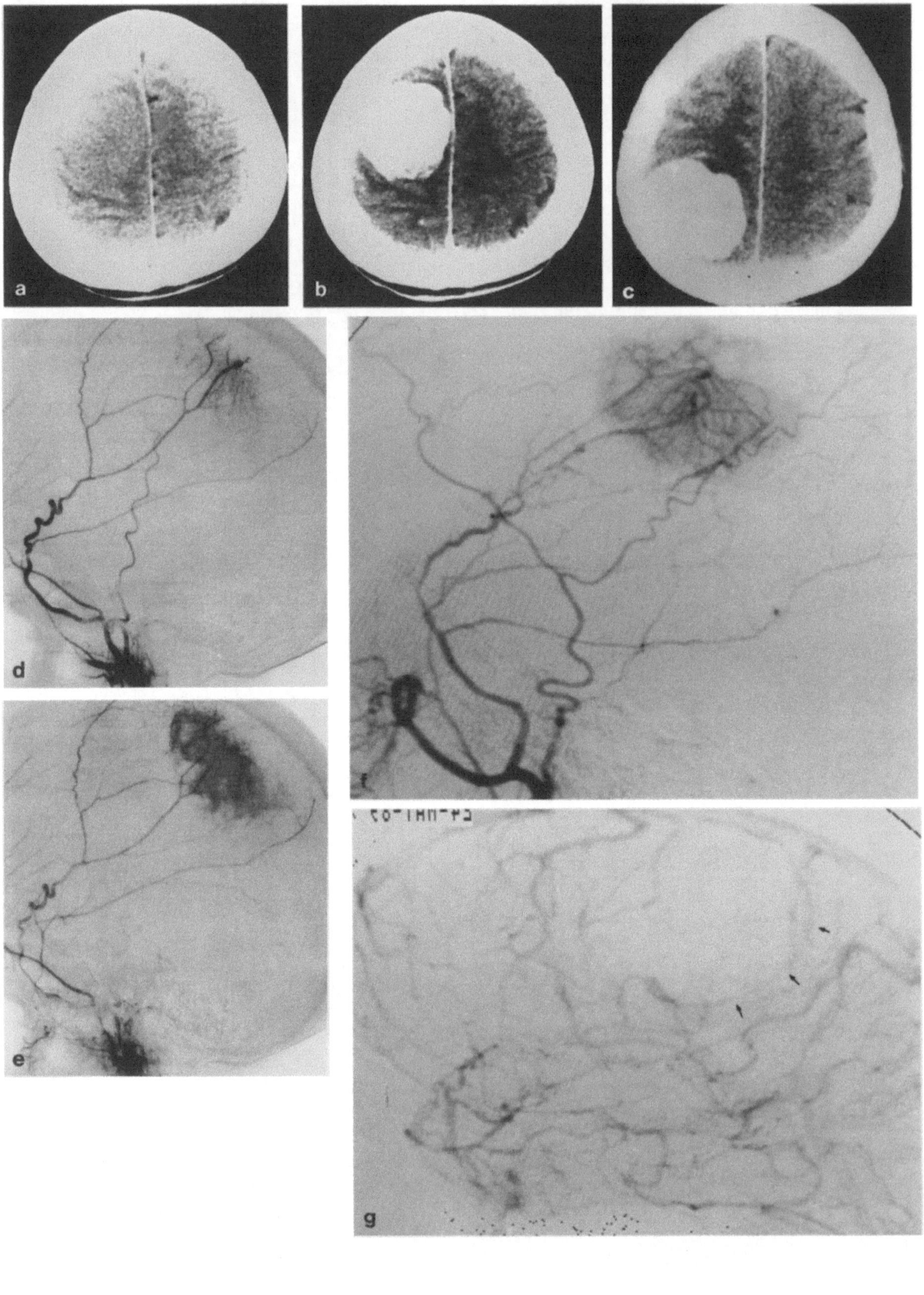
a
b
c
d
e
f
g

They appear slightly hyperdense on CT, with rich, rather homogeneous enhancement. Calcification occurs in 10% [207], that is, less frequently than in skull base and posterior fossa meningiomas. Atypical features, with low density areas corresponding to cyst formation or other degenerative processes, are frequent in this group of meningiomas (Figs. 6.8, 6.9; see also Chaps. 3, 11.1).

Bone changes are best shown by CT. Convexity and parasagittal meningiomas may induce hyperostosis of the calvarium. More rarely, they cause thinning or destruction. Hyperostosis can occur with globoid tumours (Fig. 13.1), but it is more commonly associated with en plaque lesions, which are not rare in this localization (Fig. 6.11). Ectopic meningiomas arising from arachnoid cells located within the diploë and/or outer table can also lead to hyperostosis (Fig. 6.10) [9, 58, 106, 308].

Magnetic resonance imaging is of particular use in showing the anatomical relationship between tumour and superior sagittal sinus and falx (Figs. 4.9, 4.10, 4.12, 6.12). MRI [39] can demonstrate sinus involvement in many cases (Figs. 6.12, 4.13, 4.14). Contrast medium may be necessary to show soft tissue components of en plaque tumours.

Peritumoral oedema is very frequent with these tumours. It is recognizable in CT and/or MRI, extending mainly into the corona radiata; the external and internal capsules tend to be spared (see Chap. 12).

6.3 Angiography

There is displacement of cortical vessels away from the vault or falx and, depending on tumour size, there may be stretching and contralateral shift of middle and anterior cerebral arteries. The anterior cerebral artery tends to be depressed by falx and parasagittal meningiomas, and the callosomarginal artery may be displaced ipsilaterally by the former.

The tumours are frequently richly vascularized from the internal carotid artery by leptomeningeal vessels arising from cortical branches and, in parasagittal and falx meningiomas in the frontal and parietal regions, from the anterior meningeal branch arising from ophthalmic artery (Fig. 6.3). Branches of the external carotid artery are usually involved, mainly the ipsilateral middle meningeal artery (Figs. 6.1, 6.2, 6.3, 6.6), but there is often considerable contribution from the contralateral middle meningeal artery across the midline. Meningeal branches of the occipital arteries may supply the more posteriorly situated tumours. Supply from the superficial temporal artery is uncommon and generally indicates that the meningioma has infiltrated through the bone (Fig. 13.1).

The venous phase of the angiogram should demonstrate any narrowing, filling defects within or occlusion of the superior sagittal sinus indicating tumour involvement, which occurs often with parasagittal meningiomas [89] (Figs. 6.4, 6.5). The relationship of the tumour to large cortical veins draining into the sinus is also shown (Fig. 6.2f–g).

6.4 Differential Diagnosis

Atypical features on CT are very frequent in this group of patients. They include low density areas with poor or absent enhancement, which may be within the tumour or be located adjacent to it. In these cases a misdiagnosis of glioma or metastasis may be suggested (Figs. 6.8, 6.9). The cause of these atypical findings is discussed in Chaps. 1, 3, 11). Broad contact with the dura and hypertrophied branches of the external carotid artery supplying the tumour support a diagnosis of meningioma, but occasionally the diagnosis is only established at surgery (see also Chap. 11).

Furthermore, in patients with an established or even suspected malignant neoplasm, typical meningiomas can be misinterpreted as peripheral metastases. The possibility of meningiomas should always be taken into consideration, particularly in women with cancer of the breast or of the genital organs. The association of these malignancies and meningiomas is not infrequent [128].

Primary, solitary lymphoma involving the brain adjacent to the convexity can have the CT features of a meningioma [121] (Fig. 6.13). On the angiogram, a lymphoma appears frequently as an avascular mass, and the external carotid artery is usually not in-

Fig. 6.2 a–g. Three examples of large endotheliomatous meningiomas of the parietal convexity. **a, b** CT. On the routine scan the tumour appears as a slightly hyperdense mass which displays a rich enhancement after contrast medium. There is a broad dural attachment. **c** CT. Another example of large meningioma of the convexity with rich enhancement. **d, e** Angiogram of the same case shown in **c**. There is a rich supply through the middle meningeal artery. **f–g** Angiogram in another case of convexity meningioma supplied by branches of middle meningeal artery (f). In the venous phase of internal carotid angiogram cortical veins (→) surrounding the tumour are visible

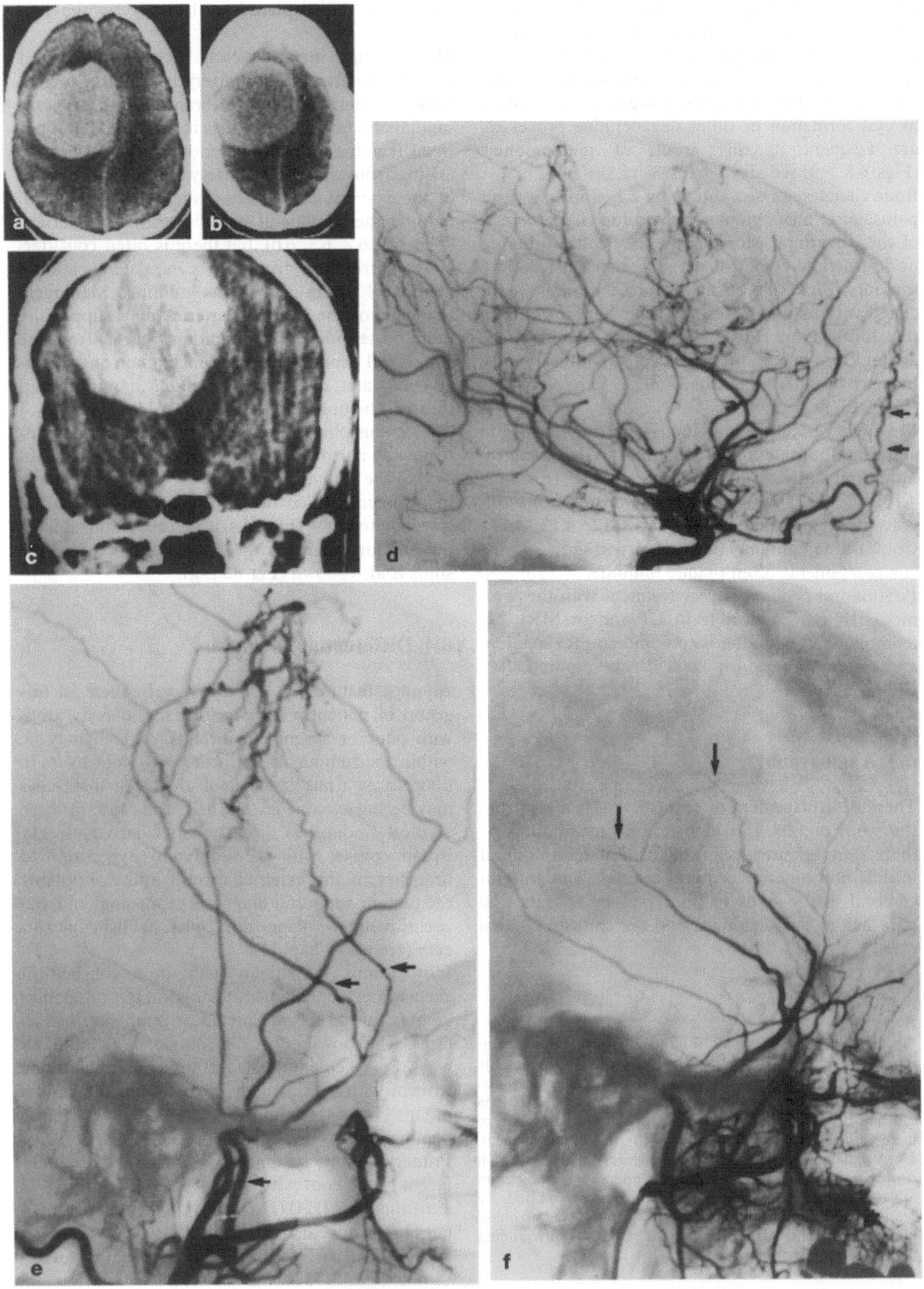

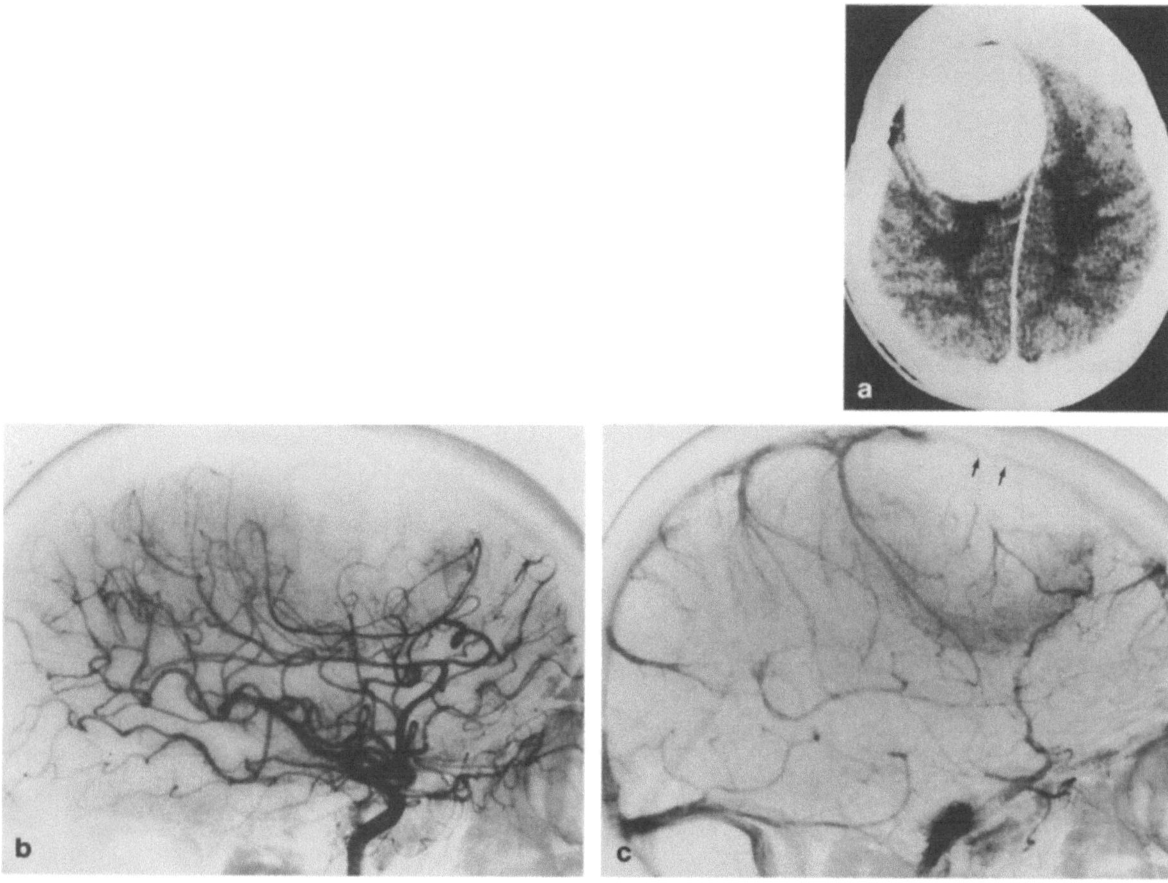

Fig. 6.4a–c. Large parasagittal meningioma. **a** CT. Very large rounded mass showing evident contrast enhancement. **b,c** Angiogram. The tumour is poorly vascularized. There is an evident downward displacement of the pericallosal and callosomarginalis arteries. The superior sagittalis sinus is infiltrated *(arrows)*. The angiogram of the external carotid artery was bilaterally normal

volved. Solitary myeloma also may simulate meningioma, but usually causes bone destruction and is commoner in elderly men.

Cryptic vascular malformations, particularly cavernous angiomas when superficial, can simulate meningioma on CT [223]. MRI, in which cavernous angiomas frequently appear as hyperintense area surrounded in all sequences by hypointense rim due to the presence of hemosiderin, can be very useful in the differential diagnosis.

Fig. 6.3a–f. Large parasagittal meningioma. **a–c** CT. The broad contact of the tumour with dura of the convexity and falx is well demonstrated on the coronal plane. **d** Angiogram of the ICA. There is an evident pathological vascularization. The tumour is supplied mainly by anterior meningeal artery *(arrows)* arising from the ophthalmic artery. **e** Angiogram of the external carotid artery (ECA), showing that the tumour is richly vascularized by branches of middle meningeal artery *(arrows)*. **f** Angiogram after embolization of these vessels *(arrows)*.

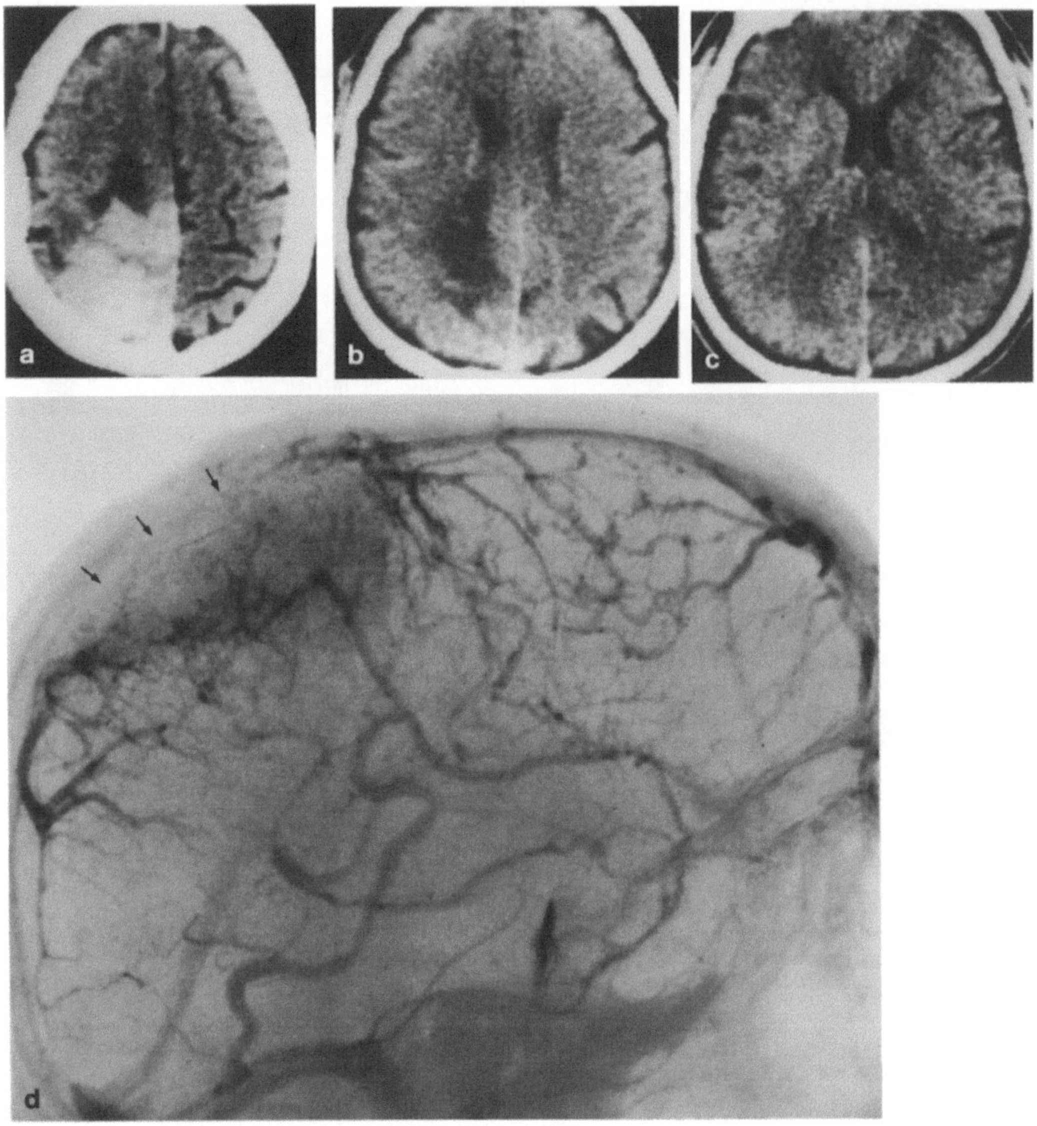

Fig. 6.5 a–d. Large parieto-occipital parasagittal meningiomas. **a–c** CT. Large enhancing mass in contact with dura of the convexity and sinus. The hypodensity in the corona radiata corresponds probably to a small area of oedema. **d** Angiogram. There is infiltration of the superior sagittal sinus (→)

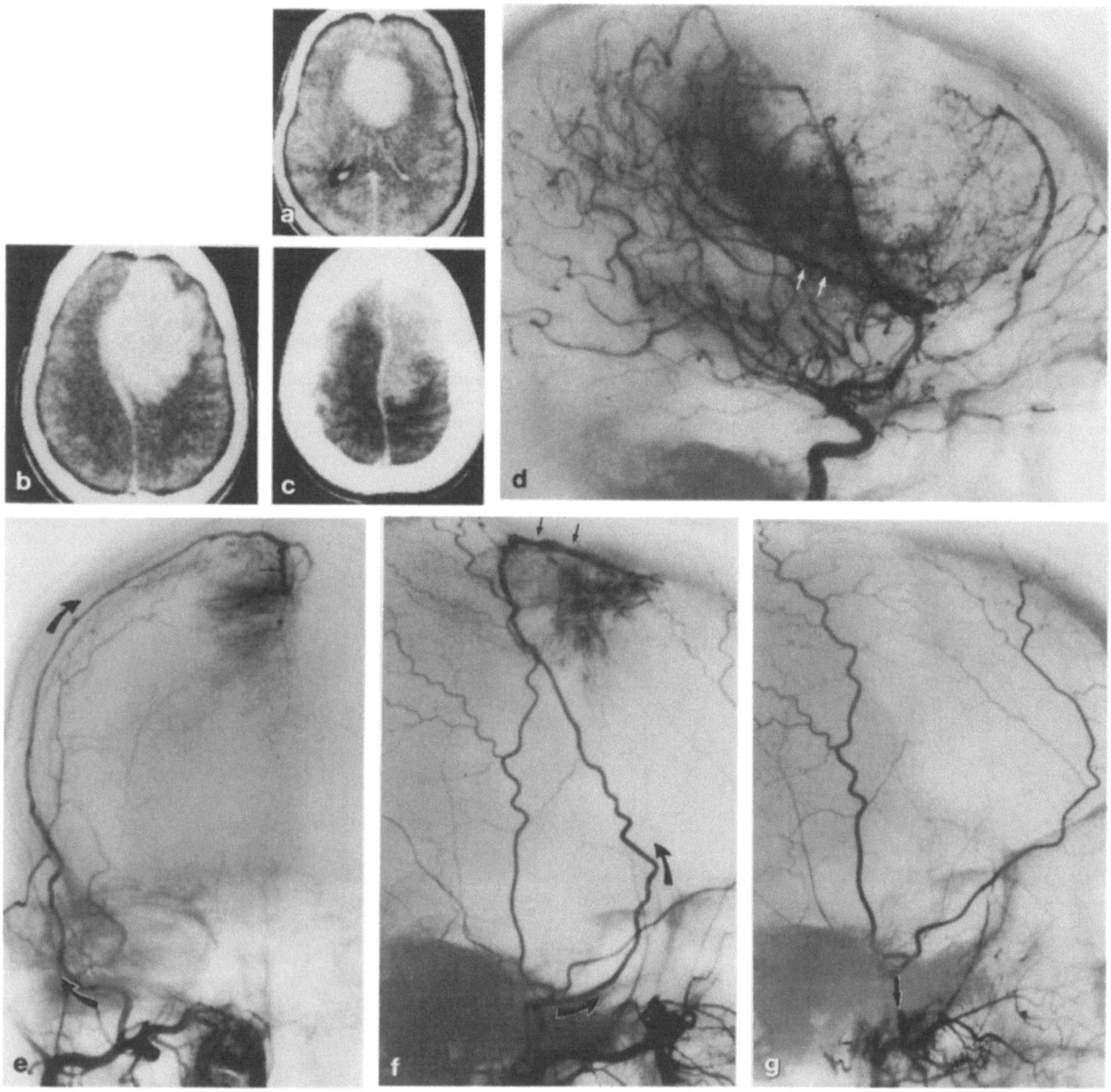

Fig. 6.6 a–g. Falx meningioma extending prevalently on the right. **a–c** CT. Very large enhanced mass in contact with the falx. **d** Angiogram of the ICA. Displaced pericallosal artery *(arrows)*. There is a pathological vascularization, too. **e–g** Angiogram of the right ECA. There is a dilatated middle meningeal artery *(large arrows)* which continues in a branch *(small arrows)* running parasagittally along the insertion of the lateral wall of superior sagittal sinus to the dura of the convexity. This gives off several small branches supplying the tumour. **g** Control after embolization of middle meningeal artery (⟶)

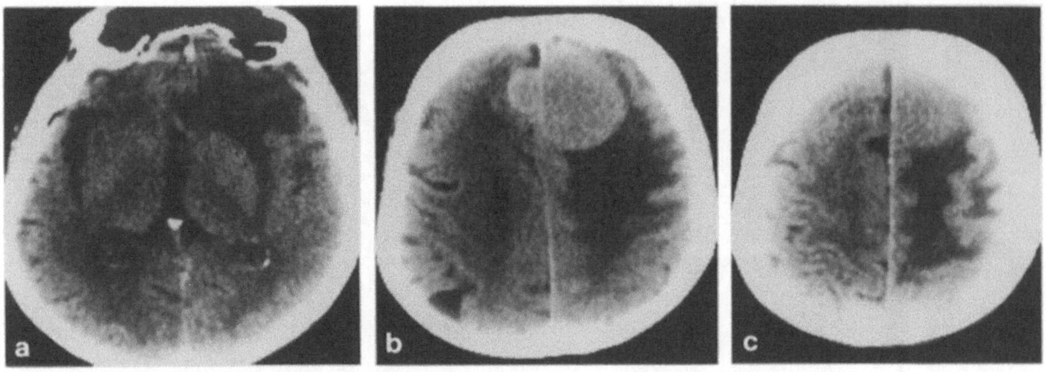

Fig. 6.7 a–c. CT. Another example of falx meningioma in the frontal area. The tumour extends prevalently on the right. There is also an evident peritumoral oedema involving the corona radiata and the external capsula. There is a small nodule on the left

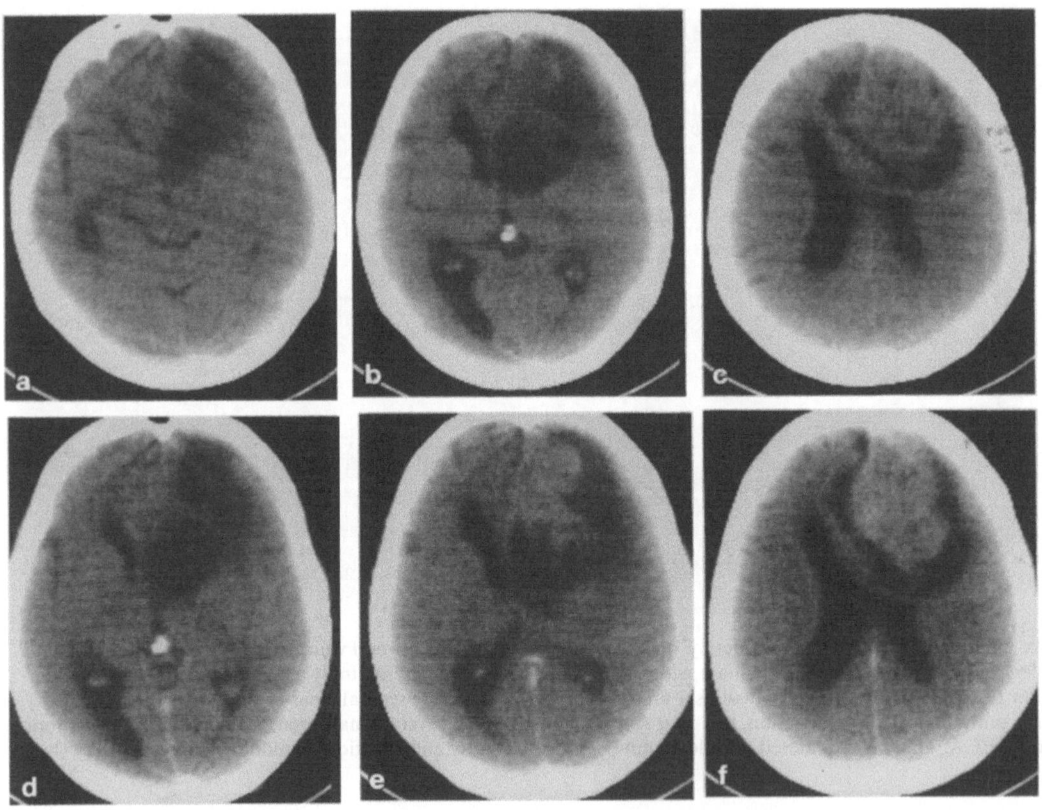

Fig. 6.8 a–f. Atypical endotheliomatous falx meningioma in the frontal area. **a–c** CT without and **d–f** CT with contrast medium. The tumour is characterized by a solid portion showing contrast enhancement and by areas of decreased density which at surgery appeared to correspond to necrotic and cystic parts of the tumour

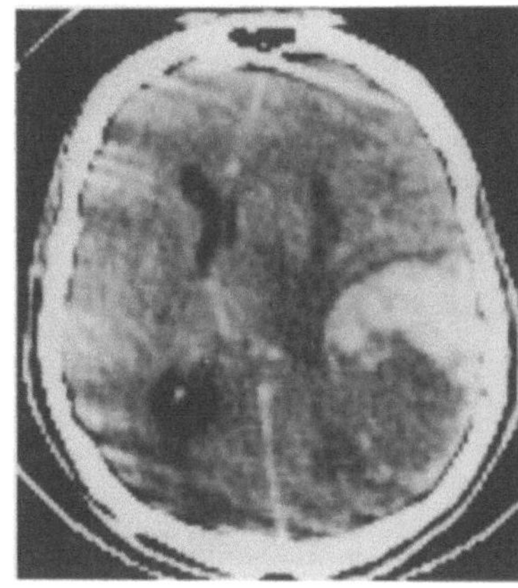

Fig. 6.9. Atypical temporoparietal endotheliomatous meningioma. CT. The tumour appears as a well-circumscribed mass with a broad dural surface. There is an evident contrast enhancement of the solid part of the tumour. The large area of hypodensity corresponded at surgery and at histological study to necrotic tissue. The peritumoral oedema is evident and involves the external and the posterior limb of the internal capsules

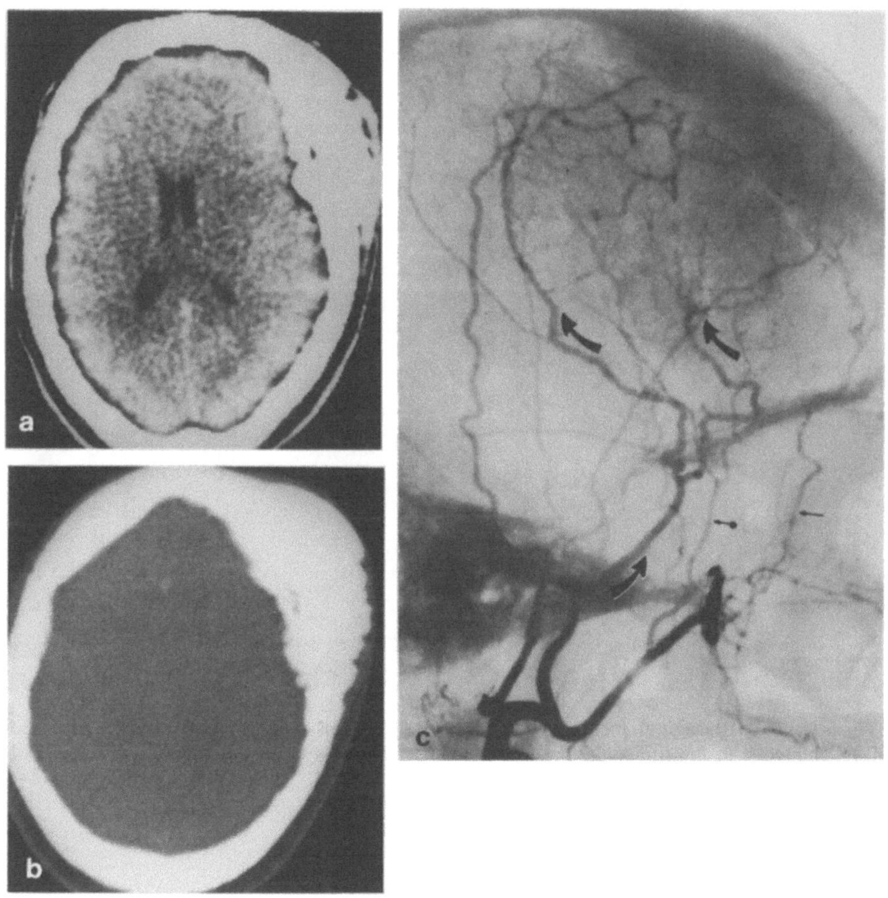

Fig. 6.10 a-c. Ectopic meningioma of the calvarium leading to hyperostosis involving the outer table, diploë, inner table and infiltrating the adjacent dura (confirmed at surgery). **a, b** CT. Hyperostosis of the bone with inward and outward bulging of the calvarium. Irregular surface of the tumour. **c** Angiogram. Hypertrophied branches of the external carotid artery supplying the tumour. Middle meningeal artery (↗). Deep temporal artery (•⟶). Anterior deep temporal (⟶)

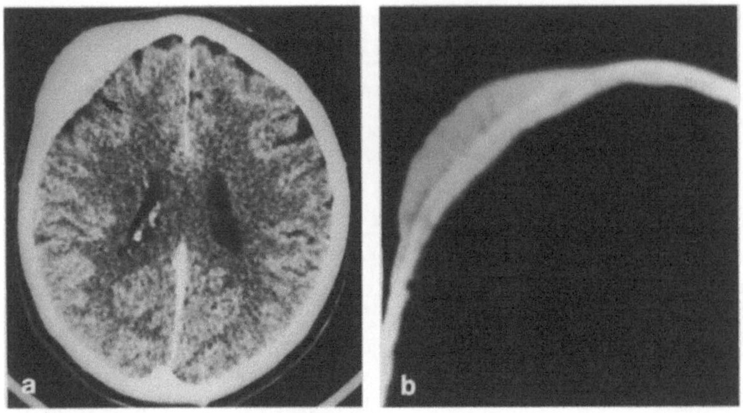

Fig. 6.11 a, b. CT. Meningioma en plaque with hyperostosis involving particularly the outer table, which is bulged outwards. There are new trabeculae perpendicular to the table. After contrast medium the small en plaque portion of the tumour is recognizable (→)

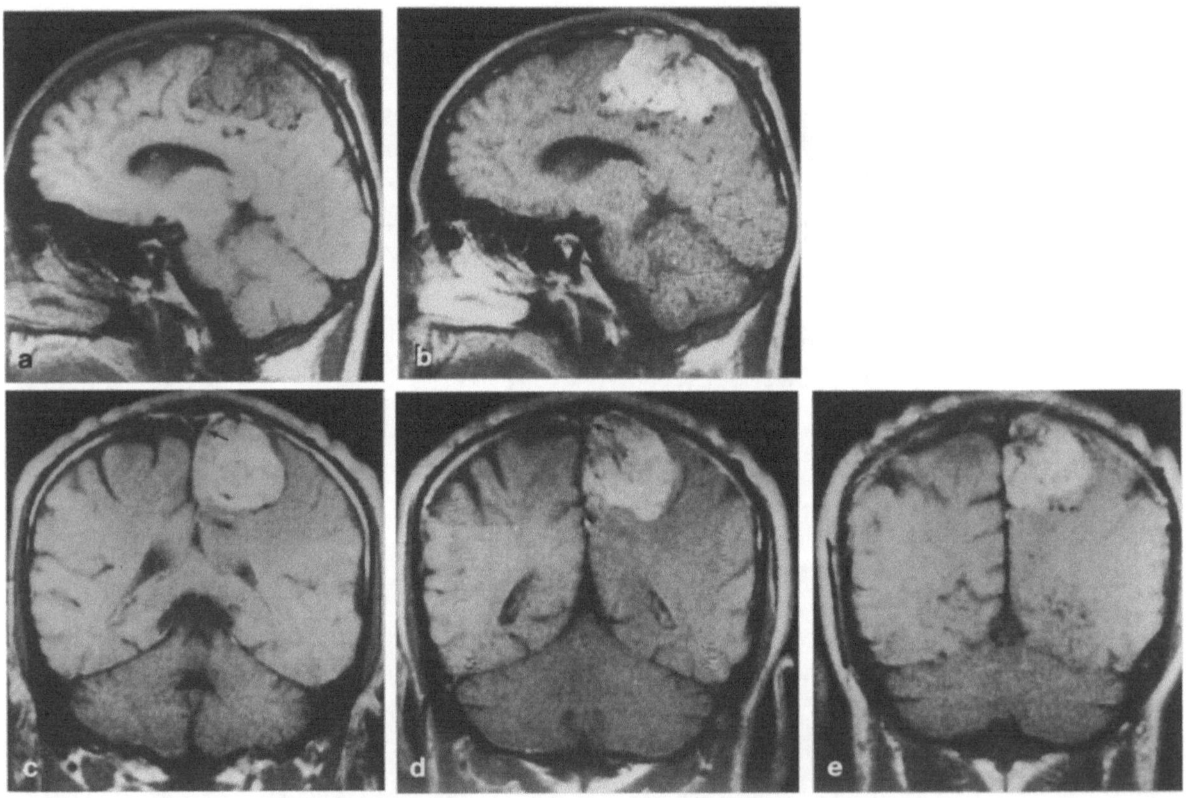

Fig. 6.12 a–e. Parasagittal meningioma. **a, b** MRI. On this T1-weighted scan the tumour appears hypointense. There is an evident enhancement after Gd-DTPA. There are several intratumoral vessels confirmed at angiography. **c–e** MRI. T1-weighted images after Gd-DTPA. There is a compression (→) of the sagittal sinus (**c**). More dorsally, the sinus (→) appears partially infiltrated (**d–e**). This was confirmed at surgery

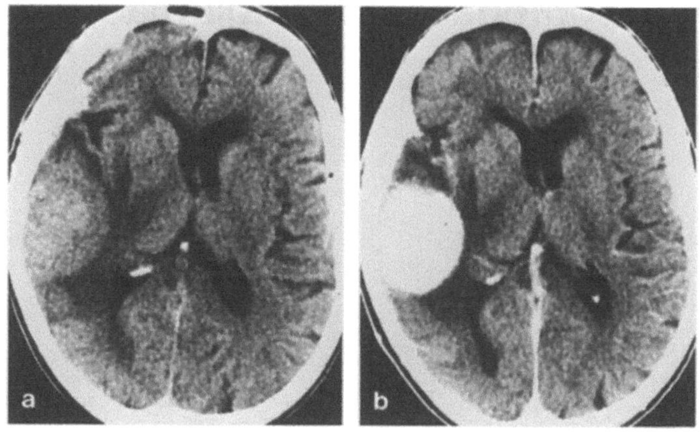

Fig. 6.13a, b. Primary lymphoma involving the tempoparietal region simulating meningioma. **a** CT without and **b** CT with contrast medium. The slightly hyperdense well-circumscribed tumour with a broad dural surface displays a rich enhancement. There is a strong peritumoral oedema. The tumour appeared in the angiogram poorly vascularized without involvement of the ECA

7 Frontobasal Meningiomas

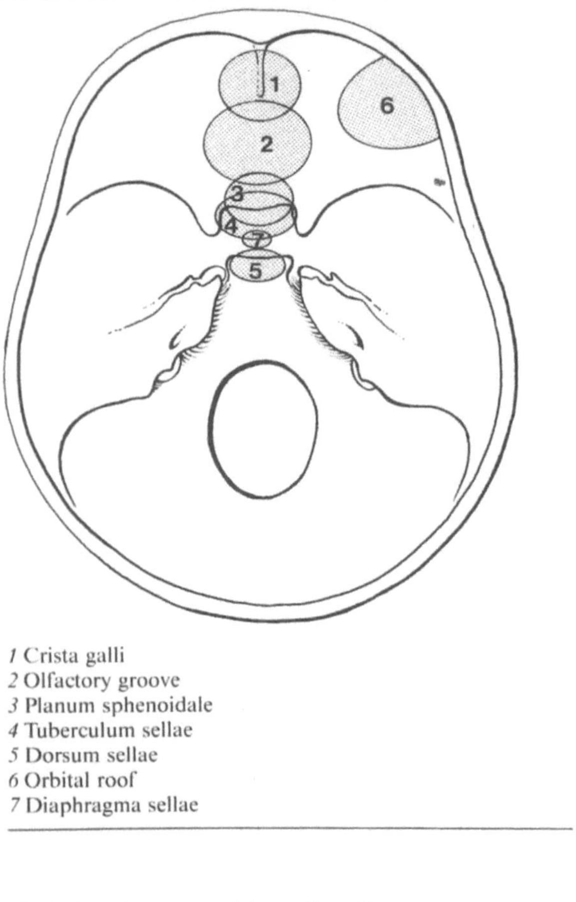

1 Crista galli
2 Olfactory groove
3 Planum sphenoidale
4 Tuberculum sellae
5 Dorsum sellae
6 Orbital roof
7 Diaphragma sellae

7.1 Incidence and Localization

Frontobasal meningiomas are relatively uncommon in comparison with other groups and constitute about 10% of all intracranial meningiomas. The incidence in women is particularly high: about 90% of the patients of Jacobs et al. [128] were women.
Frontobasal meningiomas are usually located in the midline with varying degrees of lateral extension. According to the apparent primary point of dural attachment, the following subgroups are distinguished (see diagram) as meningiomas of crista galli, olfactory groove, planum sphenoidale, tuberculum sellae, dorsum sellae, diaphragma sellae and orbital roof.
Olfactory groove, crista galli and orbital roof meningiomas are often large before the diagnosis is established. A slowly progressive psychosyndrome with or without disturbance of smell is the most frequent presenting sign.
Tuberculum sellae and planum sphenoidale meningiomas may cause compression of the optic chiasm leading to diagnostic studies earlier, when the tumours are relatively small. They may extend laterally into the optic canal and compress the optic nerve [6]. Growth into the suprasellar and sometimes into the retrosellar area may cause compression of the third ventricle or blockage of the foramen of Monro and secondary hydrocephalus.
The rare meningiomas arising from the dorsum sellae may grow in a similar fashion, but retrosellar extension is more frequent then. Meningiomas arising from the diaphragma sellae are also rare and may be difficult to distinguish from pituitary adenomas. They do not cause hyperostosis and may enlarge the sella.

7.2 Computed Tomography – Magnetic Resonance Imaging

Frontobasal meningiomas on computed tomography (CT) are generally rounded or occasionally lobulated, well-circumscribed, slightly hyperdense tumours with marked and, usually, homogeneous enhancement (Figs. 7.1, 7.2, 7,3, 7.8, 7.10). Hypodense meningiomas are rare in this region [207, 264]. Calcification is frequent: in the material of New et al. [207] it was present in 17% of cases.
The tumour can erode the skull base and spread into the paranasal sinuses (Figs. 7.2, 7.6). However, hyperostosis is more frequent in frontobasal and sphenoid wing tumours than in meningiomas elsewhere. This can be recognized easily on CT and of-

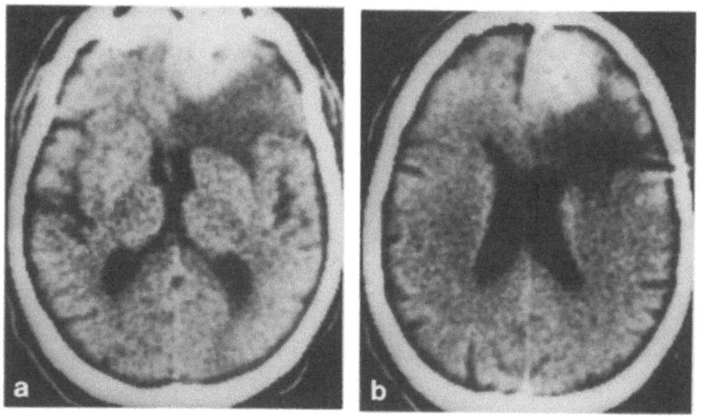

Fig. 7.1 a, b. CT. Frontobasal meningioma originating from crista galli. The tumour is partially calcified and shows rich contrast enhancement. Oedema spreads dorsally into the external capsule. The frontal horn is compressed

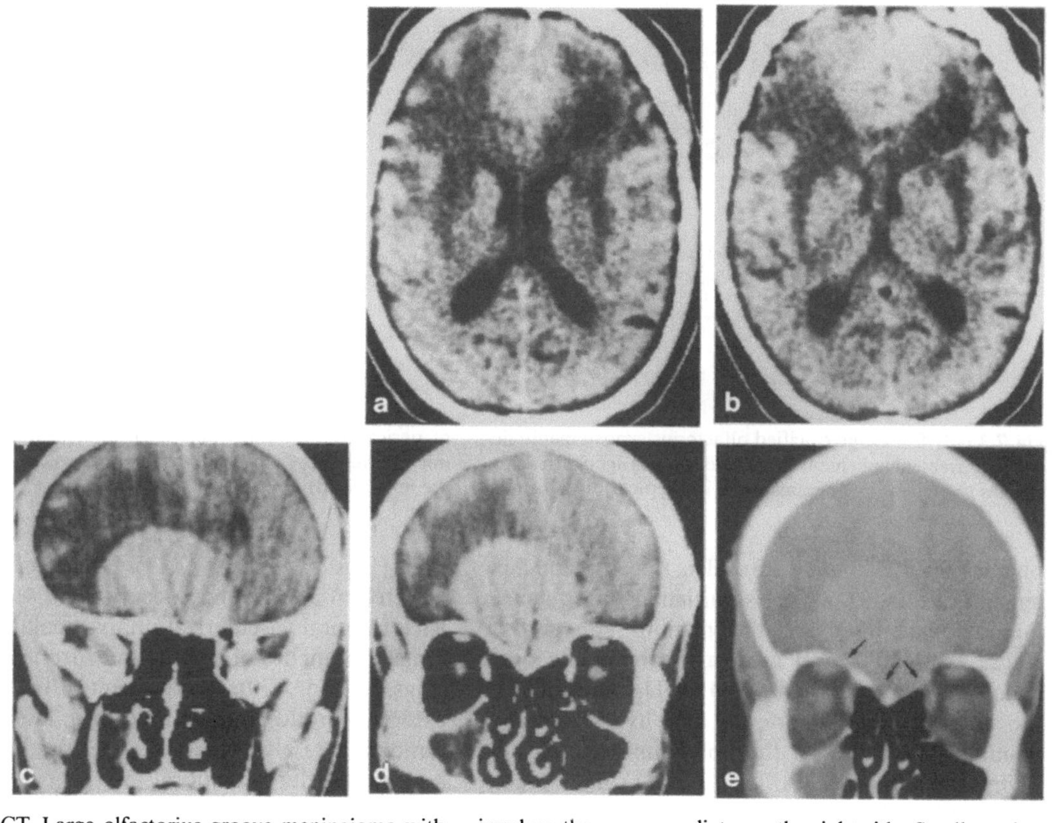

Fig. 7.2. a, b CT. Large olfactorius groove meningioma with extensive oedema involving also the external capsule bilaterally. **c–e** CT. Large olfactorius groove meningioma. Oedema involves the corona radiata on the right side. Small erosion *(arrows)* on the base of the skull

ten with MRI (Figs. 7.5, 7.9), as well as on plain radiographs.

A typical finding occurring in some meningiomas of the presellar region is upward bulging of the planum sphenoidale. This appearance is more extensively described in Chaps. 2 and 4. It is probably related to softening of the part of the wall of the sphenoid sinus infiltrated by tumour cells. Blistering, which is often associated with hyperostosis, is easily appreciated on MRI (Figs. 7.5, 7.8, 7.9). MRI has other advantages. Precise definition of the dorsal limits of the tumour and its relationship to the optic chiasm, third ventricle and pituitary gland is best shown by MRI [305], especially in the sagittal

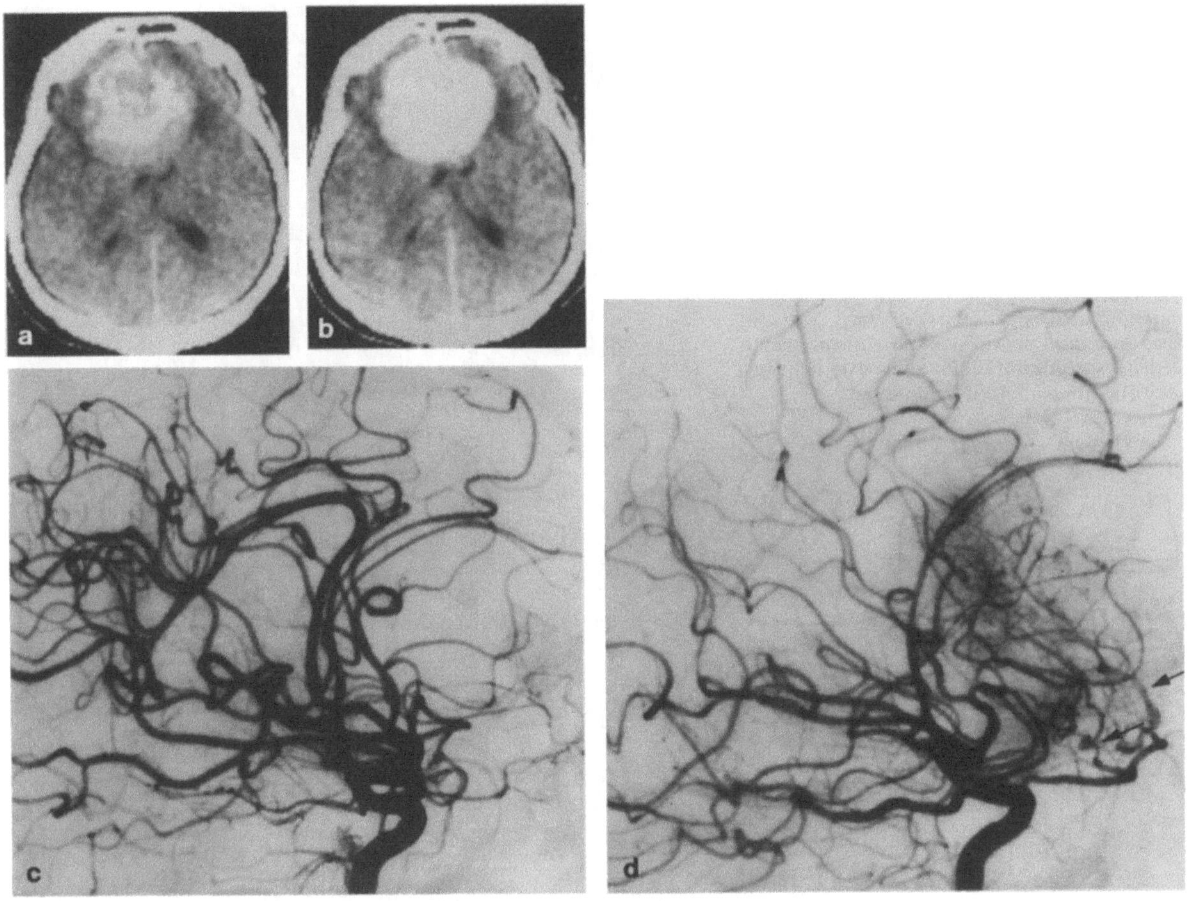

Fig. 7.3a–d. CT. Large calcified olfactorius groove meningioma with rich enhancement (**b**). There is a negligeble oedema. **c, d** On the lateral angiograms there is a typical displacement of pericallosal arteries. Meningeal branches of the ophthalmic arteries supply the tumour. That is particularly evident on the left side (d) *(arrows)*

plane (Figs. 7.5, 7.7, 7.8, 7.9). Also, the en plaque extension of tumour, which is particularly frequent in meningiomas involving the planum sphenoidale (Fig. 7.9 d), and lateral growth involving the optic canal are best evaluated by MRI. Displacement of the anterior cerebral arteries and hypertrophy of meningeal branches of the ophthalmic artery supplying the tumour (Figs. 7.5, 7.6, 7.11) can be recognized with MRI.

Peritumoral oedema is frequent in large frontobasal meningiomas, but is infrequent in the usually smaller tumours arising from the tuberculum sellae (Fig. 7.8).

7.3 Angiography

In typical cases the anterior cerebral arteries and their branches are elevated and stretched around the tumour. This is most evident on lateral projections (Figs. 7.3, 7.4, 7.5, 7.11). Encasement of anterior cerebral arteries may occur (Fig. 7.4).

Rich tumoral vascularization, particularly from meningeal branches of ophthalmic arteries, is frequent (Figs. 7.3, 7.5, 7.10). Recruitment of branches of the external carotid artery can occur in laterally located tumours (see also Chap. 5). The middle meningeal and, rarely, deep temporal arteries can be involved (Figs. 7.10, 7.11).

7.4 Differential Diagnosis

7.4.1 Pituitary Adenomas

Usually, suprasellar extensions of pituitary adenomas are in direct continuity with a visible intrasellar component enlarging and/or eroding the sella. Furthermore, the presence of endocrinological disorders are more typical of adenoma, but hyperprolac-

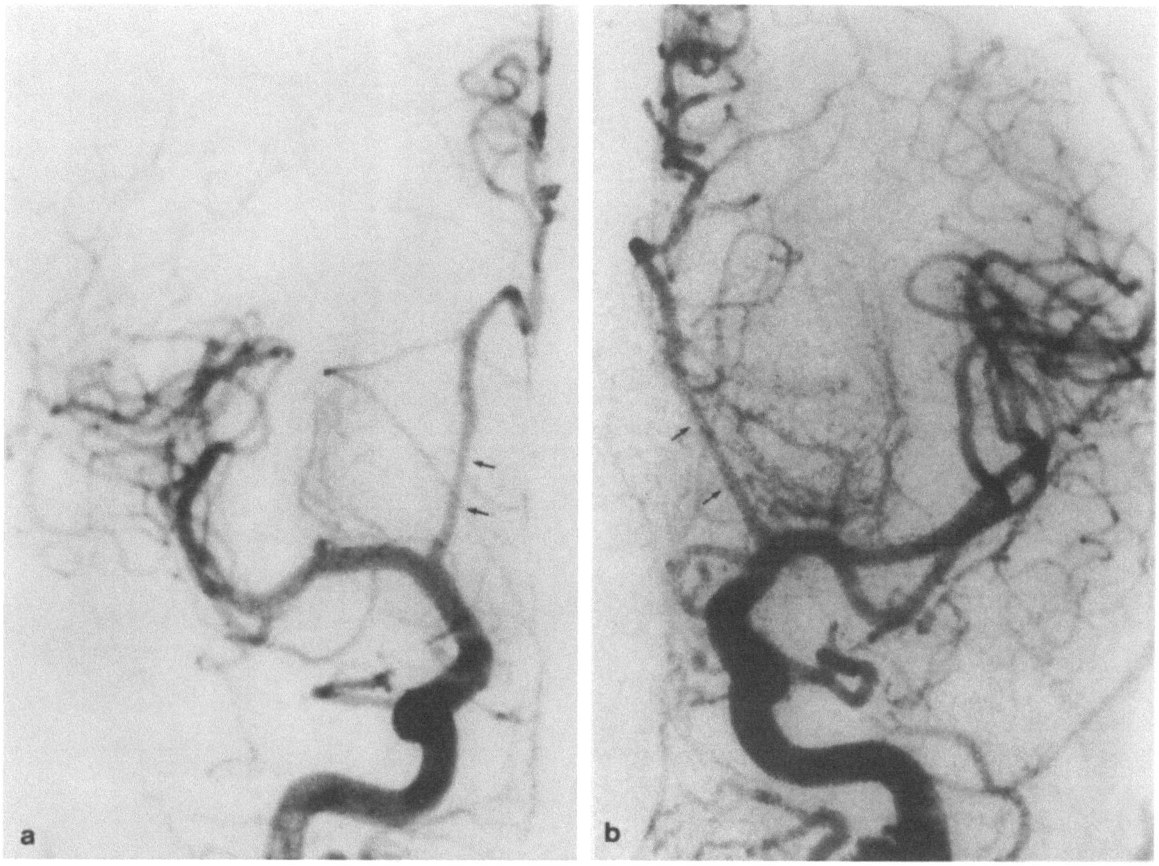

Fig. 7.4 a, b. Frontal view of carotid angiograms in another large olfactorius groove meningioma. Shifting of anterior and pericallosal arteries *(arrows)*. On the right (a), irregularities of the vessel's wall are probably due to tumoral encasement

tinaemia and hypopituitarism can occur with appropriately located meningiomas. Occasionally, when hyperostosis is not evident, it can be difficult on CT to distinguish suprasellar meningioma from pituitary adenoma. MRI, particularly in the sagittal plane, generally makes the differential diagnosis easier. The intensity of the normal pituitary gland is almost always different from that of a meningioma. The diaphragma sellae separating the two structures is frequently demonstrated as a low signal band.

7.4.2 Giant Aneurysms

Giant aneurysms in the perisellar region can usually be diagnosed with CT. They are hyperdense rounded masses, often with peripheral calcification and with marked and early enhancement of the residual lumen. MRI appearances are even more characteristic, with flow void in the patent parts and evidence of haemoglobin breakdown in intraluminal thrombus, which is often layered. Angiography will confirm and show the precise anatomy.

7.4.3 Craniopharyngiomas

Craniopharyngiomas are typically cystic and frequently calcified lesions. The enhancement after contrast medium is inhomogeneous, limited to the solid portions of the tumour. It is more frequent in young patients.

7.4.4 Other Rare Tumours

There are other more rare tumours growing into the suprasellar area which should be distinguished from meningioma. Chiasmal gliomas may have a great diversity of appearance on CT. They may show a typical tubular thickening of chiasma with occasional involvement of optic nerve and optic

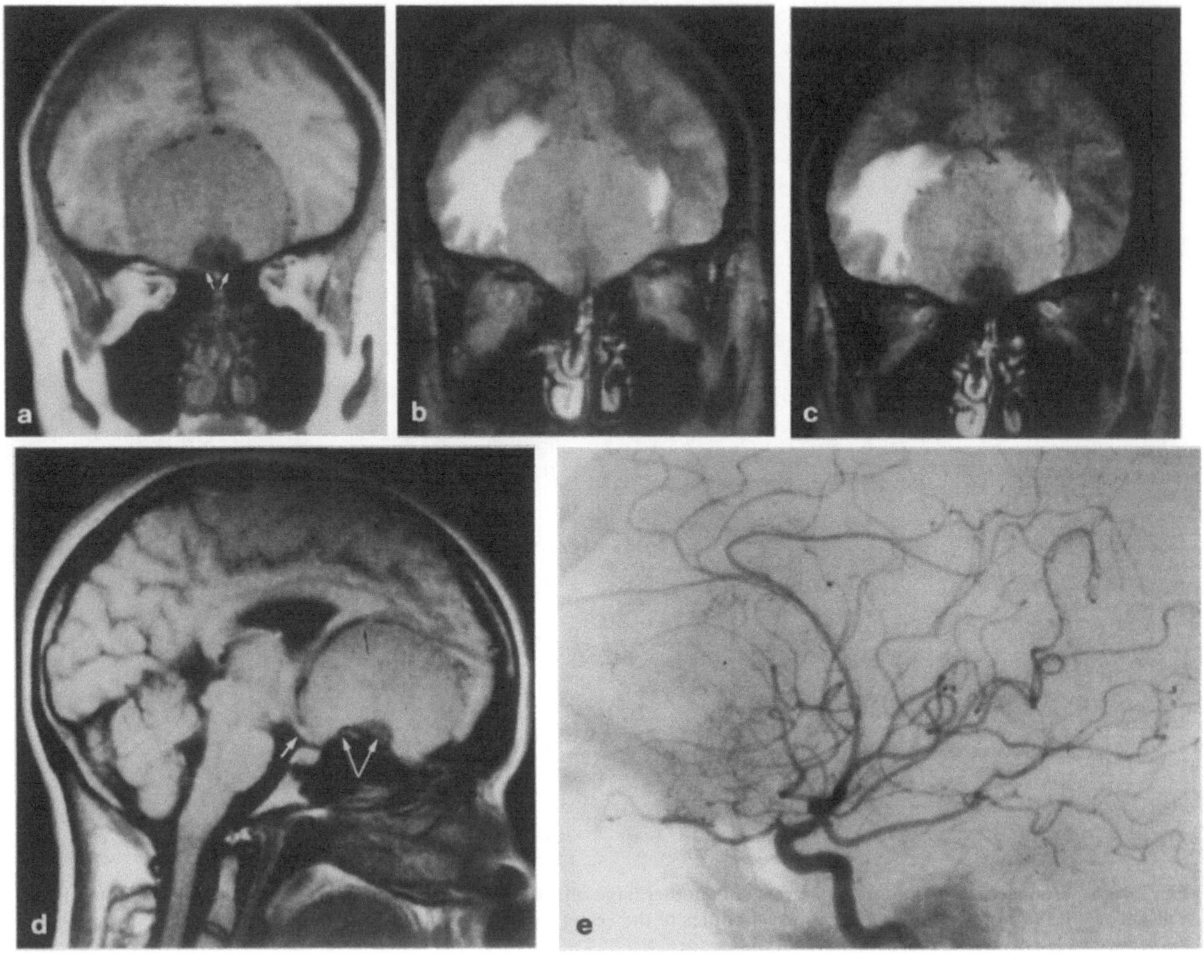

Fig. 7.5a–e. Large olfactorius groove meningioma. **a–d** MRI. **a** On this T1-weighted scan the tumour appears slightly hypointense to the normal parenchyma. The full cranial extent of the tumour as well as the basal hyperostosis *(arrows)* corresponding to the area of primary dural attachment are well demonstrated on this coronal plane. **b, c** On these T2-weighted scans the peritumoral oedema is well recognizable. It extends preferentially into the white matter on the right. **d** Sagittal plane. The displacement of the pericallosal artery *(black arrow)* is visible. There is a slight compression of the chiasma *(white arrow)*. The hyperostosis and the upward bowing of the sphenoid sinus (*double arrow;* blistering) are well recognizable. **e** Angiogram demonstrating the shifting of the pericallosal artery as already visible in **d.** There is a poor supply through the etmoidal arteries

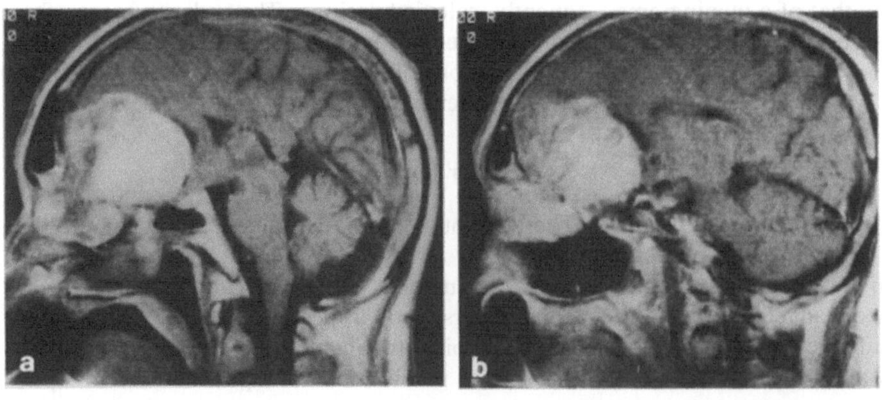

Fig. 7.6a, b. Very large olfactorius groove meningioma with widespread involvement of the paranasal and nasal cavities. **a, b** MRI, sagittal plane. Study after injection of Gd-DTPA. The tumour extends extracranially. Blood vessels corresponding to meningeal branches of ophthalmic artery supplying the tumour are recognizable

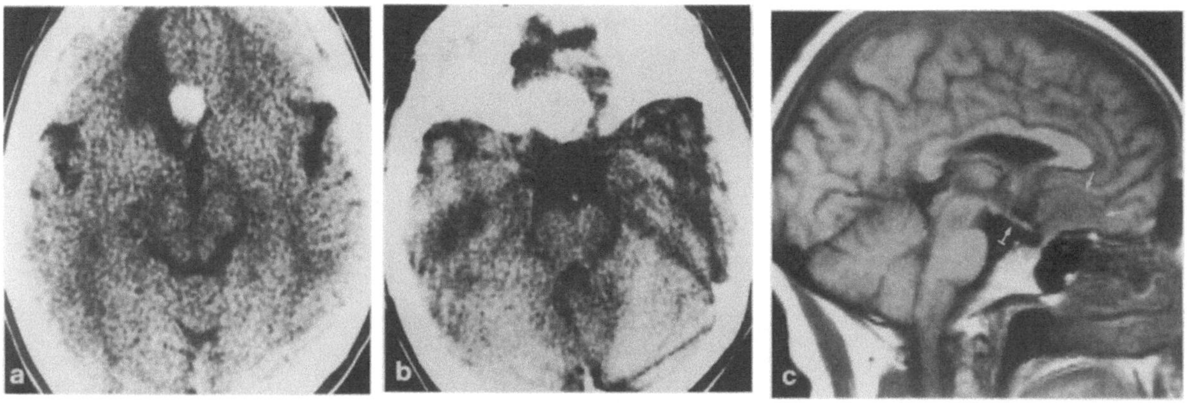

Fig. 7.7 a–c. Middle-sized sphenoid plane meningioma. **a, b** CT. Peritumoral oedema is limited to the left side. **c** MRI. The tumour *(arrows)* is characterized on this proton density-weighted scan by a signal similar to that of normal cortex. It is, however, well recognizable due to its compression of sulci. The chiasma *(arrow from line)* is well recognizable and appears normal

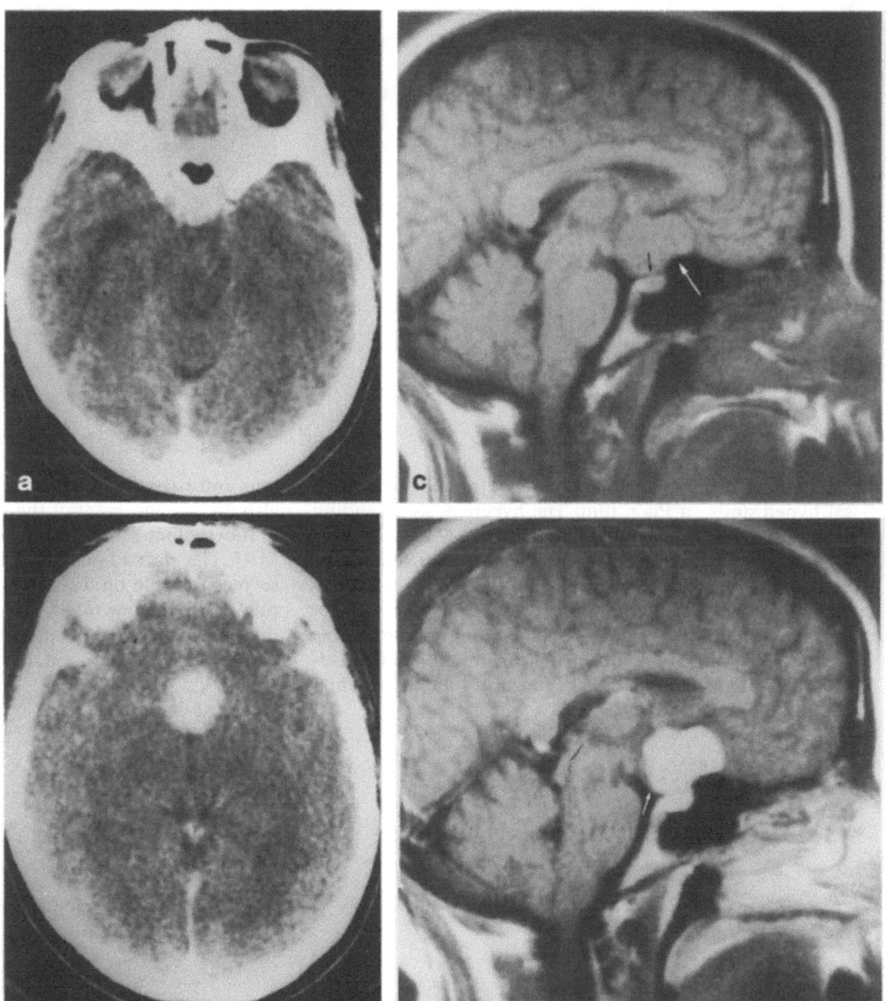

Fig. 7.8 a–d. Middle-sized tuberculum sellae meningioma. **a, b** CT. The tumour is easily recognizable after contrast medium. It is difficult to say whether it extends into the sellar cavum. There is no peritumoral oedema. **c, d** MRI. **c** On this T1-weighted scan the tumour mass is recognizable in spite of its isointensity with the normal parenchyma. The diaphragma sellae *(black arrow)* separates tumour from the pituitary gland. There is an evident upward bowing of the sphenoid sinus *(white arrow)*. **d** After injection of Gd-DTPA, there is an evident enhancement of the tumour as well as of the pituitary gland. The chiasma *(white arrow)* can be easily recognized. It appears shifted dorsally and compressed. Clinically this corresponded to a progressive visual deficit.

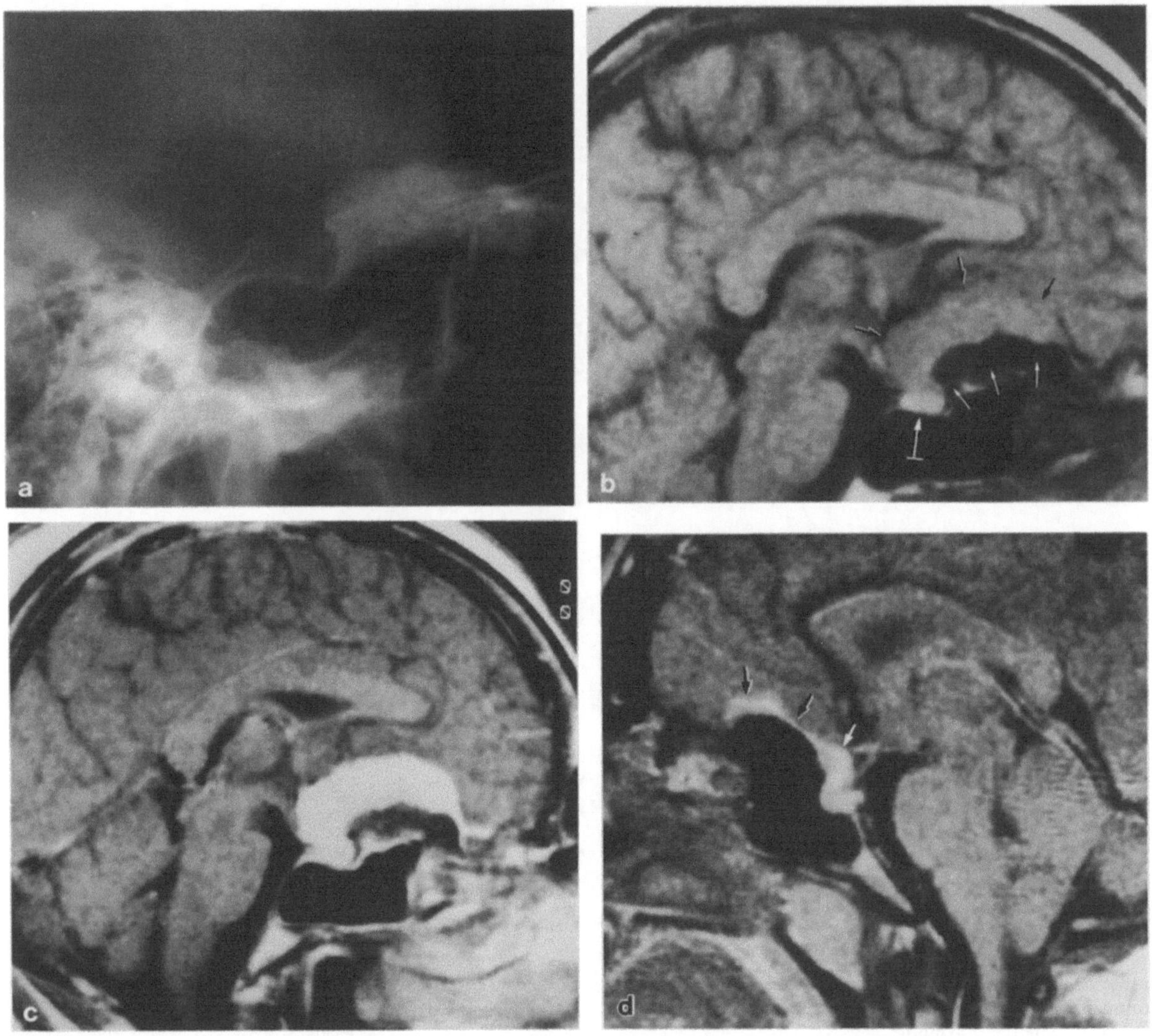

Fig. 7.9 a–d. a–c Large tuberculum sellae meningioma with basal hyperostosis. **a** Plain film. The hyperostosis extending also into the sellar cavum is visible. **b** MRI. On this T1-weighted scan the hyperostosis *(white arrows)* which also extends partially into the sellar cavum as well as the parenchymatous portion of the tumour *(black arrows)* are well recognizable. The pituitary gland is hyperintense *(arrow from line)* compared to the tumour. **c** MRI. Examination after Gd-DTPA. There is an evident enhancement in the parenchymatous and partially in the osseous portion of the tumour. Note also the enhancement of the pituitary gland.
d Tuberculum sellae meningioma with en plaque extension. MRI. The globoid portion of the tumour *(white arrow)* was also recognizable on T2-weighted images. The en plaque portion of the tumour *(black arrows)* could only be demonstrated on this T1-weighted image after Gd-DTPA. Note also the evident blistering

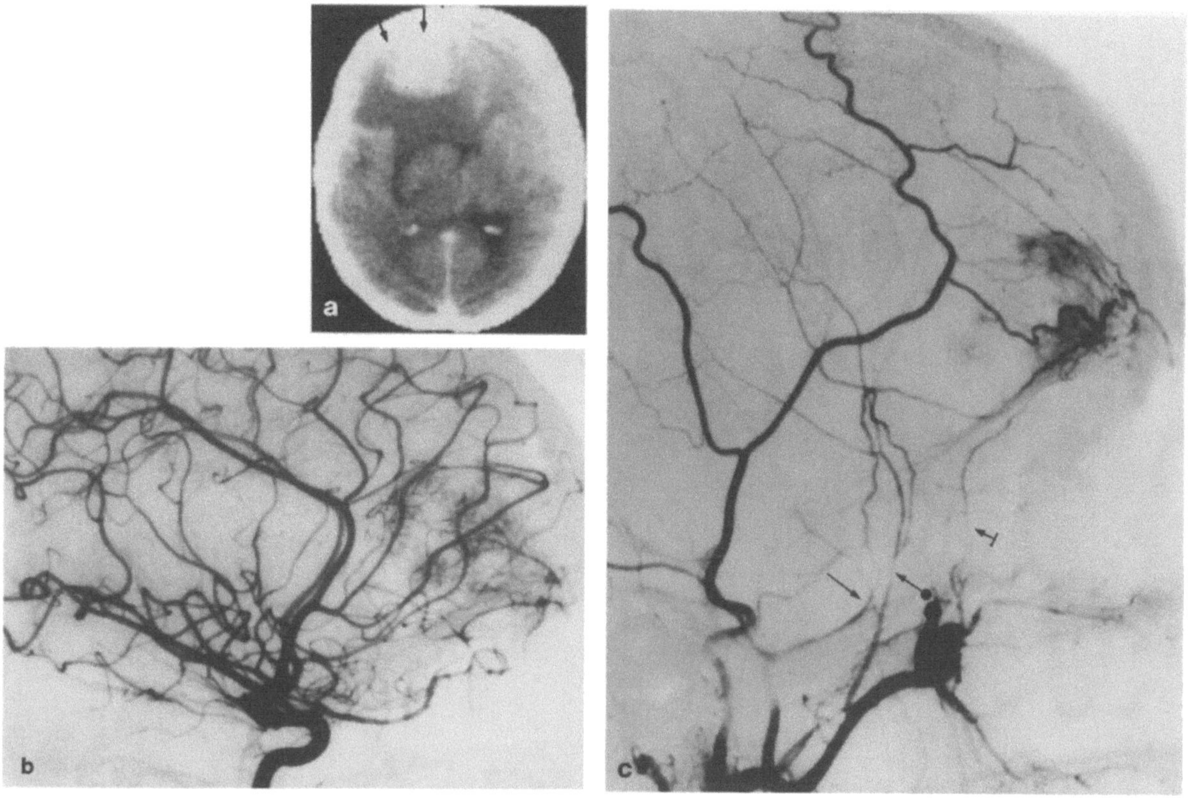

Fig. 7.10 a–c. Frontobasal and lateral meningioma. **a** CT. There is extensive oedema surrounding this middle-sized meningioma displaying rich contrast enhancement. **b, c** Angiogram. The anterior and ophthalmic arteries supply the tumour as well as branches of the external carotid artery. (Middle meningeal artery, *arrow;* deep temporal artery, *arrow from circle;* anterior deep temporal artery, *arrow from line*)

tract, sometimes bilaterally. In other cases the tumour may appear as a globular mass showing a rich contrast enhancement similar to meningioma. The association with neurofibromatosis is very frequent. This accounted for ca. 30% of the cases in the series of Fletcher et al. [87]. Chiasmal glioma is usually found in children and young adults. Two other tumours typical in children are germinomas and hamartomas. The former appear frequently as a slightly hyperdense mass with rich contrast enhancement; the latter are usually isodense showing no contrast enhancement. In all these three types of tumours MRI, particularly on the sagittal and coronal planes, is very useful in demonstrating the intra-axial location of these lesions.

7.4.5 Low Density Lesions

Low density lesions such as arachnoid, epidermoid and dermoid cysts as well as Teratomas should not present a problem in the diagnosis of meningiomas.

7.4.6 Metastases and Lymphomas

Solitary metastasis and lymphoma can sometimes simulate frontobasal meningiomas on CT. The clinical aspects and eventually angiographic findings suggesting meningioma will be helpful in the diagnosis (Fig. 7.12). (See also Chap. 6; Sect. 6.4.)

7.4.7 Paranasal Sinus Tumours

Tumours originating from the paranasal sinuses may extend intracranially: the differential diagnosis from meningioma may be difficult (Fig. 7.13). Though meningiomas may invade the frontal sinuses, extensive involvement of the ethmoid and/or sphenoid sinuses is rare at the time of initial diagnosis, though it does occur with recurrent tumour after surgery.

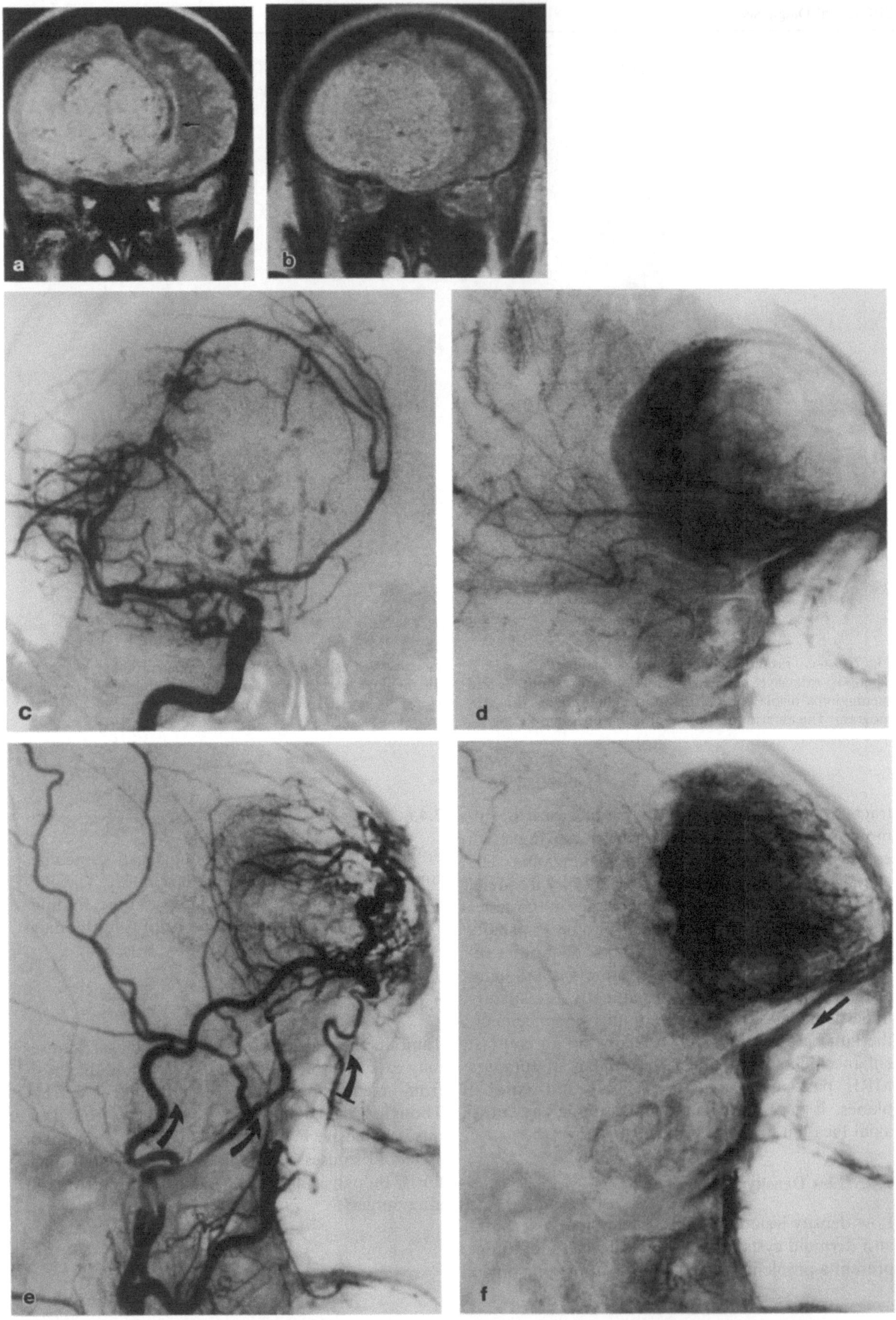
a
b
c
d
e
f

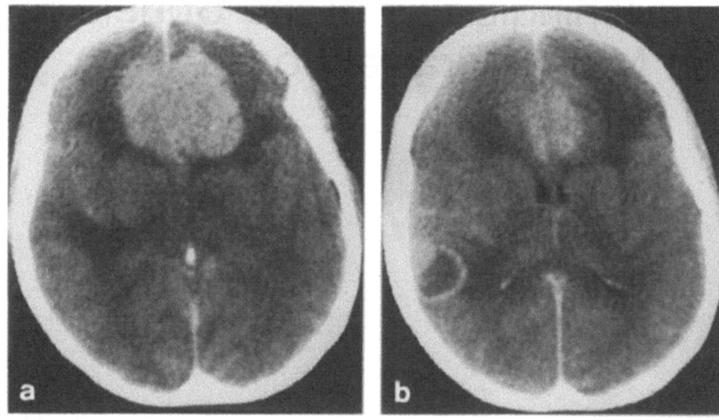

Fig. 7.12 a, b. Frontobasal metastasis in a young woman with breast carcinoma. The tumour simulates meningioma. There is, however, a second lesion in the parietal area

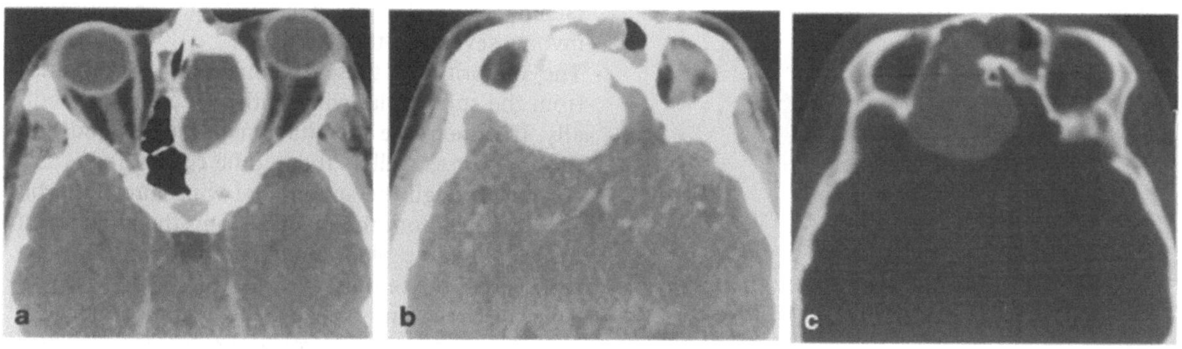

Fig. 7.13 a–c. Fibroma involving the ethmoidal cavities and extending intracranially in the frontal region. The tumour shows clear enhancement, simulating meningioma. There is no oedema

Fig. 7.11 a–f. Very large frontolateral and frontobasal richly vascularized endotheliomatous meningioma. **a, b** MRI. The tumour displays a signal of slightly increased intensity. Inside the tumour there are several linear and nodular areas with a void signal corresponding to tumoral vessels. The pericallosal artery *(arrow)* surrounding the tumour is recognizable. There is no peritumoral oedema. **c–f** Angiogram. **c** Internal carotid artery showing shifting of the pericallosal artery and pathological vessels. **d** Lateral angiogram of the internal carotid artery showing the part of the tumour vascularized by this vessel. **e** The tumour is also richly vascularized by the temporal and middle meningeal arteries *(arrows)*. The anterior deep temporal artery *(arrow from line)* is also involved. **f** Capillary-venous phases demonstrating the large venous drainage *(arrow)*

8 Meningiomas of the Sphenoid Wing and Middle Cranial Fossa

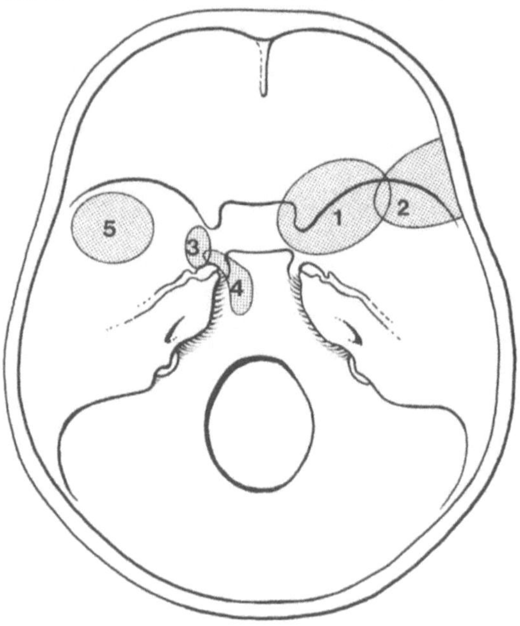

1 Medial sphenoid wing
2 Lateral sphenoid wing
3 Cavernous sinus
4 Meckel's cave
5 Temporobasal

8.1 Incidence and Localizations

This is the third most frequent site for intracranial meningiomas after the convexity and parasagittal regions, constituting about 25% of intracranial meningiomas. About 66% of them occur in women [128].

Meningiomas of this region are usually subdivided by their sites of attachment into five categories, as indicated in diagram: medial sphenoid wing, lateral sphenoid wing, cavernous sinus, Meckel's cave and temporobasal.

In small tumours and some large meningiomas with small dural attachments, it is possible to place the tumour precisely into one of these categories; often, however, the primary attachment spreads across more than one site or incorporates secondary attachments, so that the base of large tumours may involve several of the sites.

The majority of these meningiomas (80%) arise from the sphenoidal wings either laterally or medially. In either case the attachment may extend into the anterior as well as the middle cranial fossa. Extension through the sphenoidal wing into the orbit is common. From the medial group the attachment may involve the planum sphenoidale and may extend across the midline.

The cavernous sinus space is the next most frequent site of origin. In this group can be distinguished meningiomas of the cavernous sinus confined to the anterior portion of the cavernous space and meningiomas confined to the Meckel's cave. The former account for 11% of meningiomas of the middle cranial fossa and present with isolated involvement of one or more of the nerves related to the cavernous sinus at a relatively early stage. Spread through the superior orbital fissure into the orbit, laterally along the base of the middle fossa and posteriorly into the posterior fossa or along the attachments of the tentorium, is frequent. Meningiomas of Meckel's cave are comparatively infrequent (5%). The growth pattern is similar to the cavernous sinus lesions, but they more frequently extend towards the posterior fossa.

Temporobasal tumours constitute only about 4% and usually present only when large. They are an important differential diagnosis from temporal lobe malignant tumours.

Finally it should be stated that medial tentorial, clival, as well as meningiomas of the posterior surface of the petrous bone may extend into the parasellar area, and the predominant clinical sign of such tumours may mistakenly suggest an origin from the region of the cavernous sinus.

8.2 Lateral Sphenoid Wing Meningiomas

8.2.1 CT and MRI

Lateral sphenoid wing meningioma may appear as hyperostosing en plaque lesions or globoid tumours. Most of the globoid tumours are large at presentation, form well-circumscribed masses based on the lateral sphenoidal wing and pterion and occupy the anterior temporal and inferior frontal regions. The tumour margin is usually smooth, but may be lobulated. Some tumours are pedunculated, extending like a mushroom into and being engulfed by brain substance, but most have a wider attachment forming an obtuse angle with the dural surface and displace the cerebrum away from it. Many lesions extend both intracranially and intraorbitally.

On computed tomography (CT) most tumours are hyperdense, but about 15% are isodense to adjacent brain substance and may be difficult to visualize on plain CT.

Calcification is shown in about 15% of patients [207]. It may be of psammomatous type and involve most of the tumour, or floccular and located near the base of the tumour adjacent to its attachment, or peripheral and curvilinear. Contrast enhancement is almost invariable (Figs. 8.1, 8.2, 13.6).

Bony changes are almost universally present in this group of meningiomas [207] and are of great diagnostic value. These are easily demonstrated by plain radiographs, but are shown particularly well by high definition CT. The most characteristic appearance is thickening of the lesser and/or greater sphenoid wings. This may be limited to a variable amount of enostosis at the base of the tumour, but usually hyperostosis and sclerosis are diffuse, causing thickening of the anterior wall of the middle fossa and of the lateral wall of the orbit where it produces proptosis (Figs. 8.2-8.4). Even when the bony change is the predominant feature, an adjacent carpet of tumour is always present, though it may be thin and impossible to demonstrate on CT even after intravenous contrast enhancement (Fig. 8.4).

Magnetic resonance imaging (MRI) is particularly useful because of its multiplanar facility, which generally reveals the bone involvement, the extra-axial mass and the displacement of the brain substance away from the abnormal meninges (Fig. 8.4c-h).

Peritumoral oedema is frequent in meningiomas globular in shape.

8.2.2 Angiography

Internal carotid arteriography often shows typical displacement of the middle cerebral artery which is elevated and shifted medially. The predominant blood supply entering the attachment of lateral sphenoid ridge meningiomas comes from the middle meningeal artery (Figs. 8.1, 8.2, 8.4, 13.6). Other meningeal branches of the internal maxillary artery may be involved, particularly the anterior deep temporal artery as well as the ophthalmic artery and the inferolateral trunk of the C_4 portion of the intracavernous segment of the internal carotid. Accessory supply to the periphery of the tumour is frequent from displaced cortical branches of the middle cerebral artery.

8.3 Medial Sphenoid Wing Meningiomas

8.3.1 CT and MRI

Medial sphenoid wing (MSW) meningiomas may present with optic nerve or chiasmal compression when relatively small. They often extend across the midline. Large tumours may also displace the hypothalamus and third ventricle and compress the anterior horn of the lateral ventricle; they may obstruct the foramen of Monro and cause hydrocephalus. Intraorbital extension is also possible. These meningiomas are frequently calcified and are well demonstrated with CT (Figs. 8.5-8.7, 12.5, 12.13).

In most cases the optic nerve or chiasm is compressed focally by the tumour itself. In some cases the meningioma grows diffusely along the sheath of the optic nerve (Fig. 8.8), and in others the optic canal is narrowed by hyperostosis, both of which occur particularly in the en plaque forms which will be discussed later. High definition CT is mandatory for good demonstration of such features.

MRI can be particularly useful in investigating the optic nerve involvement because visualization is not hindered by signal from the sclerotic bone. Moreover, MRI can better demonstrate the relationship of the tumour to the cavernous sinus (Fig. 8.9) and arteries in the region. In particular displacement and possible encasement of the supraclinoid portion of internal carotid, anterior and middle cerebral arteries is detected (Figs. 8.9, 8.10).

Peritumoral oedema is frequent.

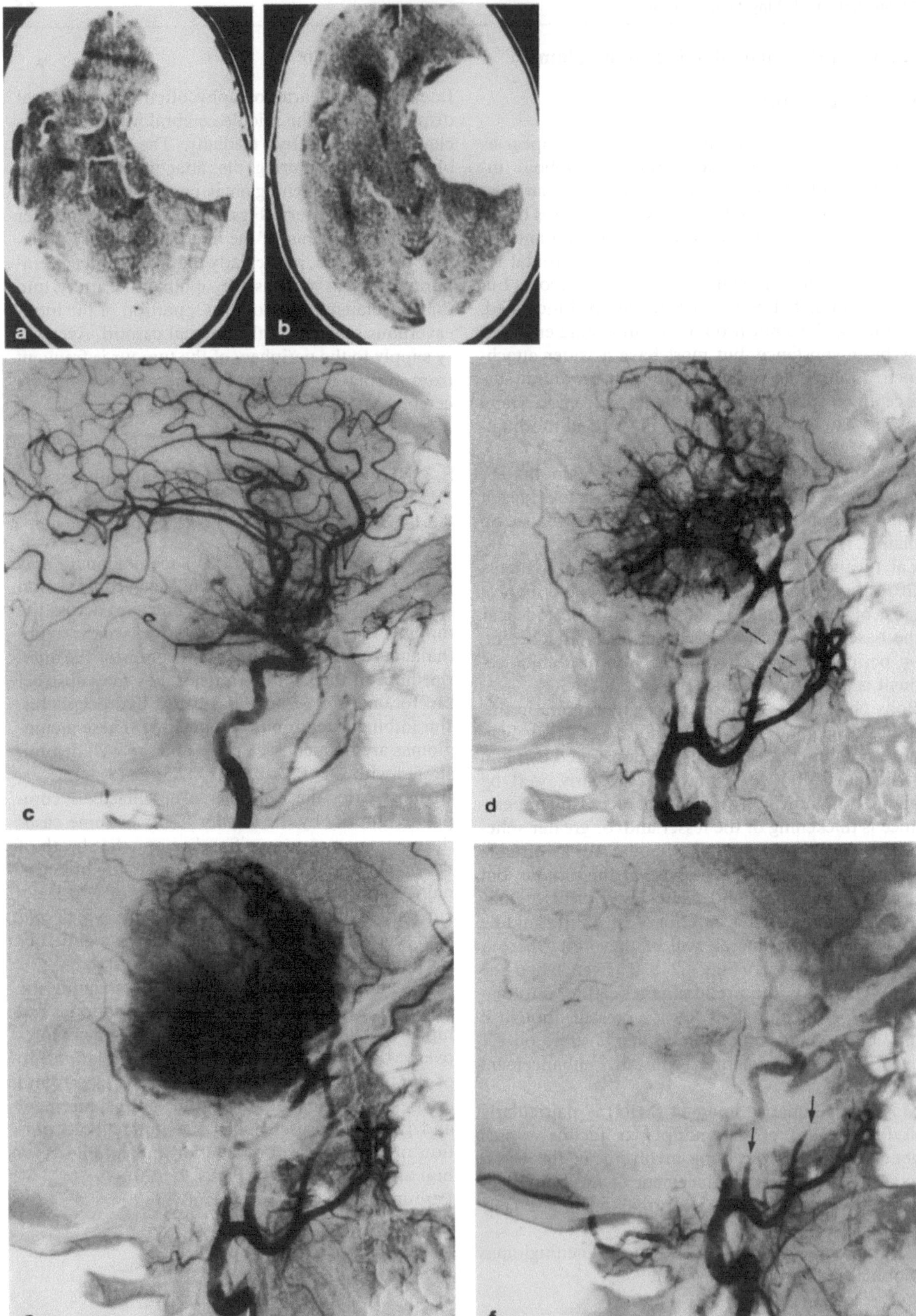
a
b
c
d
e
f

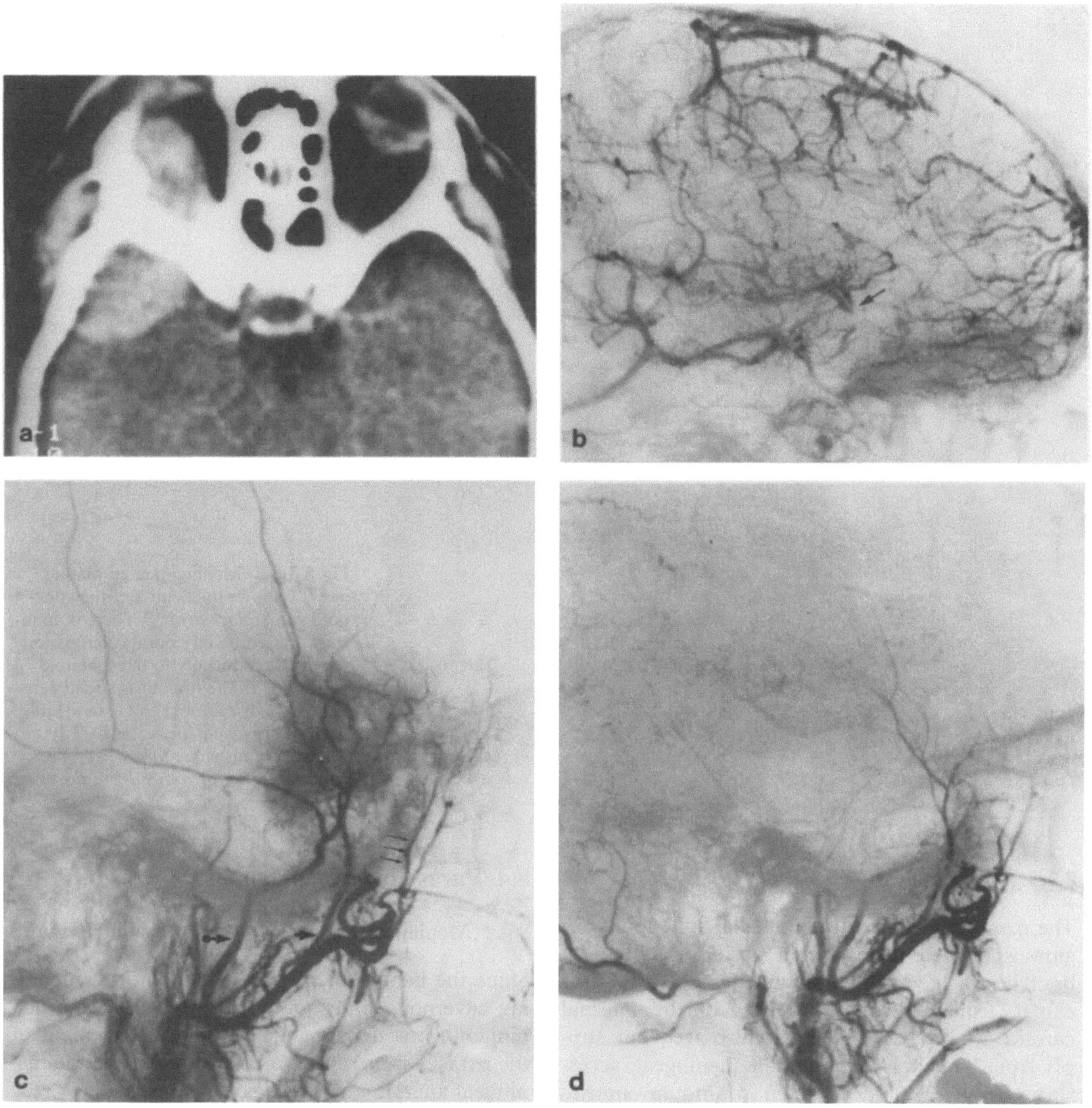

Fig. 8.2 a–d. Lateral SWM extending into the orbit. **a** CT. Thickening of the sphenoid wing infiltrated by the tumour which extends also intraorbitally. **b** Angiogram, venous phase. The superficial sylvian vein *(arrow)* is blocked. **c** Angiogram of external carotid artery. The middle meningeal *(arrow from circle)*, the deep temporal *(arrow)* and anterior deep temporal *(parallel arrows)* arteries supply the tumour. **d** Angiogram after embolization of the feeder vessels

Fig. 8.1 a–f. Large lateral SWM of angioblastic type. **a, b** CT. The meningioma shows evident enhancement. There was severe oedema in the corona radiata and into the capsulae (not demonstrated here). **c** Angiogram of common carotid artery. Lifting of the middle cerebral artery. There is evident pathological vascularization. **d, e** Angiogram of the external carotid artery (ECA). There is a large middle meningeal *(arrow)* and deep temporal *(parallel arrows)* arteries supplying the richly vascularized tumour. **f** Control common carotid angiogram after embolization *(arrows)*

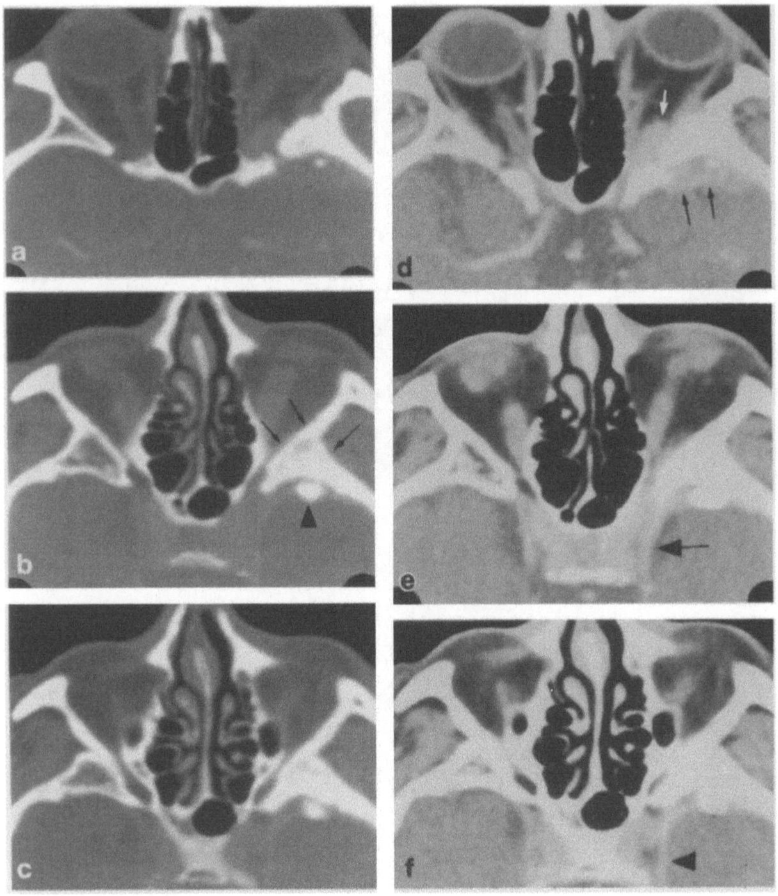

Fig. 8.3a–f. Meningioma en plaque. **a–c** CT shows thickening of the sphenoid wing *(black arrows)*. There is an intracranial, probably dural calcification *(arrowhead)* dorsally to the sphenoid wing. **d** CT. The tumour is slightly enhanced *(black arrows)* and extends intraorbitally *(white arrow)*. **e, f** CT. The cavernous sinus *(arrow)* and the Meckel's cave *(arrowhead)* are not deformed

8.3.2 Angiography

The meningeal supply to the medial sphenoidal region is derived mainly from posterior ethmoidal branches of the ophthalmic artery and, to a lesser extent, from cavernous branches of the internal carotid artery (ICA). There is also frequent supply from branches of the middle meningeal, accessory meningeal and foramen rotundum arteries (Figs. 8.5, 8.7). Large tumours may stretch the carotid siphon posteriorly, deform the ophthalmic artery and elevate the middle cerebral artery (Figs. 8.5, 8.6). Any stenosis or occlusion of the supraclinoid segment of the internal carotid artery and of middle cerebral artery caused by encasement [28, 88] is well shown, though it usually can be suspected from CT and be shown well by MRI (Figs. 8.9, 8.10).

8.4 Parasellar Meningiomas

8.4.1 Meningeal Anatomy in the Parasellar Region

Since the behaviour of parasellar tumours, including cavernous sinus space and Meckel's cave meningiomas, is dependent upon the arrangement of the parasellar meninges, a brief summary of the meningeal anatomy in this region is presented.

In the parasellar region the dura is divided into two layers: the periosteal layer, which is located medially in contact with the sphenoid bone, and the lateral layer, forming the medial wall of the middle cranial fossa. The space between these two layers has been called by Taptas [273] the "space of the cavernous sinus". This contains in its anterior portion the venous plexus of the cavernous sinus in which the ICA, and laterally to it the cranial nerves, run. According to the anatomical studies of Parkinson [217], the third and the fourth nerves lie within the dural roof of the cavernous space, the ophthalmic division of the fifth in the lateroinferior wall, and the sixth free in the cavernous space. In the posteri-

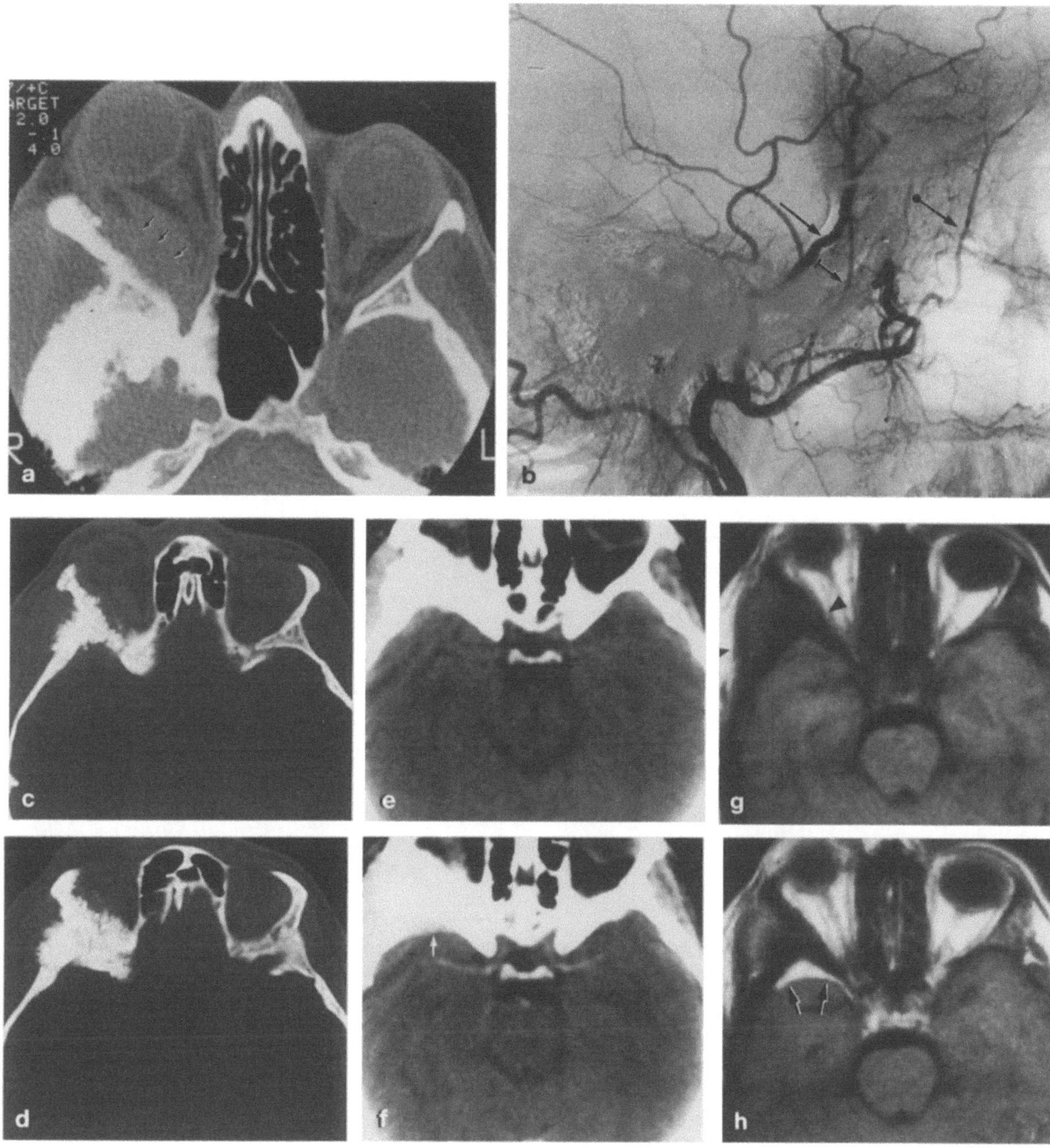

Fig. 8.4 a–h. a, b En plaque meningioma with intracranial and intraorbital components. **a** There is evident hyperostosis of the lesser and greater sphenoid wings. Tabulae interna, externa and diploë are involved and they are no longer recognizable as separated structures. The surface of the hyperostosis is irregular. There are some dural and probably tumoral calcifications, but the intracranial en plaque portion of the tumour was not recognizable after contrast medium either. Intraorbital portion of the tumour *(arrows)*. **b** Angiogram of ECA. The tumour is richly supplied by middle meningeal *(arrow)* by deep temporal *(arrow from line)* and anterior deep temporal arteries *(arrow from circle)*. **c–h** Another case of en plaque meningioma. **c, d** Hyperostosis involving lesser and grater sphenoid wings. The hyperostotic area is irregular and the tabulae externa and interna as well as the diploë are no longer distinguishable. **e, f** The en plaque portion *(white arrow)* of the tumour is only partially recognizable after contrast medium (**f**). **g, h** On MRI the hyperostosis is well recognizable *(arrowhead)*. The en plaque portion *(arrows)* is, however, only visible after Gd-DTPA (**h**)

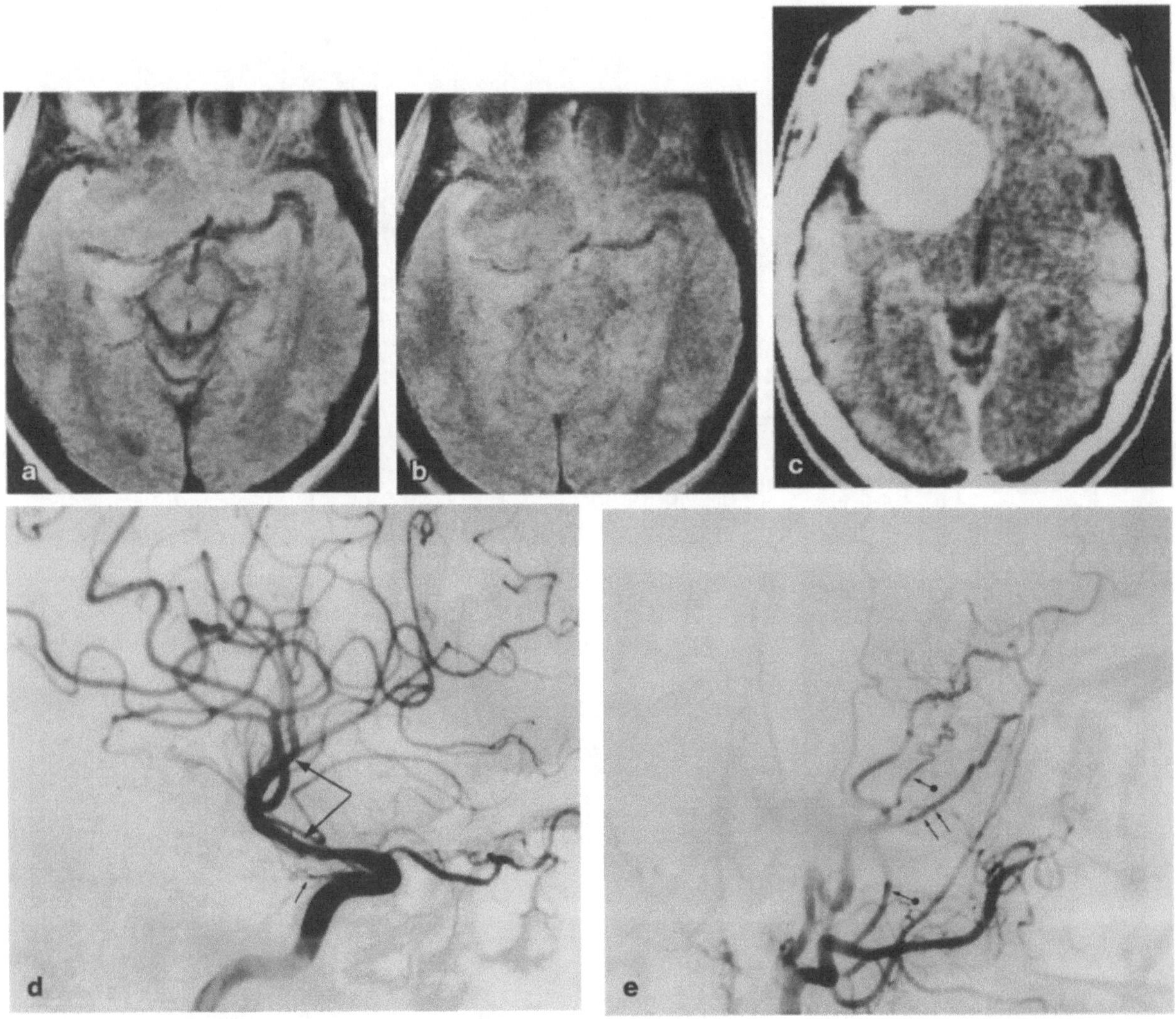

Fig. 8.5a–e. Large medial SWM in a young woman with epileptic seizures. **a** MRI, proton density-weighted scan. There is an evident shifting of middle cerebral artery as well as compression of the brainstem. The tumour, isointense, with the parenchyma is not clearly shown. **b** MRI, T2-weighted scan. The tumour remains isointense but is clearly visible against peritumoral oedema. **c** CT. The meningioma is well recognizable after contrast medium. It extends into the temporal and frontal area. **d** Angiogram of ICA. Stretching and shifting of carotid siphon and middle cerebral artery *(double arrow)*. Meningeal branches *(arrow)* of C4 portion of carotid siphon supply the tumour. **e** Angiogram of the ECA. The middle meningeal artery *(arrows)*, and the accessory meningeal artery *(arrow from circle)* supply the tumour

or part of the space is Meckel's cave, an evagination into the porus trigeminus of the dura of the posterior fossa. It contains the gasserian ganglion surrounded by the trigeminal cistern, which communicates with the rest of the subarachnoid space.

In CT, the intravenous injection of contrast medium leads to enhancement of the dura, the cavernous sinus plexus of veins and the ICA (Fig. 8.11 a–c). There is enhancement around Meckel's cave, which appears as a region of low density (Fig. 8.11 a–c), and the cave itself can be directly demonstrated at cisternography after injection of intrathecal contrast medium.

The region is well shown by MRI. In particular, the fibrous lateral wall of the cavernous sinus gives a low signal on all sequences and can nearly always be demonstrated, as can the ICA (Fig. 8.11 d–f).

8.4.2 CT and MRI

Parasellar tumours tend to present when relatively small and are characterized by a progressive cavernous sinus syndrome. On CT they appear as para-

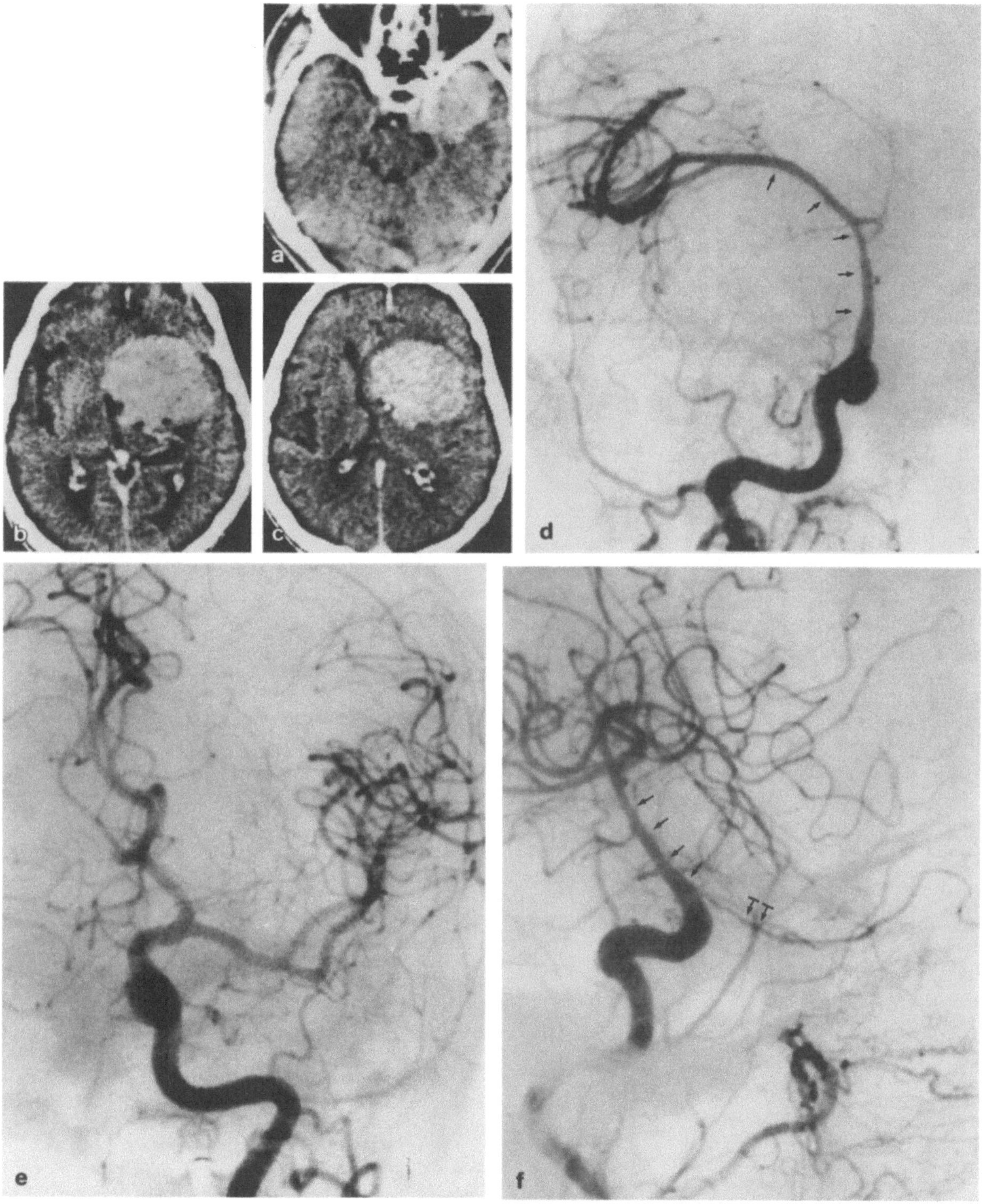

Fig. 8.6a–f. Very large medial SWM in an old woman with partial loss of vision on the right. **a–c** CT. The tumour extends into the temporal and frontal region. Compression of third and lateral ventricles which are shifted to the left. The oedema surrounding the tumour is negligible. **d, e** Bilateral carotid angiogram. Stretching and displacement of supraclinoid carotid and middle cerebral artery *(arrows)* can be seen on the right. **f** Lateral right carotid angiogram. Stretching and narrowing of the encased supraclinoid carotid *(arrows)* and deformation of the ophthalmic artery *(arrow from line)* are evident

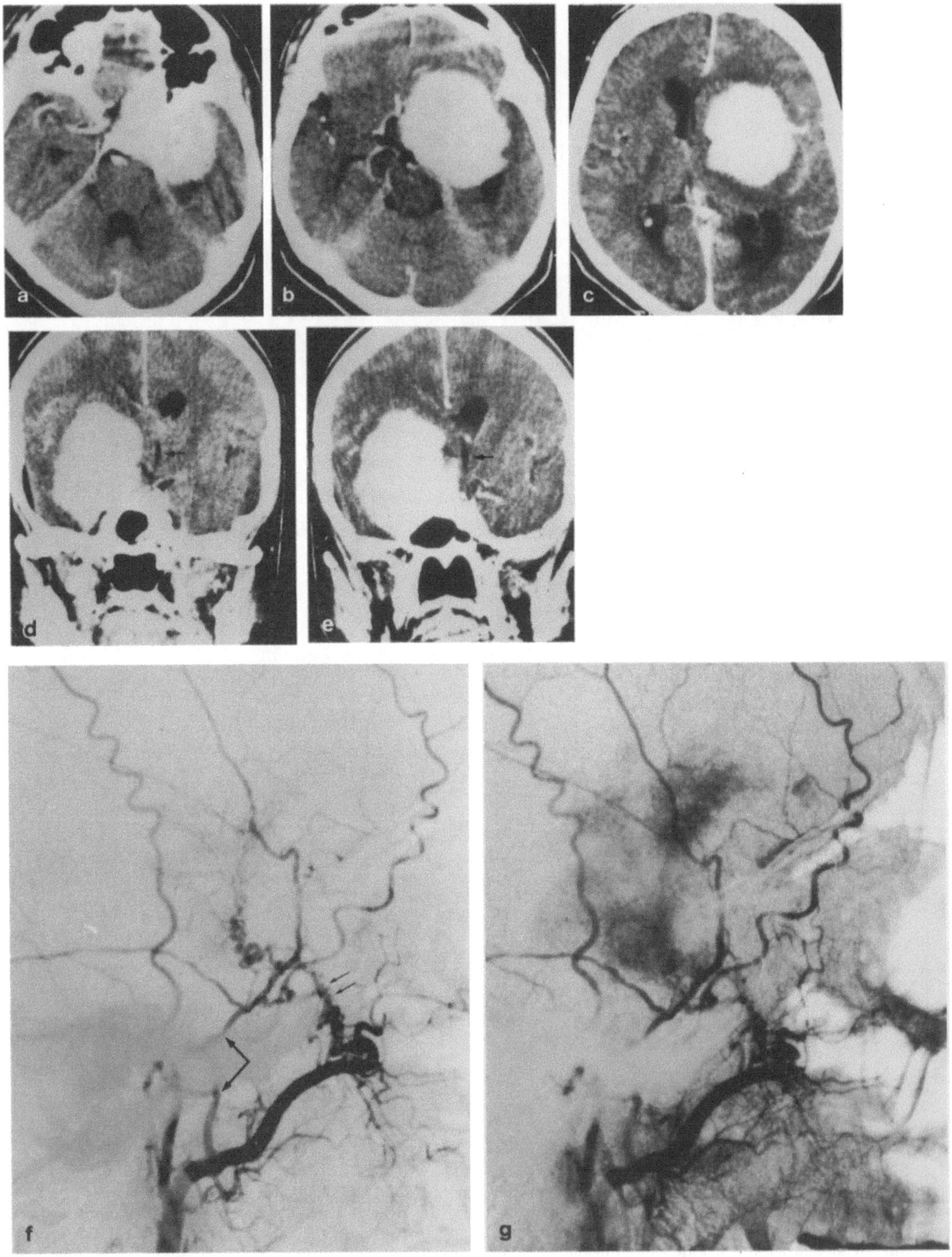

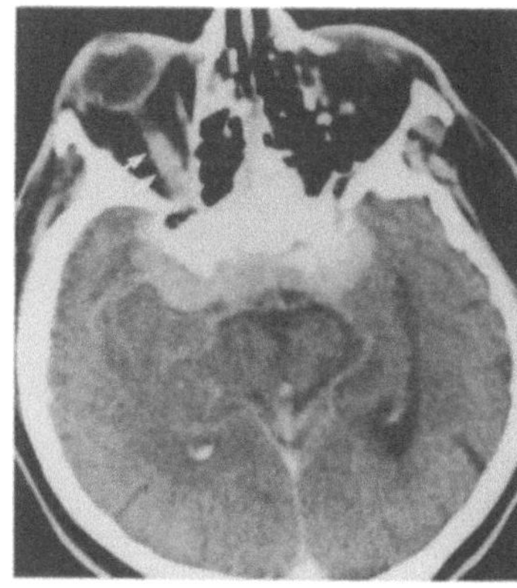

Fig. 8.8. Bilateral medial SWM and tuberculum sellae meningioma. There is spread along the sheath of left optic nerve *(arrows)*

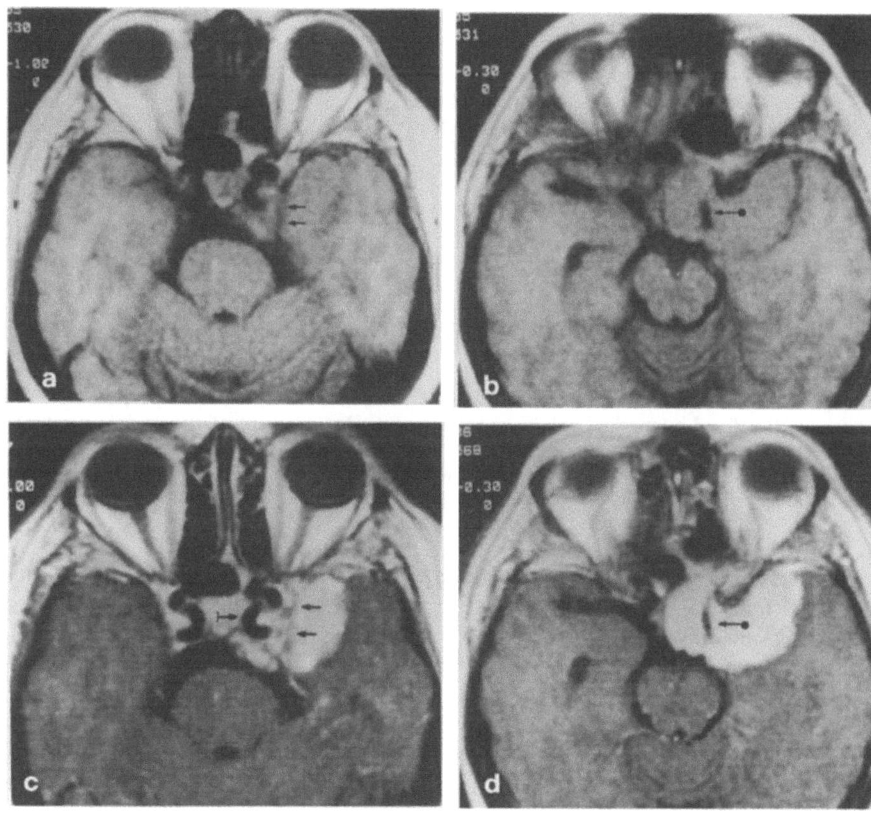

Fig. 8.9 a–d. Large medial SWM. **a, b** MRI (SE 500/50). On these T1-weighted images, the tumour displays a signal isointense with the normal parenchyma. It is located laterally to the lateral wall of the sinus *(arrows)*. In **b** the supraclinoid portion of the ICA *(arrow from circle)* is encased. **c, d** MRI. After Gd-DTPA the tumour enhances markedly. Note also that it extends into the retrosellar area. Lateral wall of the sinus *(arrow)*; normal intracavernous portion of ICA *(arrow from line)*; encased supraclinoid portion of ICA *(arrow from circle)*

Fig. 8.7 a–g. Another example of very large medial SWM in a young woman with epileptic seizures and partial loss of vision on the right. **a–e** CT, axial and coronal scans. The tumour shows rich contrast enhancement. It extends into the temporal and frontal regions and across the midline. Compression of the third *(arrows)* ventricle. The right frontal horn is compressed. The left one is dilated due to blockage of the foramen on Monro. **f, g** Angiogram of the terminal segment of the external carotid artery. The middle meningeal artery *(double arrow)*, and meningeal branches passing through the foramen rotundum *(arrows)* are involved in supplying the tumour

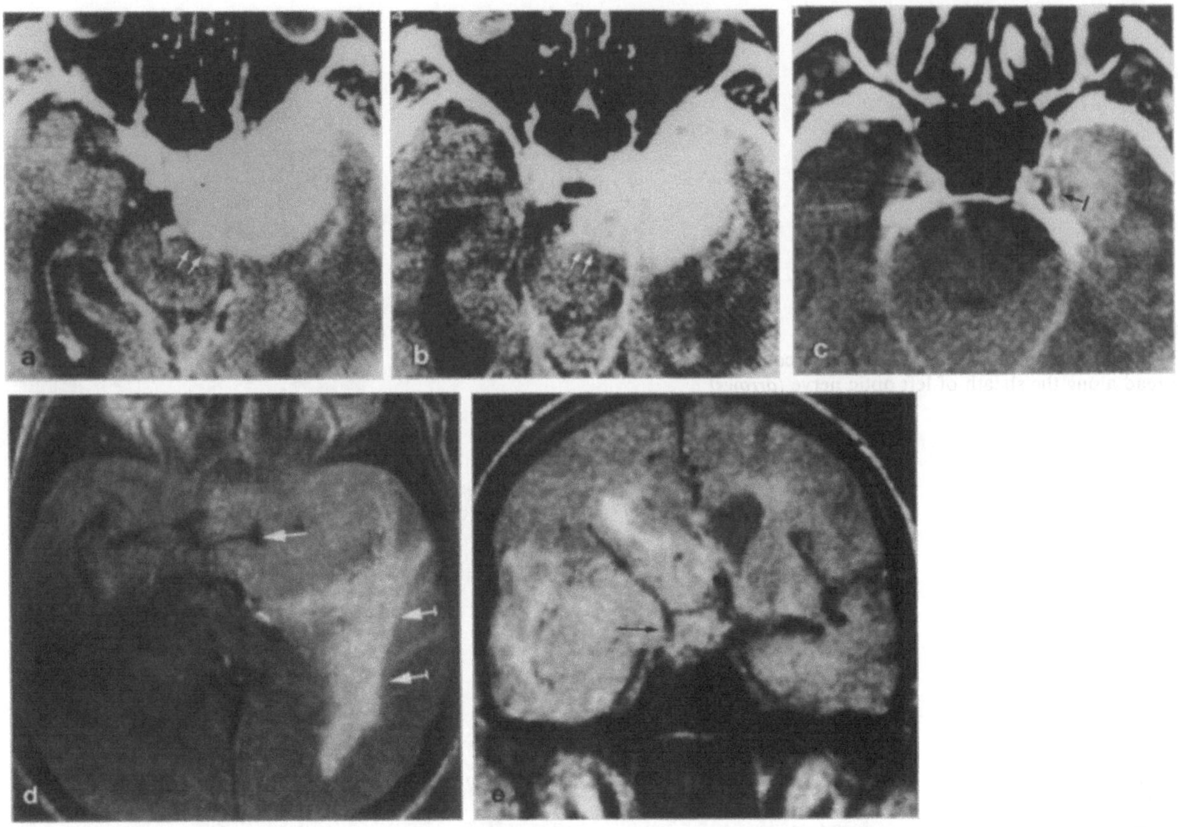

Fig. 8.10 a–e. Very large medial SWM also extending dorsally into the retrosellar area and infratentorially. **a–c** CT. The tumour is well defined by marked contrast enhancement. Dorsal extent of the tumour *(arrows)*. Note the normal Meckel's cave *(arrow from line)*. **d** MRI, axial plane T2-weighted scan. The tumour displays a slight increase of signal intensity. There is extensive peritumoral oedema *(arrows from line)*. The supraclinoid portion of the carotid siphon and the first segment of the middle cerebral artery *(arrow)* are encased. On CT the arteries can not be distinguished from the tumour. **e** MRI, proton density-weighted scan. Encased carotid siphon *(arrow)*

sellar masses (Figs. 8.12, 8.16). The lateral wall of the cavernous sinus space is bulged outwards, indicating unequivocally the presence of a mass within the sinus. This can be demonstrated with CT, but it is more conspicuous with MRI [38] (Figs. 8.13–8.16).

Cavernous sinus meningiomas can extend anteriorly into the orbit or laterally into the middle cranial fossa where they may be globular or more frequently en plaque (Figs. 8.12, 8.13, 8.14, 8.15, 8.16). The en plaque portion of the tumour may spread from the lateral wall of the sinus towards the posterior surface of the lesser and greater sphenoid wings and infiltrate the bone structures with secondary hyperostosis (Figs. 8.12, 8.15, 8.16). MRI is particularly useful in evaluating this en plaque form [38]. Cavernous sinus and especially Meckel's cave meningiomas may grow posteriorly and invade the posterior fossa. Finally, MSW meningioma can extend into the parasellar area and infiltrate the cavernous sinus, but frequently such growth seems to arrest at the dura over its lateral wall (Fig. 8.9). Meningiomas lying completely within the cavernous sinus space or having only a small or en plaque extension in the middle cranial fossa usually do not cause oedema.

8.4.3 Angiography

The blood supply of parasellar meningiomas is frequently inconspicuous (Figs. 8.12–8.16). Meningeal branches of C_5–C_4 portion of the ICA and eventually branches of the middle meningeal artery and the accessory meningeal artery can be involved. Encasement of the intracavernous portion of the ICA is frequent [166]. This can be demonstrated by angiography as well as by MRI [38] (Figs. 8.13–8.16). It is important to note that the ICA can appear normal in spite of evident encasement demonstrated with MRI.

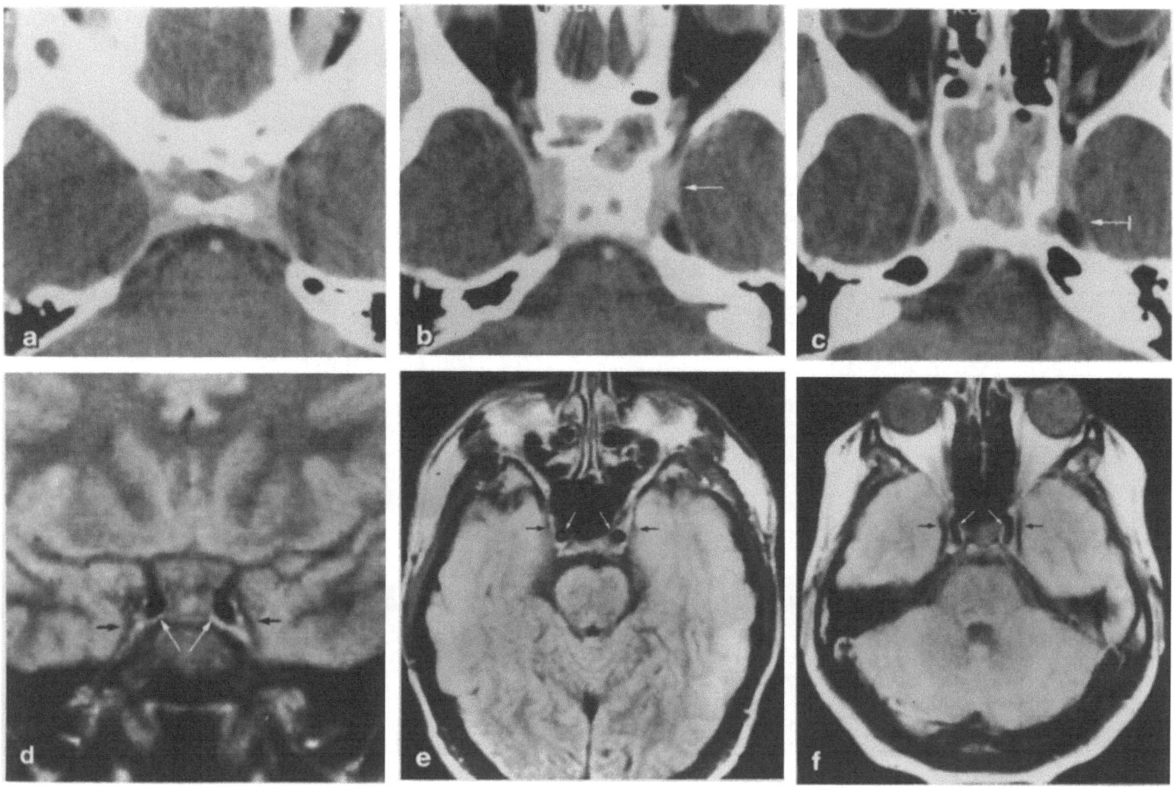

Fig. 8.11 a–f. Normal anatomical aspects of the parasellar area. **a–c** CT. Lateral wall of the cavernous sinus *(arrow)*. Meckel's cave *(arrow from line)*. **d** MRI, coronal plane. Proton density-weighted scan. Lateral wall of the cavernous sinus *(black arrows)*. The internal carotid arteries are characterized by a void signal *(white arrows)* surrounded by the venous plexus which displays a high signal. **e, f** MRI, axial planes in two diffenrent patients. The lateral wall of the cavernous sinus *(black arrows)* as well as the ICA *(white arrows)* are well recognizable

The venous anatomy of the region warrants special consideration because parasellar meningiomas frequently lead to changes in venous drainage visible on the late phases of the internal and external carotid angiograms. The cavernous sinus is best regarded as a venous plexus located in the anterolateral portion of the cavernous space, which communicates freely with the opposite cavernous sinus via intercavernous anastomoses. The most important tributaries of the cavernous sinuses are the superior ophthalmic vein and the sphenoparietal sinus, and the major drainage pathway is into the basilar and petrosal sinuses. Variations in this pattern are common [33, 35, 215, 277, 294] and include:

1. The sphenoparietal sinus draining directly into the pterygoid plexus by way of one or more veins located lateral to the space of the cavernous sinus, sometimes termed the paracavernous sinus [294]. These leave the cranial cavity via foramina in the floor of the middle cranial fossa.
2. Less frequent by a superficial sylvian vein not draining into the sphenoparietal sinus, but dorsally into the superior petrosal or lateral sinus, or, occasionally, into the superior sagittal sinus.
3. The superior ophthalmic vein draining via the paracavernous sinus [35, 277]. Since the ophthalmic vein drains tissues of the face, it is generally well filled on an external carotid angiogram.

Sphenoid wing, cavernous sinus and Meckel's cave meningiomas may block the superficial sylvian or ophthalmic veins (Figs. 8.2, 8.12), or blood from the superficial sylvian veins may be diverted into the ophthalmic vein and carried by inversion of flow towards the facial veins (Fig. 8.17). It is important to establish whether the cavernous sinus space is also occupied by the tumour. The absence of filling of the cavernous plexus of veins in the venous phase of carotid angiography, though suggesting infiltration, can be caused by external compression rather

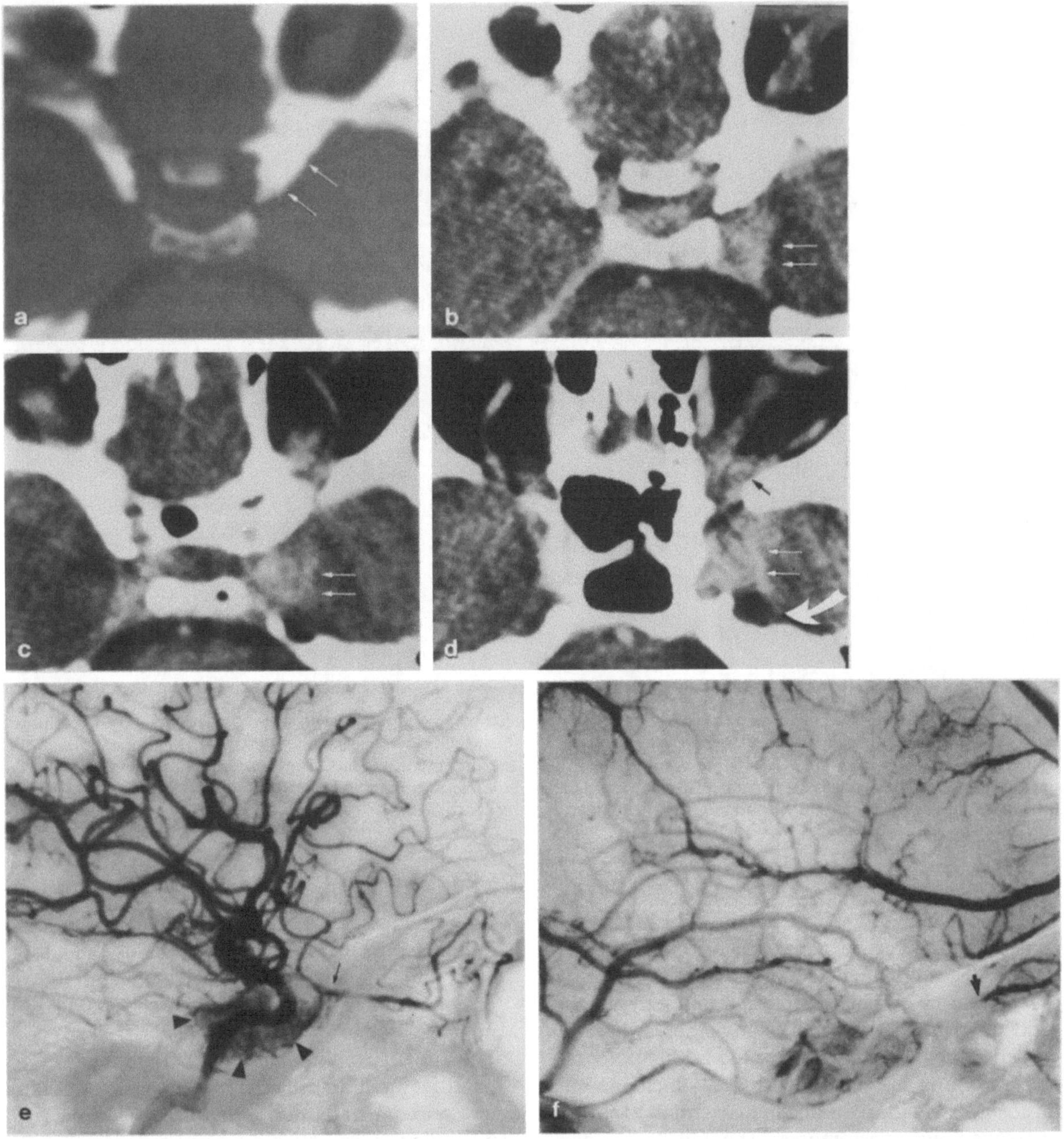

Fig. 8.12a–f. Cavernous sinus meningioma with en plaque extracavernous portion. **a** CT shows thickening of the sphenoid wing *(white arrows)*. **b–d** After contrast medium the tumour is recognizable as an enhanced mass in the area of the cavernous sinus *(white arrows)*. The tumour spreads intraorbitally *(black arrow)*. Meckel's cave *(large white arrow)* appears slightly deformed. **e, f** Internal carotid angiogram shows pathological vascularization *(arrowheads)*, stretching of the ophthalmic artery *(arrow)*, and in the venous phase (**f**) blockage of the superior ophthalmic vein *(arrow)*. *At the operation*, the en plaque portion of the tumour along the lateral wall of the cavernous sinus was confirmed. Tumour along the posterior surface of sphenoid wing was also detected, which was not visible on CT

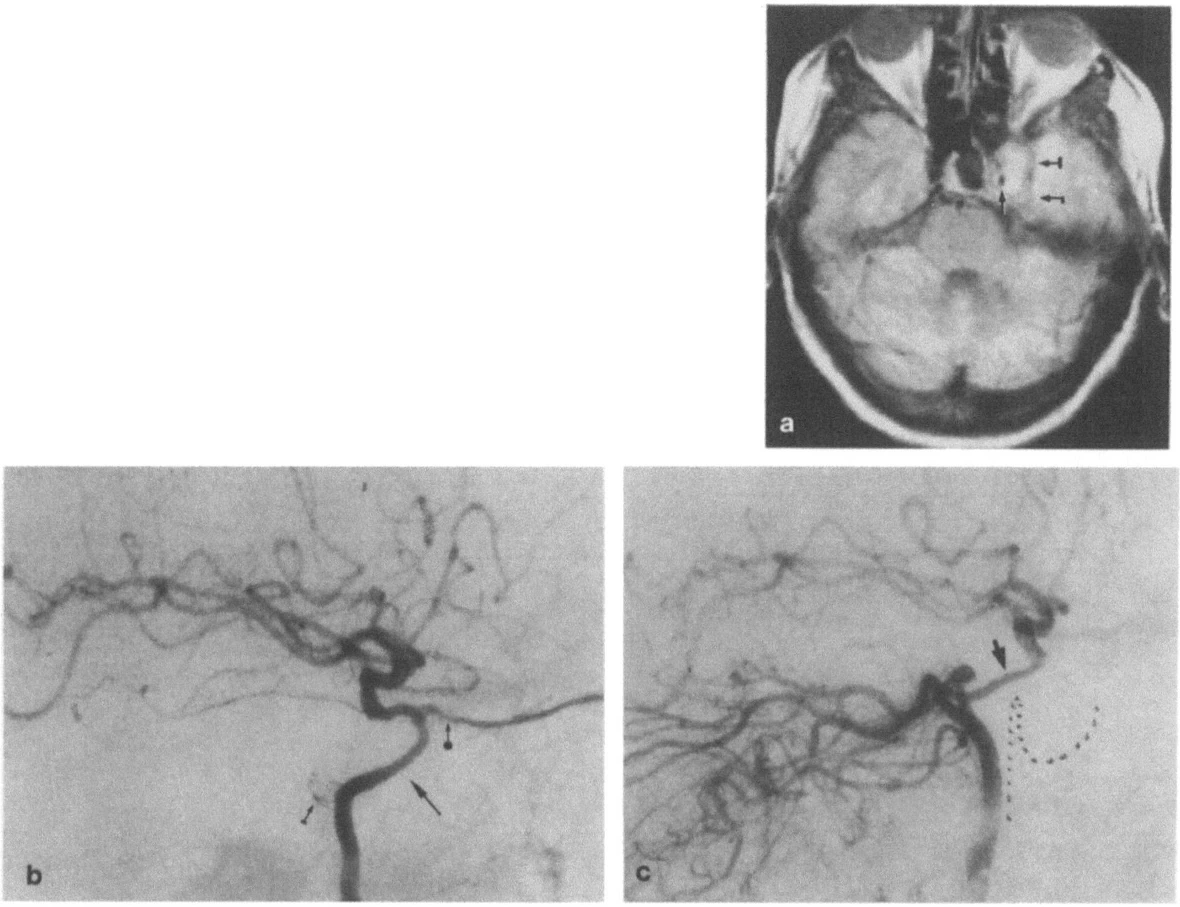

Fig. 8.13a–c. Cavernous sinus meningioma. **a** MRI, proton density-weighted scan. The tumour well demonstrated on CT appears slightly hyperintense to the brain parenchyma. The right cavernous sinus appears very large. Its lateral wall is bulged outward *(arrows from line)*. The intracavernous portion of ICA is small *(arrow)*. **b, c** Angiogram shows narrowing due to encasement of the intracavernous portion of ICA *(arrow)*, irregularities of the ophthalmic artery *(arrow from circle)*, and meningeal branches of C5 portion of the carotid siphon *(arrow from line)* supplying the tumour. In **c** collateral circulation through the posterior communicans artery *(arrow)* is evident

than invasion. Concomitant angiographic signs of encasement, such as narrowing or distortion of the cavernous portion of the carotid siphon, are useful in making the distinction, but a normal appearance of the parasellar portion of the internal carotid does not exclude infiltration of the cavernous sinus space (Fig. 8.16). The parasellar veins may be well demonstrated by dynamic CT [29]. Asymmetry between the two sides is the rule, but marked distortion and lack of filling is suggestive of invasion of the sinus. The demonstration of encasement of the ICA or of enlargement of the cavernous sinus space on MRI, with outward bulging of its lateral wall, is reliable evidence of invasion of this space (Figs. 8.13–8.16).

8.5 Meningioma En Plaque

Meningioma en plaque can be found elsewhere, but as already described is particularly frequent in lesions on the lateral wall of the cavernous sinus space, extending from a cavernous sinus origin, and in lesions spreading behind the posterior surface of the sphenoid wings. These meningiomas extend like a carpet along the skull base where they infiltrate both dura and bone. Intraorbital extension is relatively common either through the bone or superior orbital fissure or optic canal. Proptosis and involvement of the optic nerve are frequent.

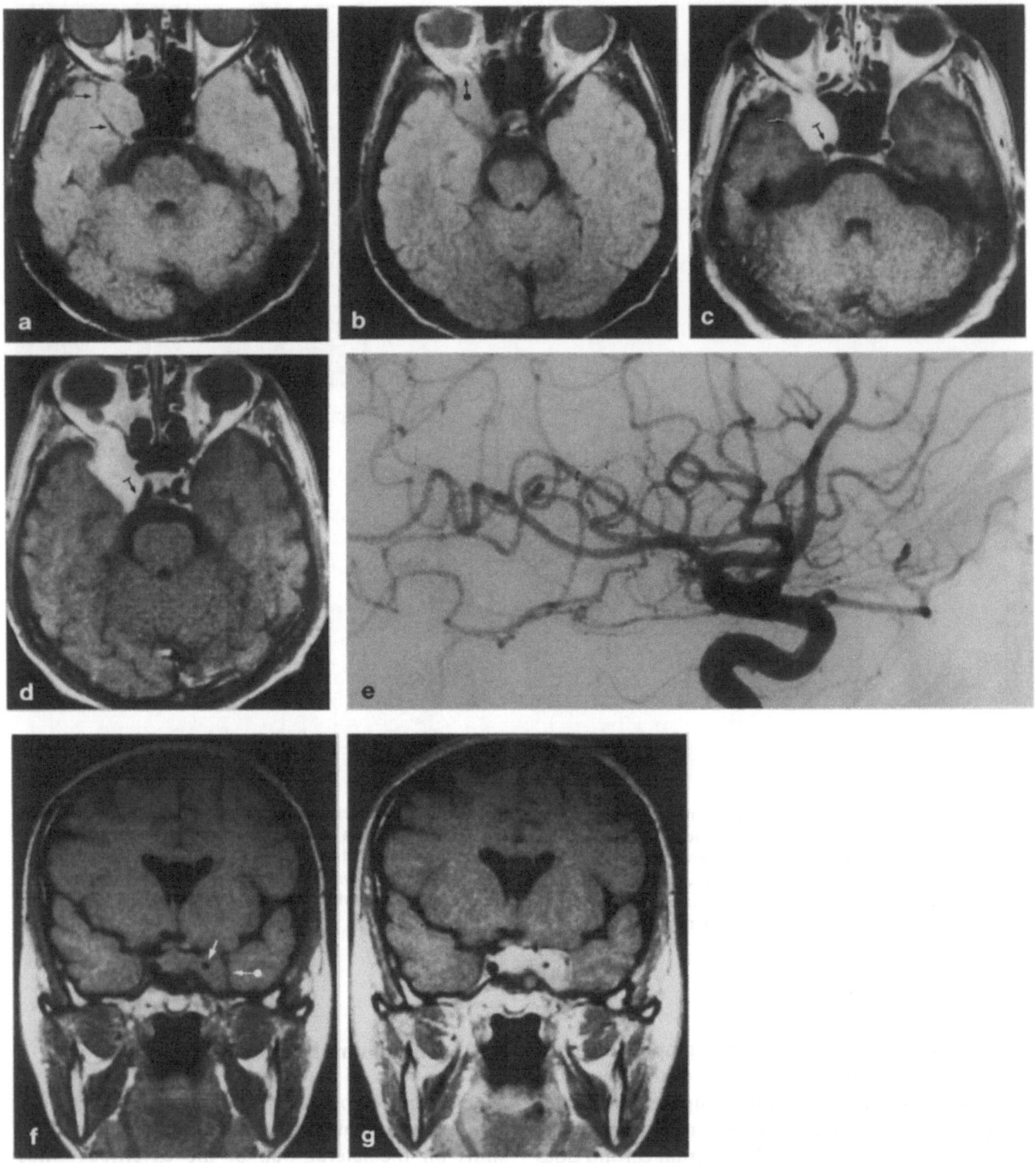

Fig. 8.14a–e. Cavernous sinus meningioma. **a, b** MRI (SE 1600/50). The tumour which appears isointense with normal brain parenchyma, completely fills the space of the cavernous sinus and extends intraorbitally *(arrow from circle)*. The lateral wall of the sinus is bulged outward *(arrows)*. **c, d** MRI (SE 500/50). After Gd-DTPA there is an evident tumoral enhancement. There is a very small part *(arrow)* of the tumour growing outside of the sinus. In the same area the lateral wall of the sinus (**a**) appeared interrupted. The compression of the optic nerve is well shown. The ICA *(arrow from line)* is slightly displaced medially, but its lumen is normal. **e** Angiogram. Normal aspect of the intracavernous portion of the ICA
f, g Another case of cavernous sinus meningioma. MRI (T1-weighted images. Coronal planes). The tumour appears isointense with the normal brain parenchyma (**f**). The lateral wall of the sinus (•⟶) is bulged laterally. The ICA (→) is narrowed due to tumoral encasement. After Gd-DTPA (**g**) the tumour is clearly recognizable. There is a small en plaque portion outside of the sinus

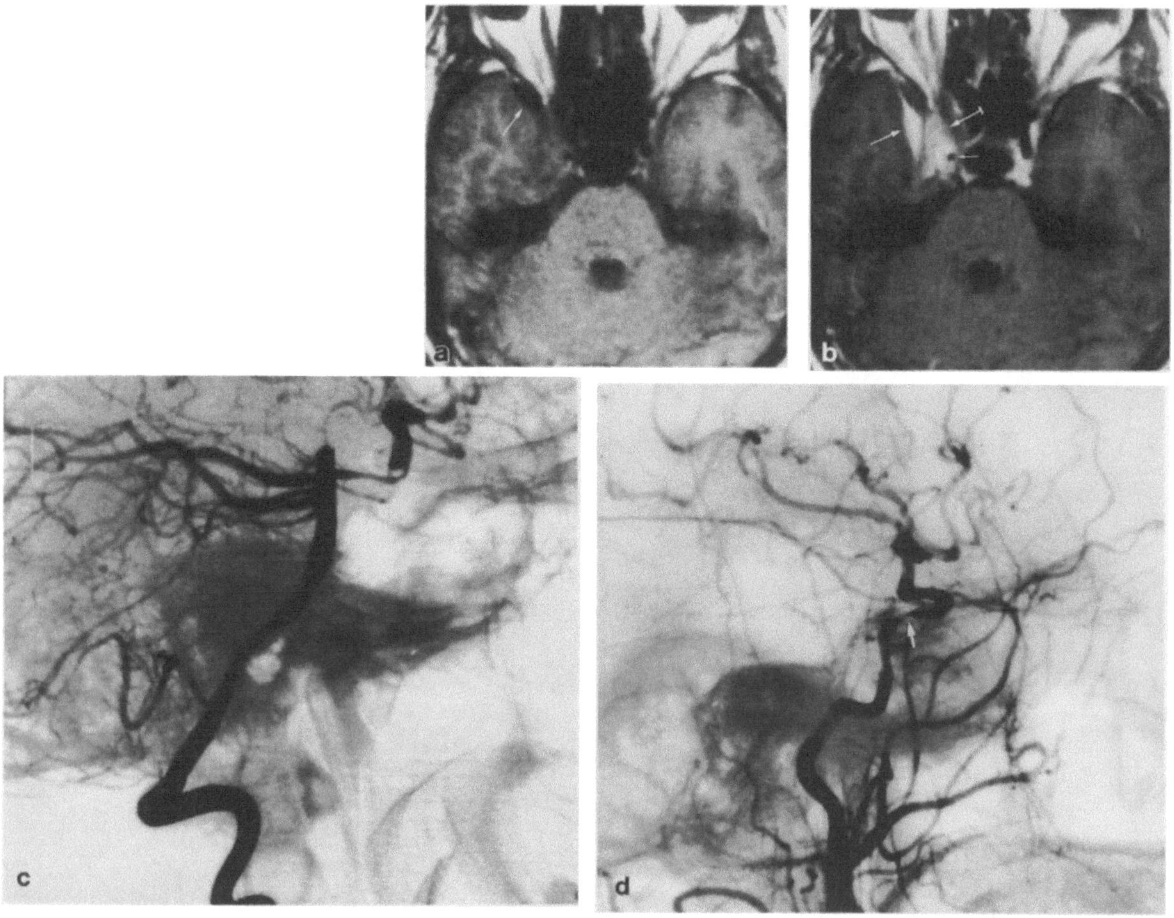

Fig. 8.15 a–d. Cavernous sinus meningioma with an en plaque extracavernous portion. **a, b** MRI, T1-weighted scans, without and with contrast medium. **a** The tumour is not recognizable. Only a thickness of the left sphenoid wing is visible *(white arrow)*. **b** There is evident enhancement after contrast medium. The intracavernous *(white arrow from line)* and the en plaque extracavernous *(white arrow)* portions of the tumour are demonstrated. The lateral wall of the cavernous sinus is bulged outward. The intracavernous portion of the carotid siphon is very small *(small white arrow)*. **c–d** Angiogram shows narrowing due to encasement *(white arrow)* of the intracavernous portion of the internal carotid artery. On the vertebral angiogram a collateral circulation with injection of the carotid through the posterior communicating artery is already present

8.5.1 CT and MRI

Thickening of the lesser and greater sphenoid wings as well as narrowing of the optic canal is frequent [28, 62], usually marked and extensive (Figs. 8.3, 8.4, 8.12, 8.16).
The tumour may be visible as an area of increased density in the parasellar region or as a shallow rim behind the surface of the sphenoid wing, frequently with an intraorbital component (Figs. 8.3, 8.4). The presence of tumour can also be inferred on the basis of obliteration or distortion of Meckel's cave [60, 134] but in many cases the soft tissue component cannot be distinguished from hyperostosis on CT (Fig. 8.4). MRI usually shows the tumour as a thin rim of high signal intensity on T2-weighted images (Fig. 8.16), and particularly well on T1-weighted images performed after intravenous injection of Gd-DTPA (Figs. 8.4, 8.14, 8.15, 8.16).
Peritumoral oedema is uncommon in this group of tumours.

8.5.2 Angiography

The angiographic findings depend upon extent and localization of the tumour. Occasionally the internal carotid arteriogram appears normal, or abnormalities are seen only in the venous phase. The external carotid artery is frequently involved, especially in lateral sphenoid wings lesions (Fig. 8.4), and a ho-

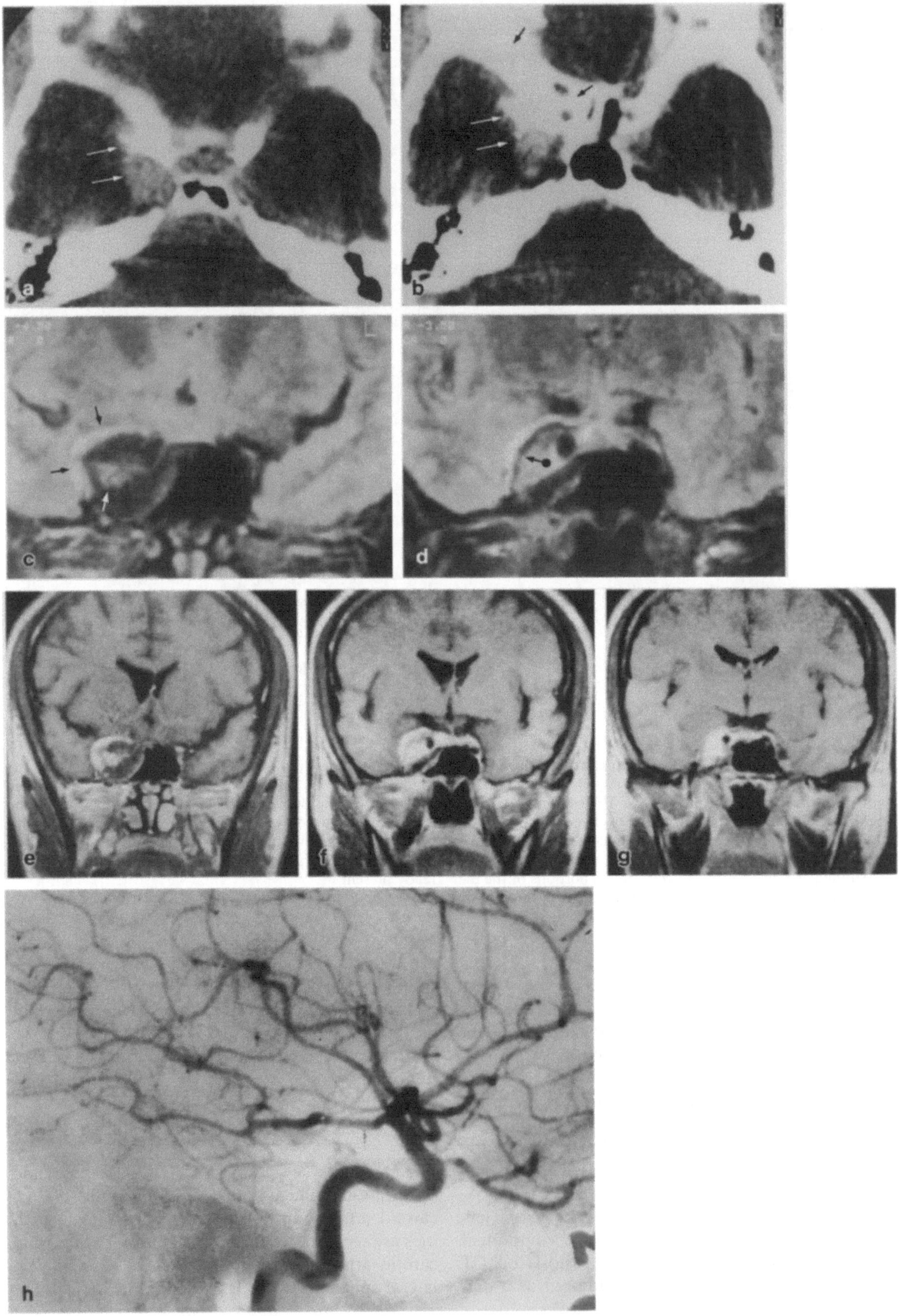
a
b
c
d
e
f
g
h

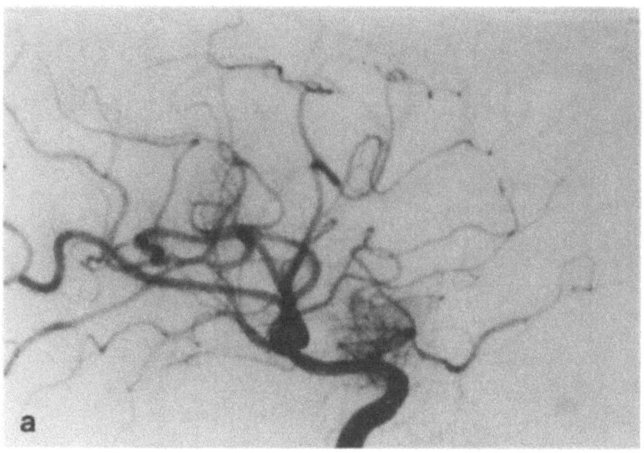

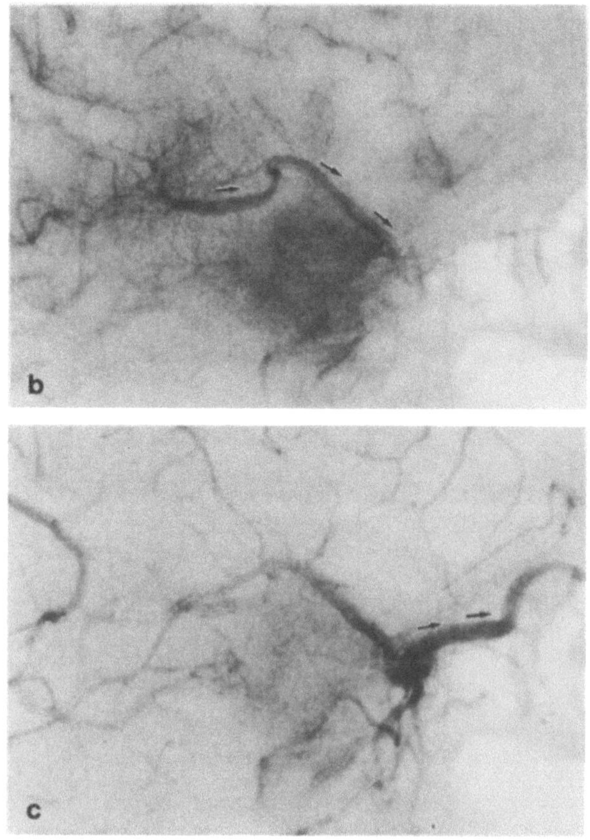

Fig. 8.17 a–c. Large medial SWM. The drainage of the sylvian veins into the cavernous sinus is blocked. Diversion of the drainage into the ophthalmic vein *(arrows)*

mogeneous capillary blush often involving the entire area of the hyperostosis usually indicates meningioma.

8.6 Temporobasal Meningiomas

Temporobasal meningiomas, uncommon lesions, typically invaginate into the temporal lobe and become enclosed in brain tissue. The dural attachment lies in the same plane as axial CT or MRI sections, and if the lesion possesses atypical features such as low CT attenuation or lobulation or is pedunculated, the resemblance to a temporal lobe glioma, metastasis or lymphoma can be close. Coronal imaging on CT, or better on MRI, should identify the dural attachment, however. Angiography usually provides a diagnosis, showing typical tumour circulation supplied mainly by arteries of the dura mater (Fig. 8.18).
Peritumoral oedema is frequent.

◄

Fig. 8.16 a–h. Cavernous sinus meningioma with an en plaque extracavernous portion. **a, b** CT. Enhanced mass in the parasellar area *(white arrows)*; Hyperostosis of the sphenoid wing *(black arrows)*. **c, d** MRI, coronal planes, proton density-weighted scans. The *black area* corresponds to the hyperostosis of the bone structures involving the sphenoid and the sphenoid wing. The *white areas* correspond to tumoral tissue *(arrows)*, which have an en plaque growth along the lateral wall of the sinus. The lateral wall of the cavernous sinus is bulged outward *(arrow from circle)*. The ICA appear slightly lifted but otherwise normal. **e–g** MRI, coronal planes, T1-weighted scans after Gd-DTPA. There is an evident tumoral enhancement outside and inside of the cavernous sinus. **h** Angiogram. There are only slight irregularities of the intracavernous portion of ICA which otherwise appears normal. The ophthalmic artery is narrowed at its origin

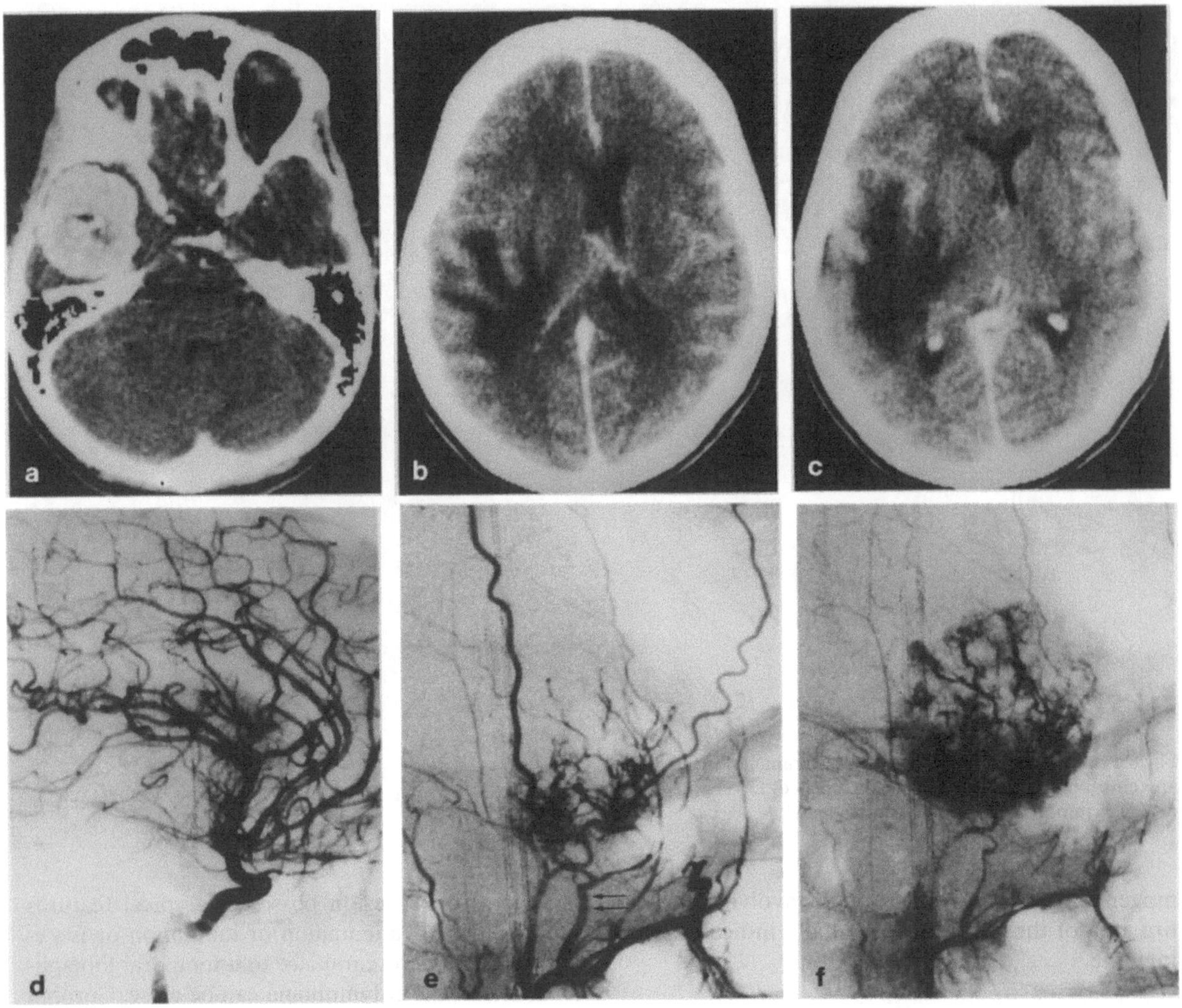

Fig. 8.18a–f. Richly vascularized endotheliomatous temporobasal meningioma. **a–c** CT. There is evident peritumoral oedema involving the corona radiata, the capsula externa and the posterior limb of the capsula interna. **d** Internal carotid angiogram demonstrates lifting of the middle cerebral artery. There is no pathological vascularization. **e, f** Angiogram of the external carotid artery. The tumour is richly vascularized by branches of the middle meningeal artery (arrows)

8.7 Differential Diagnosis

8.7.1 Metastases

The major differential diagnosis is from other extra-axial masses. Malignant involvement of bone, such as by metastases from carcinoma of the breast or prostate, usually produces destruction as well as sclerosis of bone, with little soft tissue mass. Knowledge of the primary tumour or evidence of metastases elsewhere may be a useful pointer to the correct diagnosis, although breast cancer and meningiomas may occur simultaneously in the same patient (Chaps. 1, 6).

8.7.2 Fibrous Dysplasias

Fibrous dysplasia may simulate sphenoid wing meningiomas (see Chaps. 2, 3).

8.7.3 Giant Aneurysms

Giant aneurysms can sometimes closely simulate globular meningiomas in the parasellar and suprasellar region. Usually they are partly thrombosed, and on CT the residual lumen enhances after intravenous contrast like other vascular structures and less persistently than meningioma; curvilinear calcification is often shown in the wall. Laminated

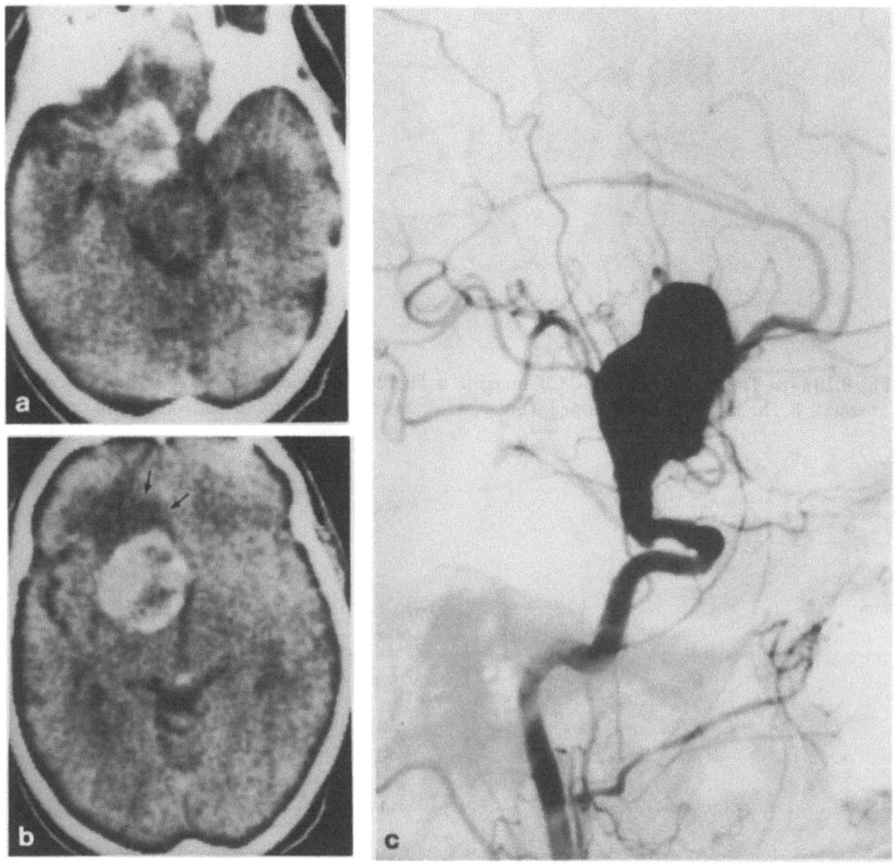

Fig. 8.19 a–c. Giant aneurysm of ICA. **a, b** CT. The aneurysm, which is partially calcified and thrombotic, is surrounded by oedema *(arrows)*. **c** Angiogram

thrombus is usually characteristic on MRI. Only occasionally is angiography needed for confirmation (Fig. 8.19).

8.7.4 Pituitary Adenomas

Pituitary adenoma infiltrating one cavernous sinus can sometimes be difficult to differentiate from meningioma in this site on CT. Encasement of ICA is more frequent in meningioma, but can also occur in adenoma [38, 250]; in adenoma the artery is usually displaced laterally, while in meningioma it is medially displaced. This is usually well demonstrated on MRI. Furthermore, adenoma usually yields a more intense signal on T2-weighted images; it occupies the pituitary fossa, which is nearly always enlarged, and endocrine disorders are more frequent. Very occasionally, however, meningioma can grow into and expand the pituitary fossa to become indistinguishable from pituitary adenoma.

8.7.5 Trigeminal Neuromas

Trigeminal neuroma typically causes erosion without sclerosis of the apex of the petrous pyramid and erosion of the foramen ovale (Fig. 8.20) [34, 134]. Very large neuromas can destroy the middle cranial fossa in the parasellar area (Fig. 8.21). Bone destruction is uncommon even with massive meningiomas. Trigeminal neurinomas are frequently characterized on MRI by a high signal on T2-weighted images due to large cystic and necrotic components, and they usually appear inhomogeneous on CT and MRI. After intravenous injection of iodinated or paramagnetic contrast, neurinomas frequently appear inhomogeneous (Figs. 8.20, 8.21).

8.7.6 Craniopharyngiomas

Craniopharyngiomas mainly affect young patients. They appear typically as partly calcified and cystic suprasellar masses, causing erosion without sclerosis of the dorsum sellae.

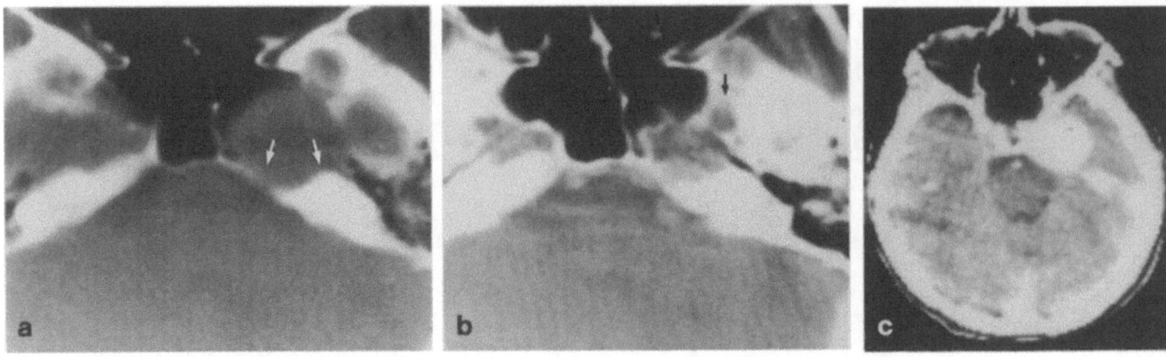

Fig. 8.20 a–c. Trigeminal neuroma, CT images. **a** There is an evident concave impression of the apex of the petrous pyramid *(arrows)*. **b** The foramen ovale appears enlarged *(arrow)*. **c** The tumour shows evident enhancement

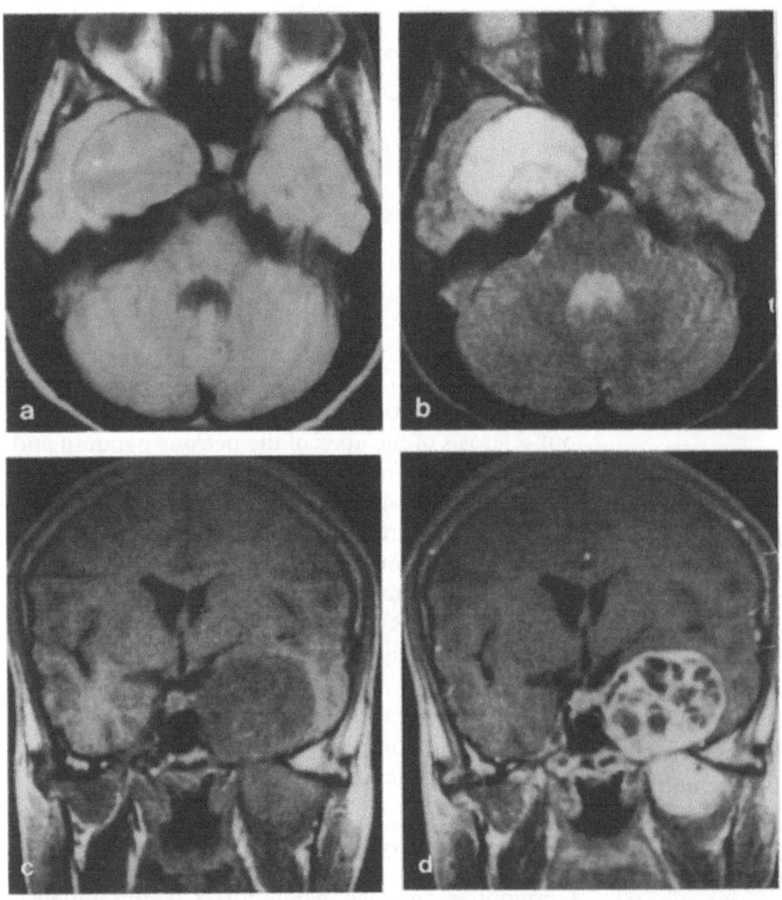

Fig. 8.21 a–d. Trigeminal neuroma. **a, b** MRI. The tumour is separated from cerebral parenchyma by a hypointense rim as in meningioma. The tumour itself appears isointense on **a** proton density-weighted image, but displays a very high signal on **b** T2-weighted image. **c, d** MRI, T1-weighted images without and with Gd-DTPA, coronal plane. The extracranial extension of the tumour is clearly demonstrated, as its inhomogeneous enhancement

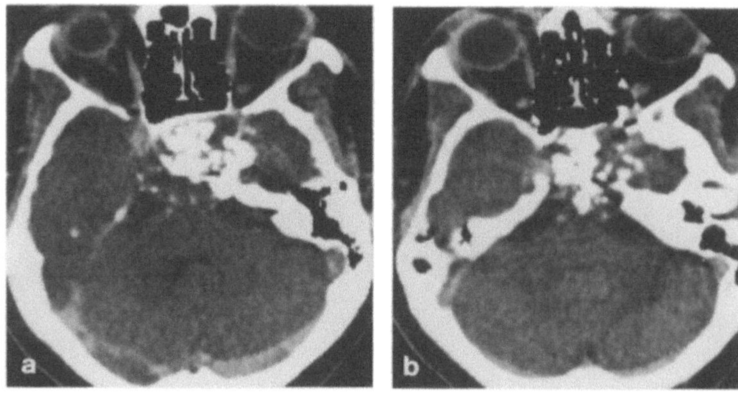

Fig. 8.22 a, b. Parasellar chondroma, CT images. The tumour, which is richly calcified, has destroyed the adjacent bone

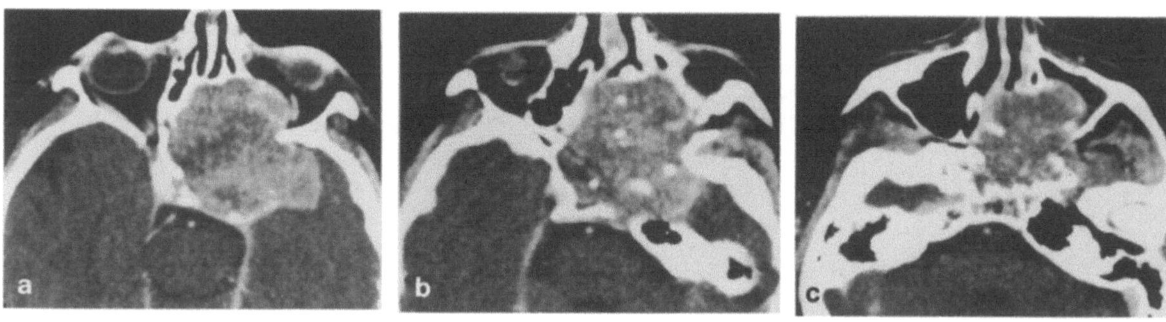

Fig. 8.23 a–c. Chordoma of the parasellar area infiltrating also the nasal cavity and the orbit, CT images. The tumour is partially calcified. There is evident bone destruction

8.7.7 Chondromas and Chordomas

Chondromas are frequently extensively calcified or ossified (Fig. 8.22). Chordomas appear as inhomogeneous, partially calcified masses on CT. They show inconsistent, usually patchy enhancement after intravenous contrast on CT and MRI and are frequently associated with extensive destruction of the skull base (Fig. 8.23).

8.7.8 Cystic Lesions

Cystic lesions like arachnoid cysts and epidermoid-dermoid tumours should not present a problem in differential diagnosis.

8.7.9 Gliomas

Well-circumscribed gliomas of the temporal lobe may be confused with temporobasal meningiomas showing atypical features.

9 Tentorial Meningiomas

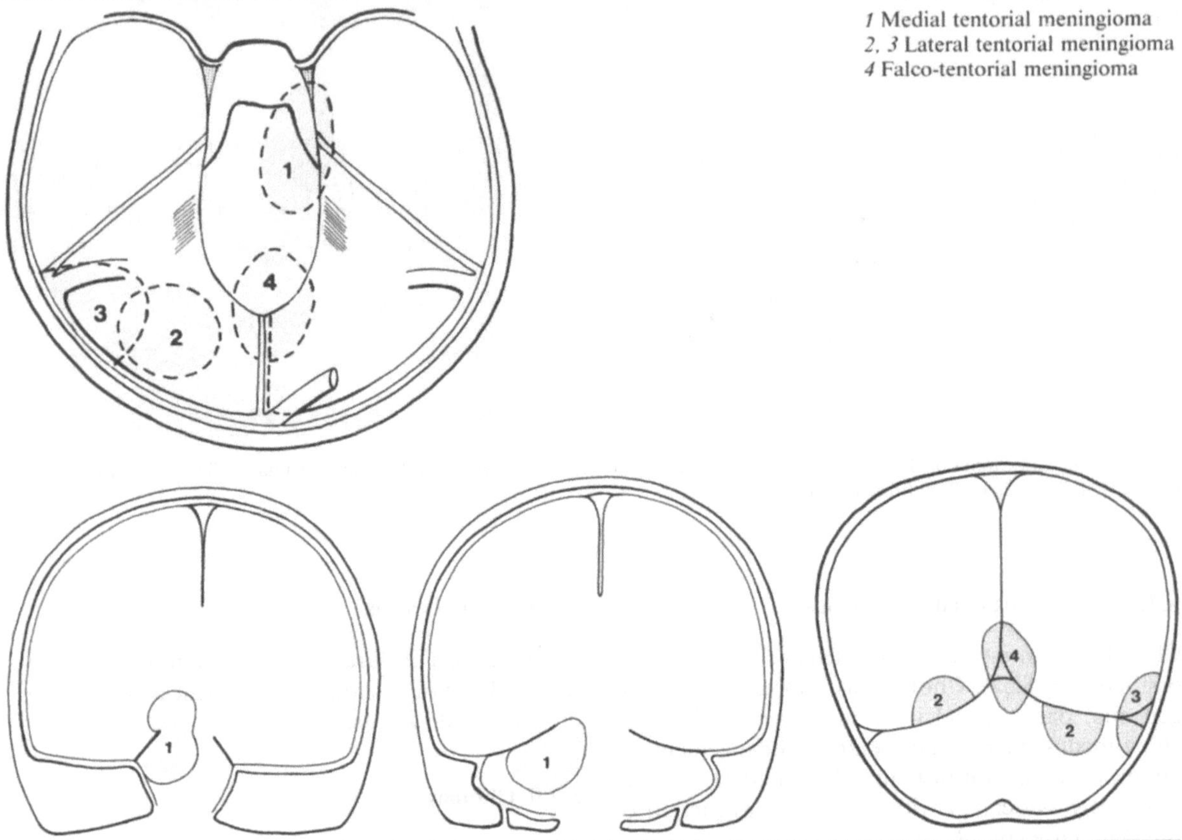

1 Medial tentorial meningioma
2, 3 Lateral tentorial meningioma
4 Falco-tentorial meningioma

9.1 Anatomical Considerations

At the anterolateral border the tentorium is attached to the petrous ridge, where it separates to include the superior petrosal sinus. The posterolateral border is attached to the temporal and occipital bones and includes the transverse sinus and the torcular. The medial borders are free and form the margins of the tentorial incisura. They join posteriorly at the midline, at the apex of the tentorium, and, immediately behind this, the tentorium fuses with the falx. The falx-tentorial junction contains the straight sinus, draining Galen's vein and the inferior sagittal sinus.

The anterior end of each free edge is attached to the petrous apex, the posterior and anterior clinoid processes. According to the anatomical study of Ono et al. [214], these attachments form three dural folds: the anterior, which extends from the petrous apex to the anterior clinoid process, the posterior, from the petrous apex to the posterior clinoid process, and the interclinoid fold, between the posterior and anterior clinoid processes. Finally, from its anterior part, the free edge of the tentorium continues laterally downward to form the lateral wall of the cavernous sinus.

9.2 Incidence and Localization

Tentorial meningiomas are uncommon; they account for 2%-3% of all intracranial meningiomas [17, 54, 190]; the proportion of women is high (70%) [108, 252].

These tumours tend to be large when diagnosed. In the material of Sekhar et al. [252] about 80% of the tumours were more than 5 cm in diameter. This, coupled with the relatively difficult operative approach, explains the high frequency of tumour recurrence and the high operative mortality [108, 252]. Refined radiological diagnostic techniques such as high definition computed tomography (CT), magnetic resonance imaging (MRI) and selective angiography will help detect these tumours at an earlier stage and should contribute to improving the surgical results.

According to the primary site of attachment, we can distinguish three subgroups: medial tentorial, lateral tentorial and falco-tentorial meningiomas (see diagram).

9.2.1 Medial Tentorial Meningiomas

Medial tentorial meningiomas (MTM) account for about 50% of all tentorial meningiomas. Their most frequent area of origin is at the attachment of tentorium to the petrous apex and medial petrous ridge (petrous ridge-tentorial meningiomas). Medial extension of the tumour with secondary attachment to the clivus, as well as growth into the cerebellopontine and/or parasellar area with infiltration of the cavernous sinus are frequent. These tumours often spread both above and below the tentorium: this was present in more than 60% of patients in one large series [252]. Compression and displacement of the brain stem is usual, and the third ventricle is frequently narrowed, causing hydrocephalus.

9.2.2 Lateral Tentorial Meningiomas

More laterally located meningiomas may also be both supra- and infratentorial, but more frequently they grow into one compartment only. Lateral tentorial convexity meningiomas may infiltrate the calvaria and the adjacent transverse sinus.

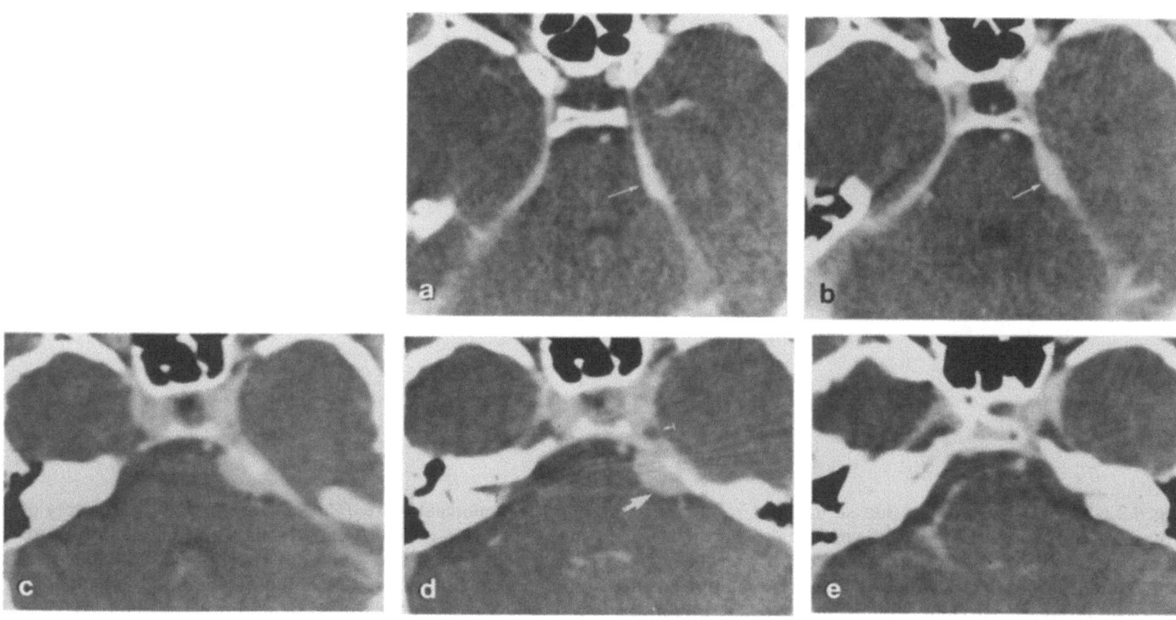

Fig. 9.1 a–e. Small MTM. CT images show attachment of the tumour to the tentorium *(thin white arrows)* and to the petrous apex *(thick white arrow)*. Meckel's cave seems to be slightly compressed *(arrow from line)*. On a slice 2 mm lower, Meckel's cave appears normal

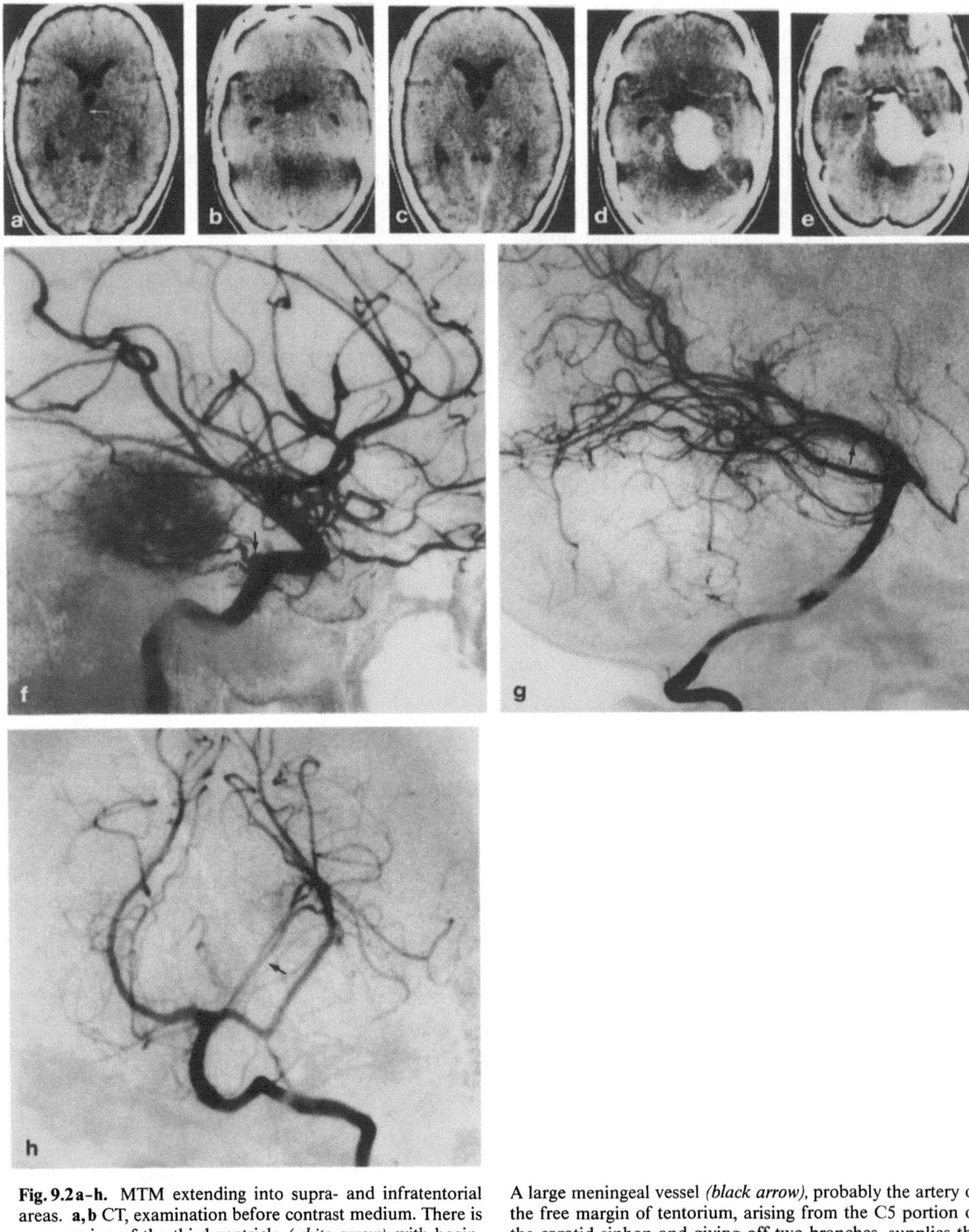

Fig. 9.2 a–h. MTM extending into supra- and infratentorial areas. **a, b** CT, examination before contrast medium. There is compression of the third ventricle *(white arrow)*, with beginning supratentorial hydrocephalus (note the dilatation of the temporal horn). The circumpedoncular cisterns are no longer recognizable. There is a distortion of the brain stem. **c–e** CT, tumoral enhancement after contrast medium. **f** Angiogram. A large meningeal vessel *(black arrow)*, probably the artery of the free margin of tentorium, arising from the C5 portion of the carotid siphon and giving off two branches, supplies the tumour. **g, h** Both the left posterior cerebral and left superior cerebellar arteries are elevated *(black arrows)*. On the AP view (**h**) the posterior cerebral artery and superior cerebellar artery *(black arrow)* are shifted medially

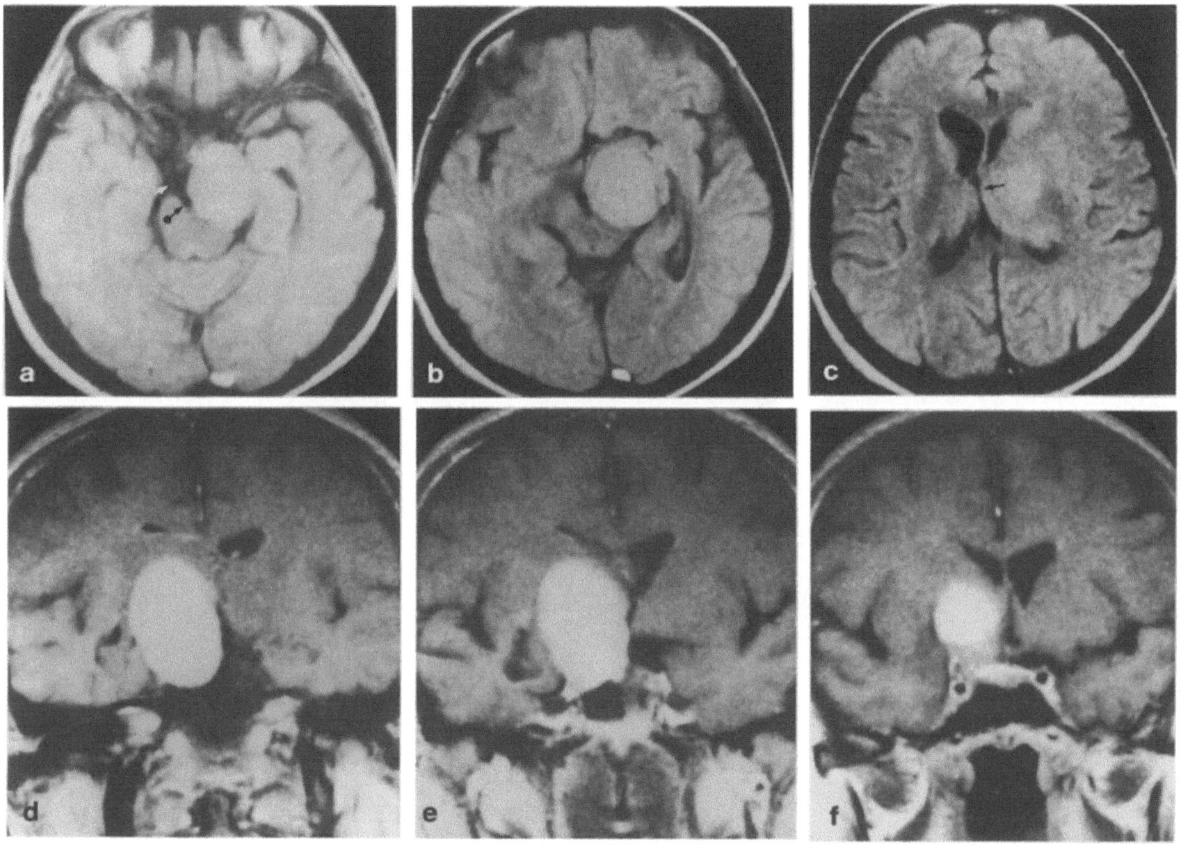

Fig. 9.3a–f. Right MTM with clearly prevalent growth in the supratentorial area. **a–c** MRI, proton density-weighted scans. The tumour is slightly hyperintense. There is evident compression of mesencephalon and diencephalon with shifting of the third ventricle *(black arrow)*. The basilar artery *(black arrow from circle)* runs close to the tumour. The opposite III° cranial nerve is well recognizable *(white arrow)*. **d–f** MRI, T1-weighted images after Gd-DTPA. On these coronal planes the prevalent extent of the tumour supratentorially is evident

9.2.3 Falco Tentorial Meningiomas

Falx tentorial meningiomas may be unilateral, extending into the parieto-occipital region, or may grow on both sides of the falx. Rostral spread may compress the mesencephalon, the third ventricle and, eventually, the aqueduct, causing supratentorial hydrocephalus. Infiltration of the straight sinus and/or Galen's vein also occurs.

9.3 Computed Tomography - Magnetic Resonance Imaging

Demonstration of symptomatic tumours with CT is generally simple since they are rarely small (Figs. 9.1, 9.14). They are frequently isodense or only slightly hyperdense and recognizable only indirectly by compression and distortion of surrounding cerebral structures (Fig. 9.2). After contrast medium there is commonly marked homogeneous enhancement (Fig. 9.2).

Since these tumours tend to be relatively large, MTM located near the petrous apex often cannot be distinguished by radiology from petrosphenoidal clival meningiomas or those arising from the posterior surface of the petrous bone extending into the supratentorial area.

Erosions of the clivus and of the petrous tip may occur in MTM, but are usually very limited and not recognizable even with high definition CT. Lateral tentorial lesions can infiltrate the calvarium and cause hyperostosis (Fig. 9.13).

It is not always possible with CT to define precisely the supra- and/or infratentorial extent of a tumour (see also Chap. 10). MRI, by demonstrating the meningioma in three orthogonal planes, shows its relationship to the tentorium and the frequent extensions into the pontocerebellar, retroclival, supra- and parasellar regions, including any involvement

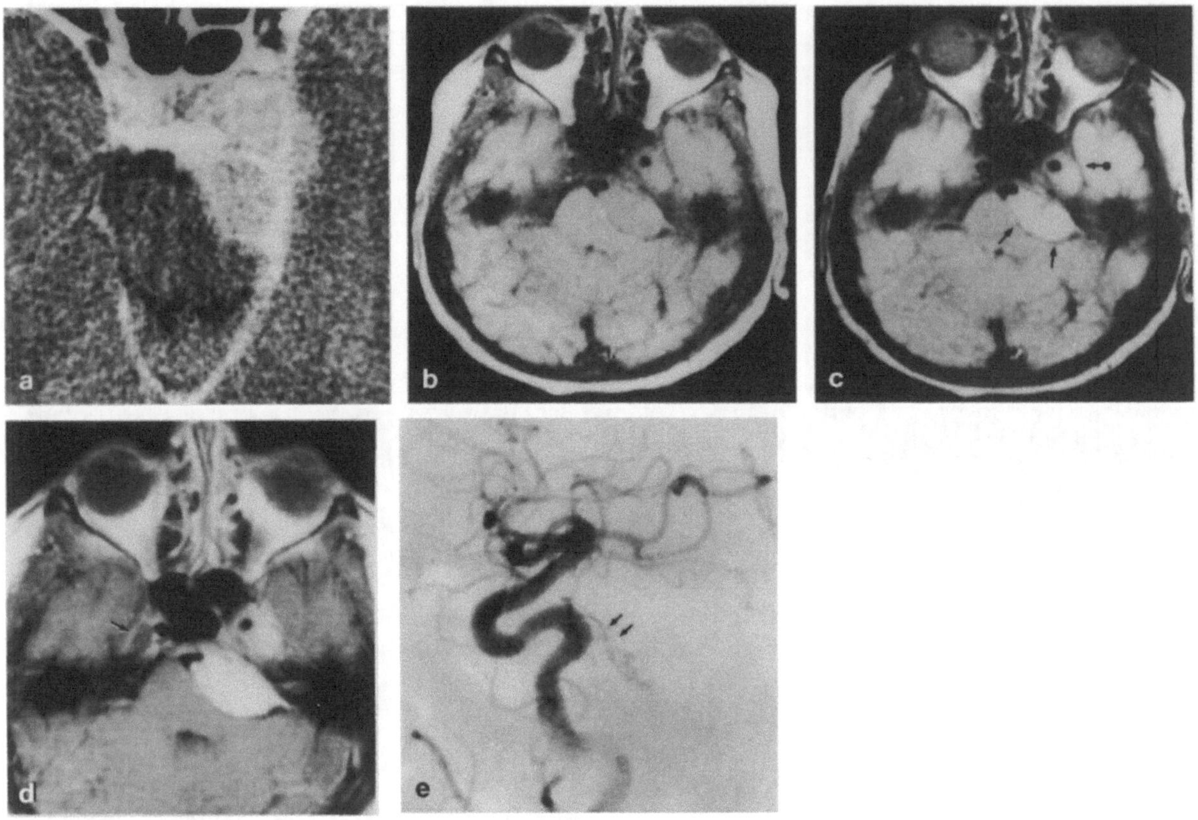

Fig. 9.4a–e. MTM extending into the pontocerebellar area and infiltrating the cavernous sinus. **a** CT. The meningioma showing evident enhancement extends far into the posterior fossa and parasellar area. **b,c** MRI. The tumour appears isointense on **b** the T1-weighted image, but displays hyperintense signal on **c** the proton density-weighted image. On the two sequences the meningioma is well separated from the pons by a black rim *(arrow)*, probably corresponding to vessels. The tumour has extended into the cavernous sinus whose lateral wall *(arrow from circle)* is bulged outwards. In spite of the cavernous sinus infiltration, the ICA appears normal. **d** MRI after Gd-DTPA. There is evident tumoral enhancement. On the *left* we can recognize the Meckel's cave *(arrow)* which is no longer visible on the *right*. The lateral borders of the tumour are irregular due to extension outside the cavernous sinus. **e** Angiogram, normal ICA. Meningeal branches *(arrows)* supply the tumour

of the cavernous sinus. The degree of displacement and distortion of the brain stem and of major vessels, especially the basilar artery, can be recognized (Figs. 9.3–9.6; 9.9–9.11).

Peritumoral oedema will be discussed in a separate chapter, but, generally, MTM do not induce much oedema; falx tentorial and lateral tentorial tumours tend to induce more (Figs. 9.8, 9.9, 9.13, 9.14).

9.4 Angiography

9.4.1 Arteries

The arteries running near the free margin of the tentorium (anterior choroidal, posterior cerebral and superior cerebellar arteries) may be encased by the tumour. These vessels tend to be elevated and deviated medially (Fig. 9.2), and there is frequent upward displacement of the middle cerebral artery also due to either the supratentorial growth or hydrocephalus. Infratentorial tumours will deviate the superior cerebellar artery and its branches inferiorly, away from the posterior cerebral artery and its temporal branches (Fig. 9.6), and displacement of the basilar artery is often evident, sometimes with encasement.

Tentorial meningiomas, particularly when medially located, are almost always supplied by meningeal branches of the C_4–C_5 portion of the carotid siphon (see Chap. 5; Figs. 9.2, 9.4, 9.6, 9.10). The petrosquamous branches of the middle meningeal (Fig. 9.7) as well as branches of ascending pharyngeal artery also frequently contribute. Falx tentorial and lateral tentorial tumours may also be supplied from the occipital artery (Fig. 9.10). Branches of the

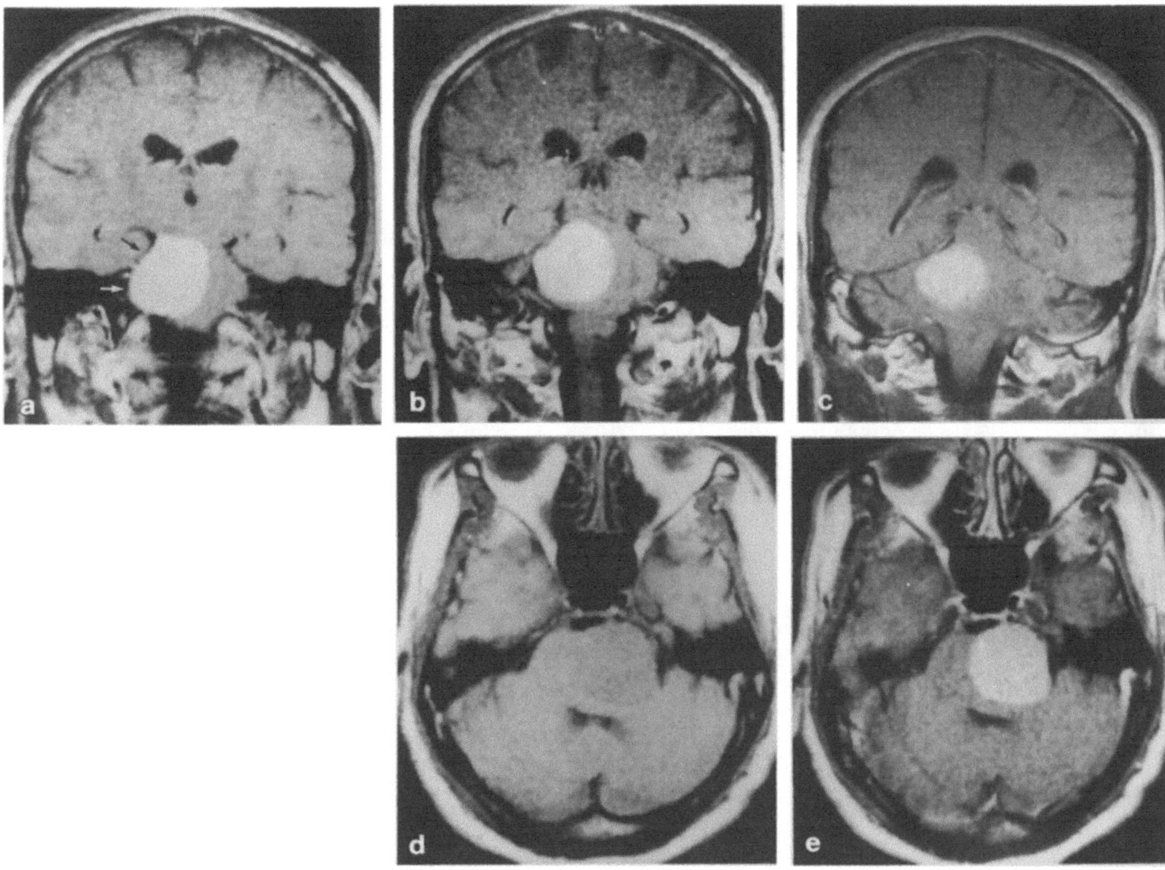

Fig. 9.5 a–e. MTM prevalently extending into the pontocerebellar area. **a–c** MRI, T1-weighted images after Gd-DTPA, coronal planes. Tentorium *(black arrow)*; petrous bone *(white arrow)*. **d, e** MRI, axial planes. Examination **d** before and **e** after Gd-DTPA. There is evident compression of the fourth ventricle

posterior cerebral and superior cerebellar arteries may also supply adjacent tumour (Fig. 9.10).

9.4.2 Venous Sinuses

Involvement of venous sinuses is frequent [108, 252]. Falco-tentorial meningiomas may infiltrate the straight sinus and Galen's vein (Fig. 9.12), the superior petrosal sinus may be involved in tentorial petrous ridge tumours and lateral tentorial meningiomas may invade the transverse sinus (Figs. 9.13, 9.14). A transverse sinus can be safely resected together with the tumour, provided that there is good communication with an adequate opposite transverse sinus, demonstrated by angiography (Figs. 9.13, 9.14), and the cortical venous drainage, particularly from the temporal region, can also be accommodated by anastomotic veins (see Chap. 10).
MRI can demonstrate tumoral infiltration of venous sinuses: currently it is a good complement to angiography and may well replace it in future (Figs. 9.9, 9.11).

9.5 Differential Diagnosis

Brain stem gliomas are commonly low density lesions with inhomogeneous or no enhancement and can also be easily distinguished from meningiomas by their central position. Some gliomas are hyperdense and/or grow exophytically, and these may simulate meningiomas. Evidence of attachment to the tentorium and extension into the parasellar region, frequent in MTM, is useful in differential diagnosis, and blood supply from meningeal branches of internal carotid artery (ICA) and/or external carotid artery (ECA), though it is not specific, suggests meningioma.

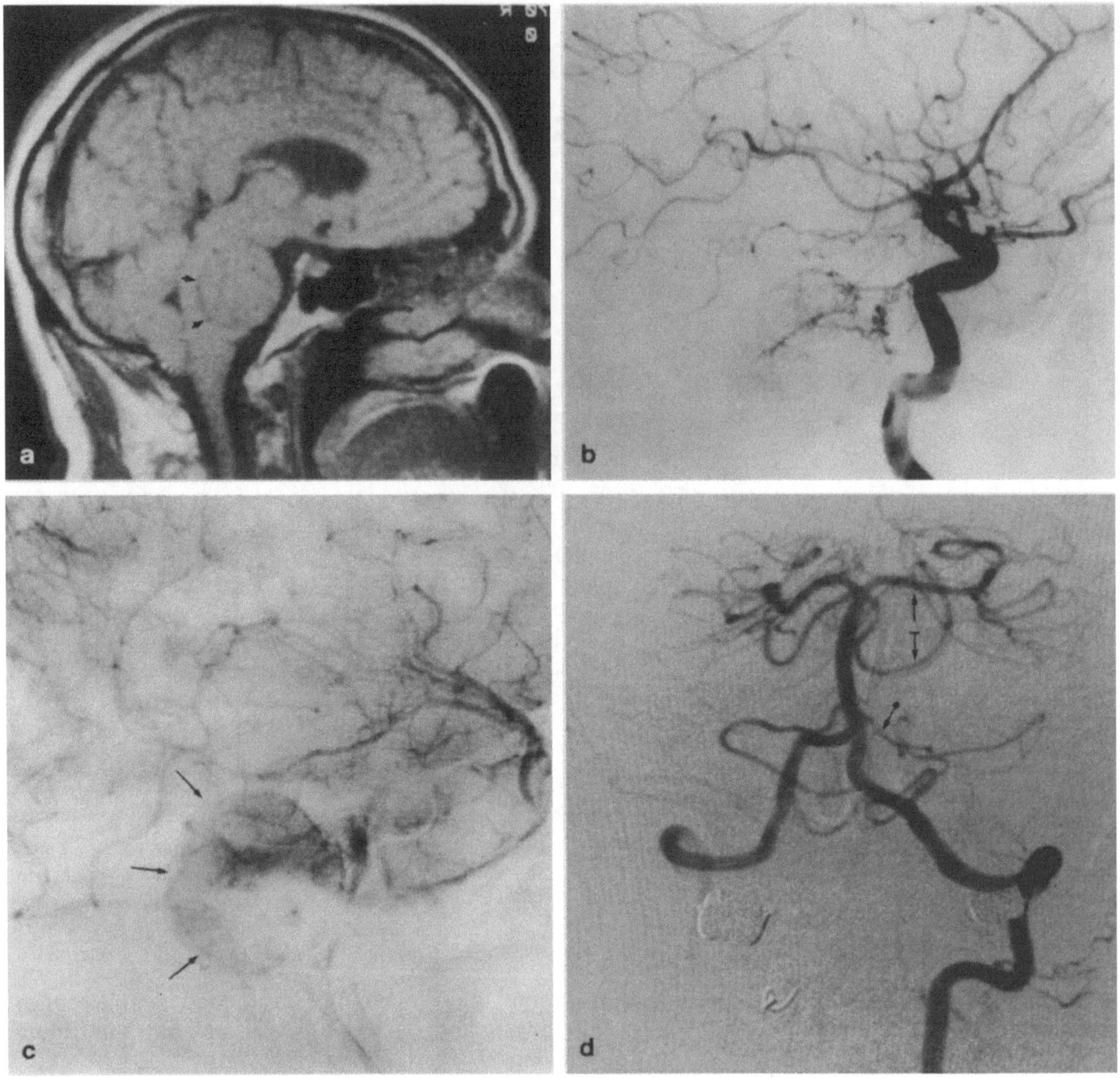

Fig. 9.6 a–d. Additional images of the patient from Fig. 9.5. **a** MRI, sagittal plane, T1-weighted image. The meningioma is isointense with cerebral parenchyma. On the inside and on the periphery *(arrows)* of the tumour, there are nodular and linear structures characterized by a hypointense signal corresponding to vessels. **b, c** Angiogram. **b** Meningeal branches of C5 portion of the carotid siphon supply the tumour. **c** In the venous phase the peripheal veins *(arrows)* also visible on MRI are recognizable. **d** Angiogram. Typical slight upward shifting of posterior cerebral artery *(arrow)*, while the superior cerebellar artery is displaced downward *(arrow from line)*. Stretching of middle cerebellar artery *(arrow from circle)*

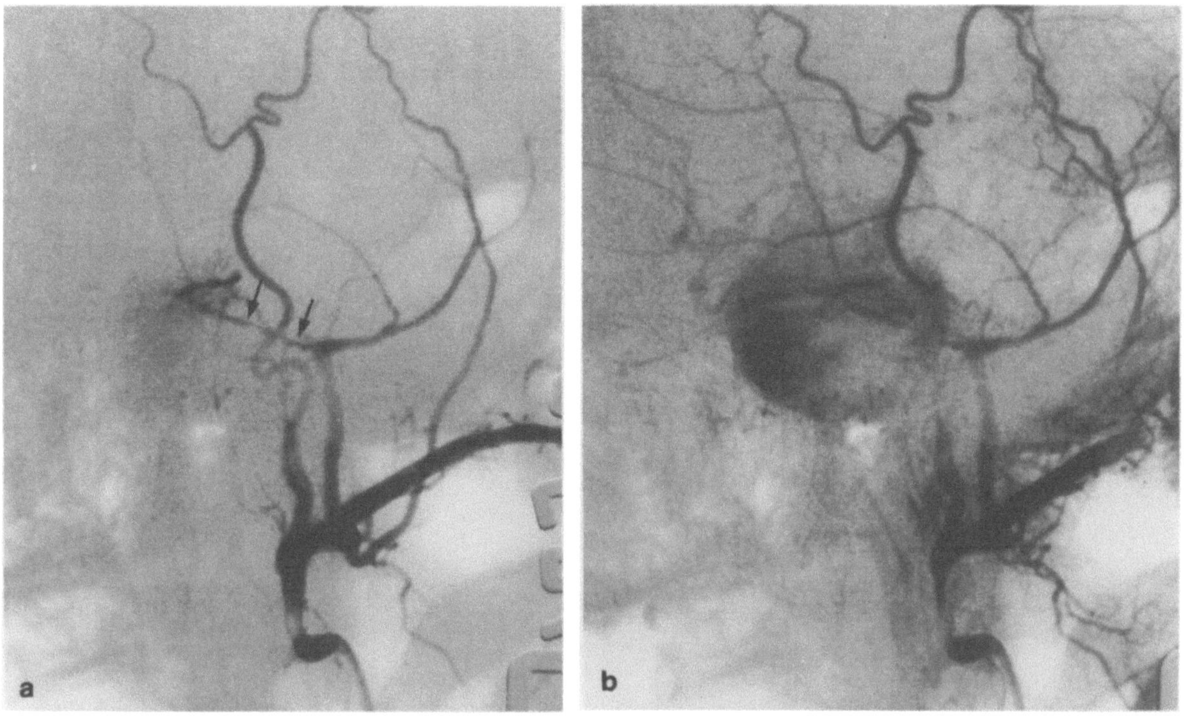

Fig. 9.7 a, b. MTM prevalently extending into the pontocerebellar area. This case similar to this of Figs. 9.5 and 9.6, demonstrates the possible supply of the tumour by the petrosquamous branch of the middle meningeal artery *(arrows)*

Other intra-axial tumours, including germinomas, medulloblastomas and haemangioblastomas (Figs. 3.2, 3.3, 3.4), may occasionally simulate meningioma, particularly if they adhere to the dura.

Metastasis or lymphoma can simulate meningiomas. Lateral tentorial meningiomas infiltrating the calvarium usually cause hyperostosis, whereas in metastases bone destruction is more typical.

Chordomas are generally partly calcified tumours with bone destruction. Contrast enhancement is usually slight and inhomogeneous on CT and MRI (see also Chap. 10).

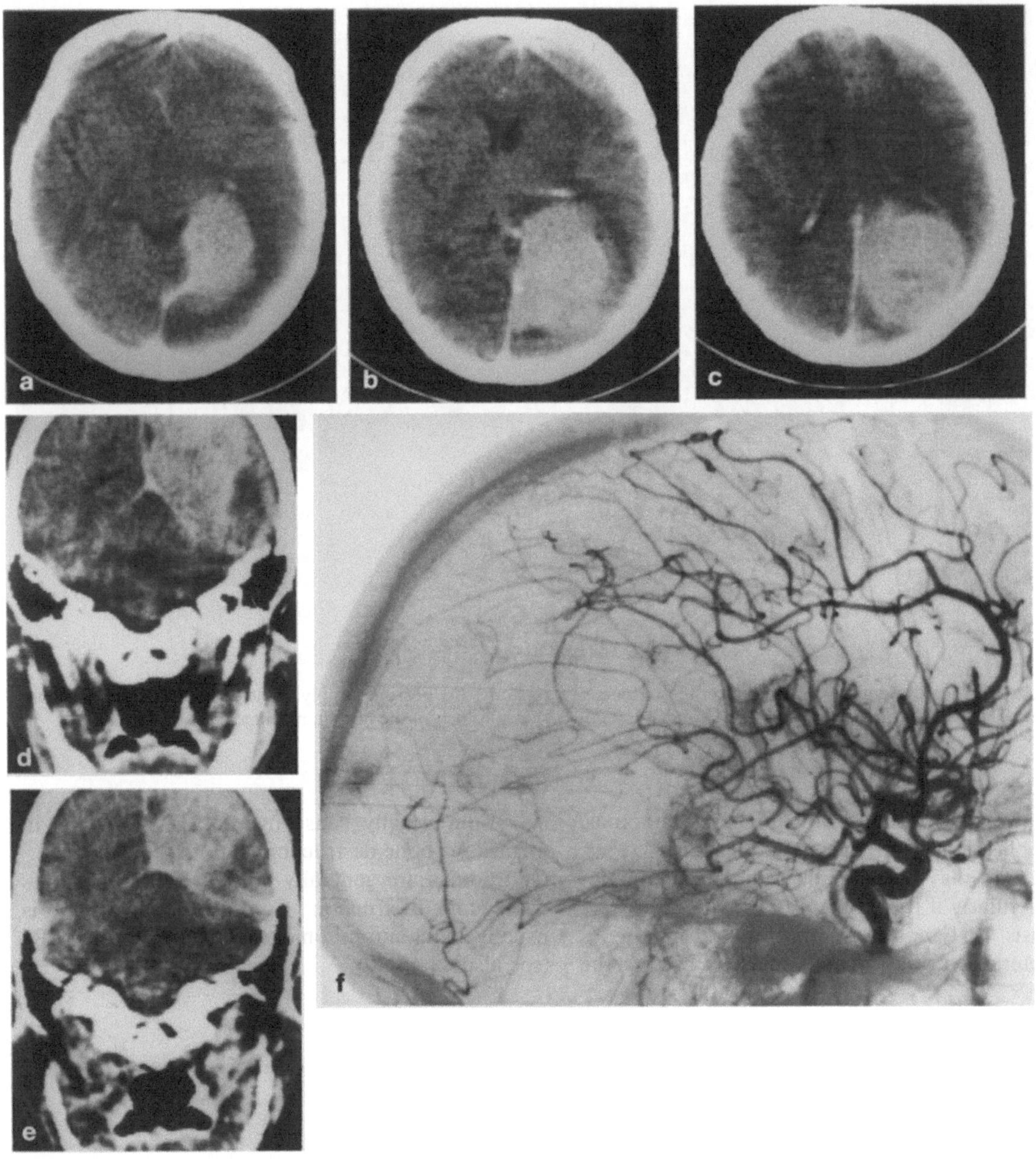

Fig. 9.8 a–f. Falco-tentorial meningioma. **a–e** CT, axial and coronal planes. The tumour which displays a rich contrast enhancement, grows unilaterally in the occipital and parietal regions and extends rostrally, reaching the trigonum area. **f** Common carotid angiogram. The tumour is poorly vascularized

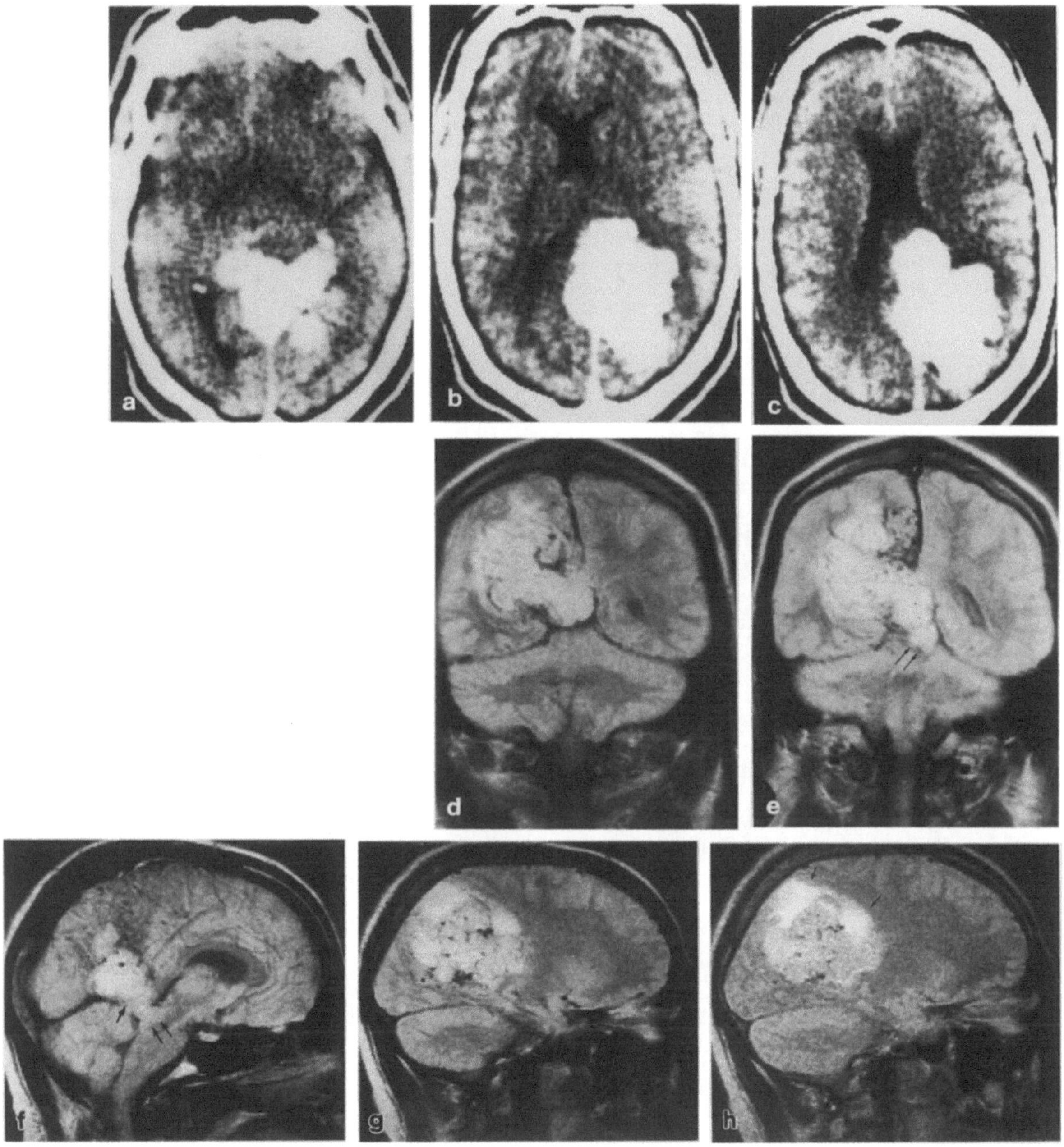

Fig. 9.9 a–h. Falco-tentorial meningioma. **a–c** CT. The tumour which shows evident contrast enhancement extends dorsally into the right occipital region and rostrally on both sides of the falx and the area of Galen's vein. **d, e** MRI, coronal planes, proton density-weighted scans. The tumour spreads on both sides of the falx and partially along the tentorium into the right infratentorial area *(parallel arrows)*. **f–h** MRI, sagittal planes, proton density-weighted scans. **f** On the scan on the midline, tumoral *(arrow)* compression or infiltration of the proximal part of the straight sinus, of the Galen's vein and of the terminal portion of the internal cerebral vein is well recognizable. The tumour *(parallel arrows)* extends rostrally, fills the upper part of the Galen's cistern and compresses the aqueduct. **g, h** On the paramedian scans the large mass of the richly vascularized tumour as well as peritumoral oedema *(arrows)* are demonstrated

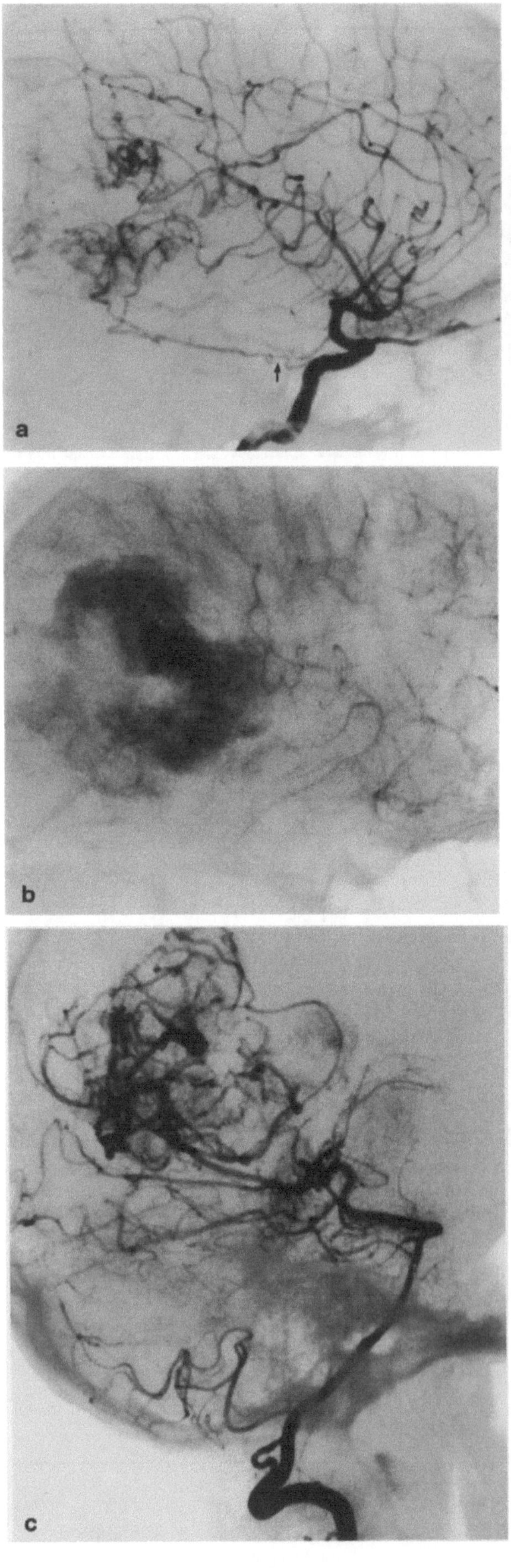

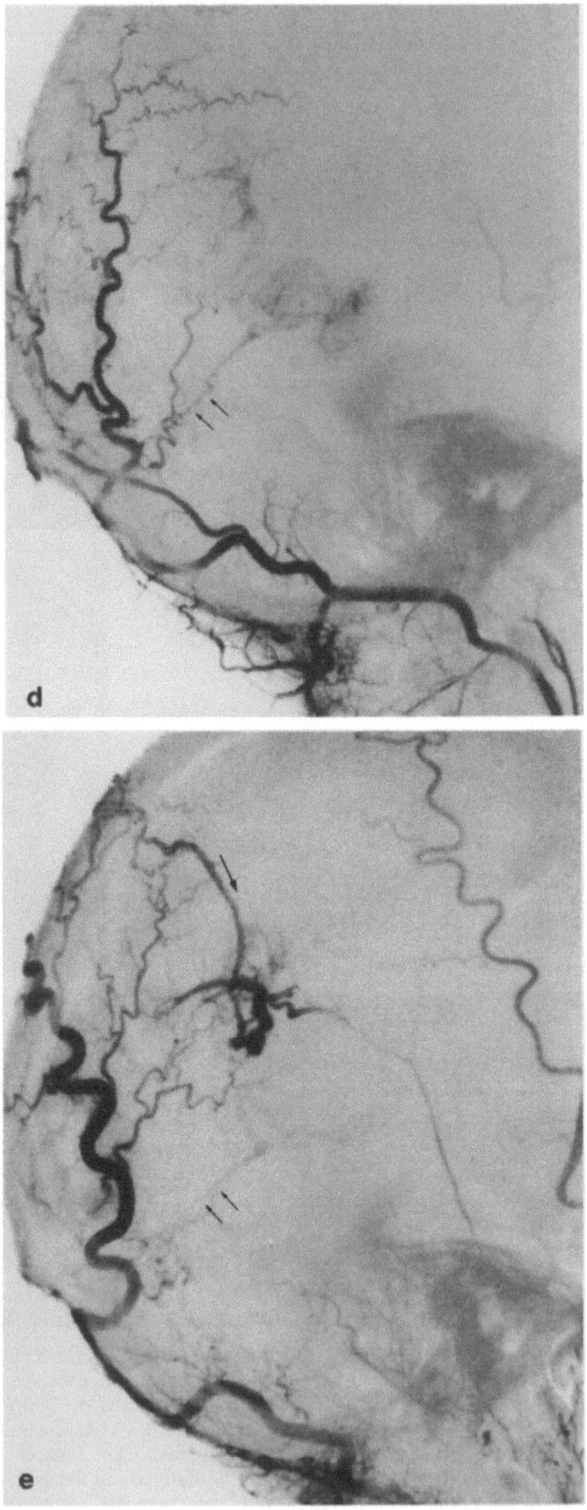

Fig. 9.10 a–e. Additional images of the patient from Fig. 9.9. **a–c** Angiograms of the carotid and vertebral arteries confirmed the presence of a richly vascularized meningioma. In **a** a large artery of the free margin of tentorium supplying the tumour *(arrow)* can be seen. **d, e** On the bilateral angiogram of the occipital artery, meningeal branches running along the straight sinus *(parallel arrows)* and supplying the tumour are recognizable. **e** In addition, meningeal branches running along the falx *(arrow)* are also shown

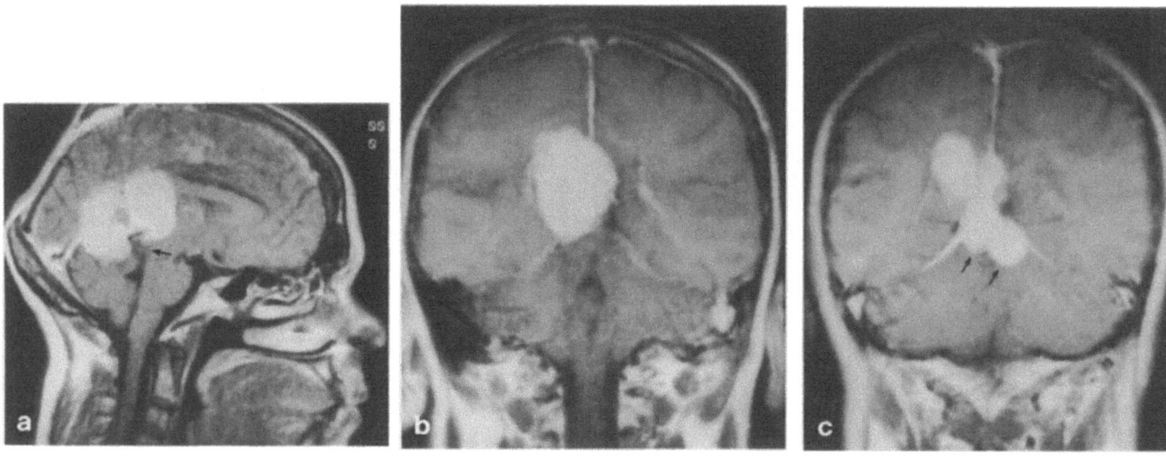

Fig. 9.11 a–c. Falco-tentorial meningioma (recurrence). **a** MRI sagittal plane, T1-weighted scan performed after injection of Gd-DTPA. The tumour, localized in the area of Galen's vein, extends rostrally and compresses the diencephalon and mesencephalon. The aqueduct is interrupted *(arrow)*. There is also evident extension into the infratentorial area. Galen's vein and the proximal portion of the straight sinus are no longer recognizable, they have been infiltrated by the tumour. **b, c** MRI coronal planes. The infratentorial portion of the tumour is evident (→)

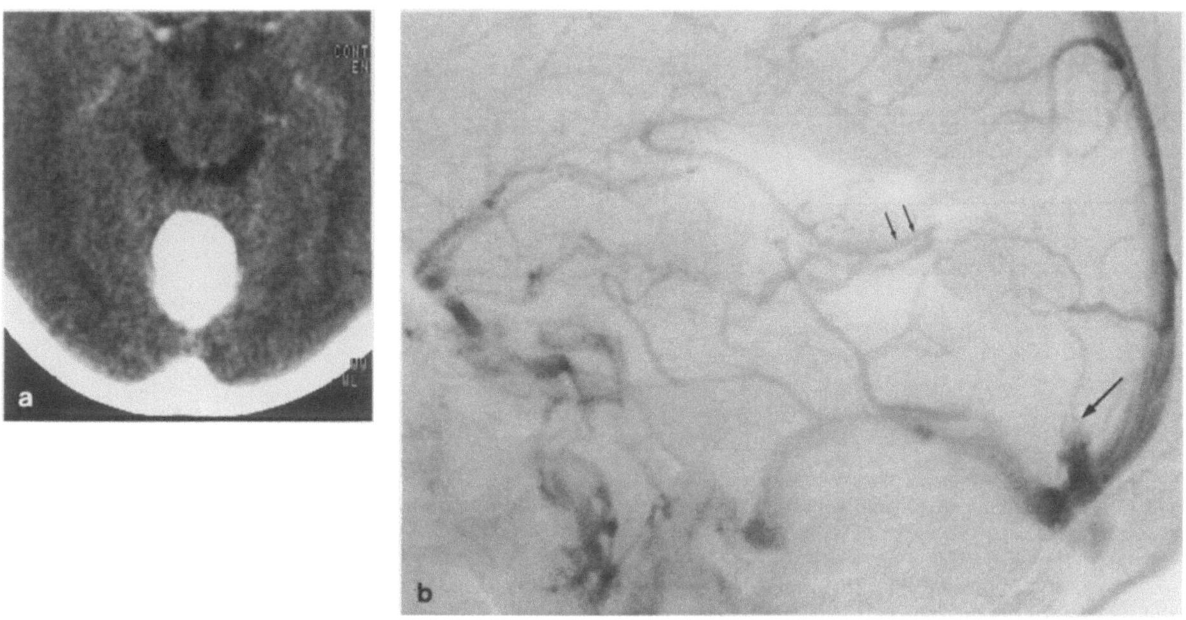

Fig. 9.12 a, b. Falco-tentorial meningioma. **a** CT. The tumour is heavily calcified. **b** Angiogram. The meningioma is poorly vascularized. The straight sinus infiltrated by the tumour is visible only in its terminal part *(arrow)*. Galen's vein *(parallel arrows)*

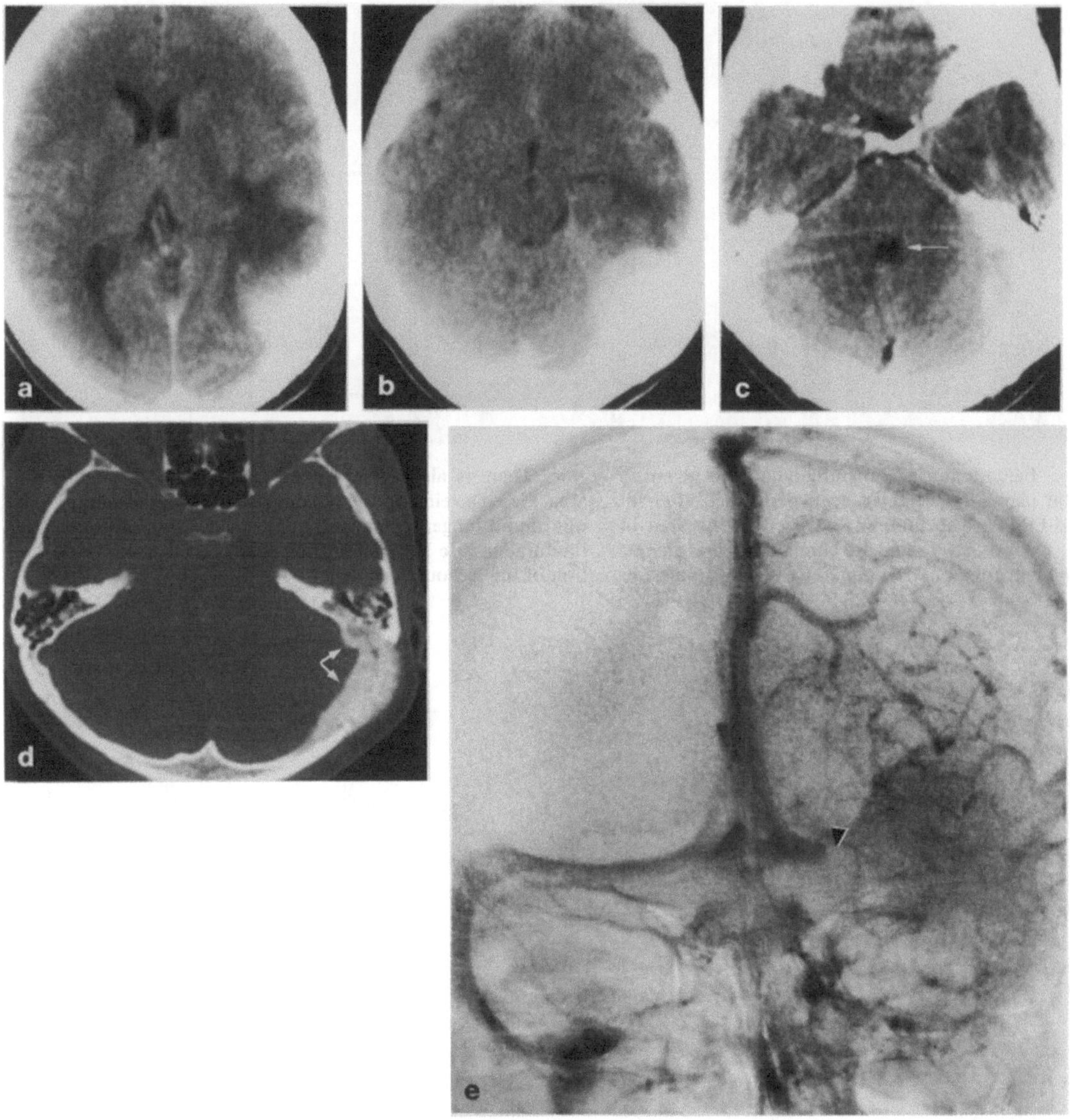

Fig. 9.13 a–e. Lateral tentorial convexity meningioma. **a–d** CT. The tumour extends into supra and infratentorial areas. Note the extensive oedema in the supratentorial area and a compression of the fourth ventricle *(white arrow)*. There is hyperostosis involving the petrous and occipital bone *(double white arrow)*. Inner and outer tables as well as diploë are no longer distinguishable. **e** Angiogram. Infiltration of the transverse sinus *(black arrowhead)*

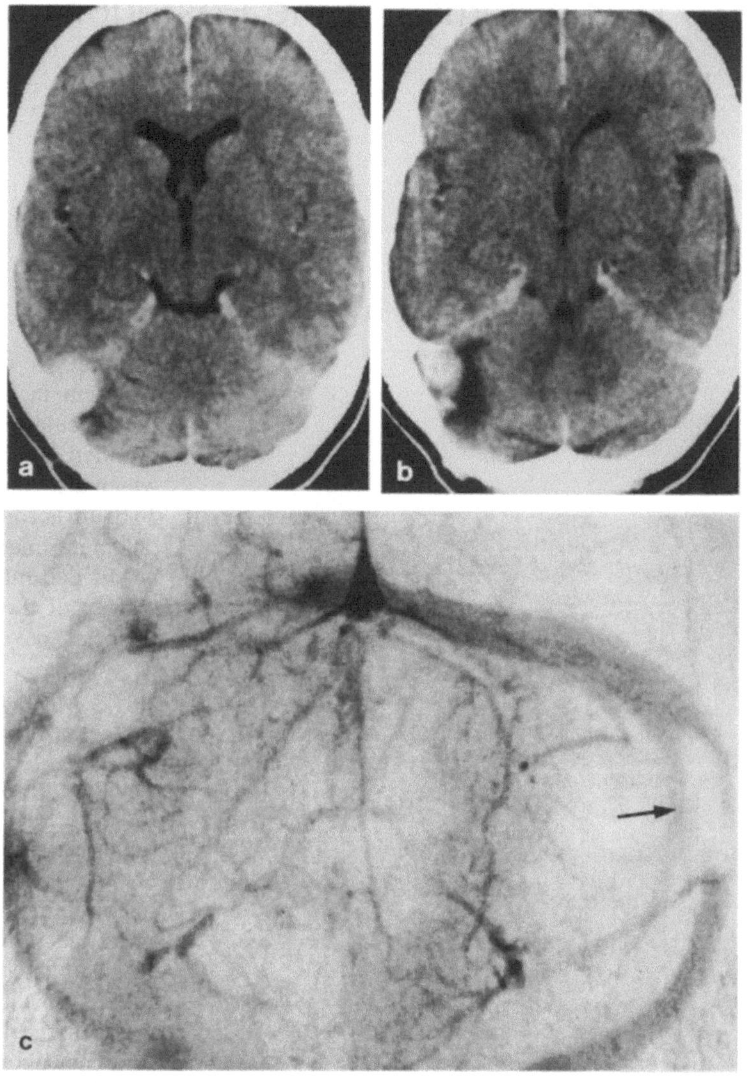

Fig. 9.14 a–c. Small lateral tentorial convexity meningioma. **a, b** CT. The tumour extends infratentorially. There is an oedematous reaction around the tumour. **c** Angiogram shows infiltration of the transverse sinus *(arrow)*

10 Meningiomas of the Posterior Fossa

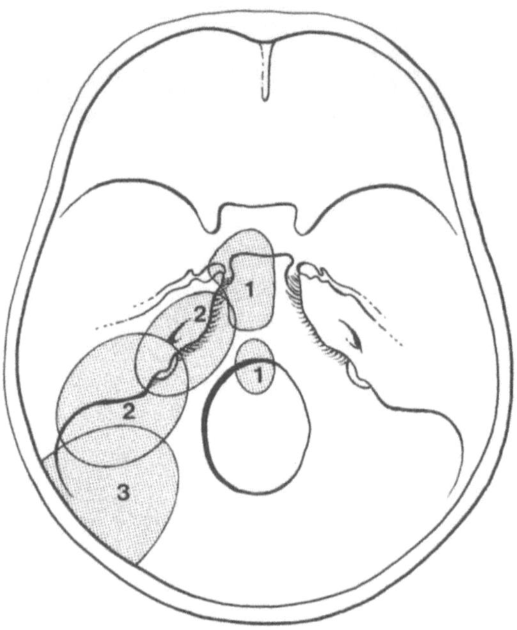

1 Clivus
2 Posterior, surface of the petrous bone
3 Convexity

10.1 Incidene and Localization

About 10% of all intracranial meningiomas occur in the posterior fossa and over 70% are found in women [303]. A higher frequency in children was described which has not been confirmed in more recent studies [68]. The cells of origin are probably the arachnoid cell clusters found embedded in the dura mater of the basilar regions, near the exit foramina of the cranial nerves, especially of the trigeminal and vestibuloacoustic, and in relation to the dural sinuses, especially the inferior petrosal and sigmoid [67, 303]. Meningiomas of the posterior fossa are usually at least 3 or 4 cm in size when diagnosed, and their precise site of origin can be difficult to determine. In some cases a relatively small base 1-1.5 cm in diameter is definable which contains the vascular pedicle, although usually this is surrounded by a wider area of secondary attachment which also may be traversed by vessels [54, 189, 251, 303]. In accordance with site of primary dural attachment, meningiomas of the posterior fossa can be divided into the following subgroups: posterior surface of the petrous bone, clivus, convexity and tentorial (see diagram).

10.1.1 Meningiomas of the Posterior Surface of the Petrous bone

The most frequent meningiomas of the posterior fossa are those of the posterior surface of petrous bone, constituting about 40% [54, 282, 303]. They are the second most common tumour of the cerebellopontine angle, constituting about 6.7%-9.5% of lesions in this location [54, 141, 282]. The microsurgical dissections of Yasargil et al. [303] have indicated that about 50% originate inframeatally lying between the internal auditory meatus and jugular foramen, about 20% originate anterior to the meatus, lying between it and Meckel's cave and the remainder have either suprameatal or postmeatal origins. The most posterior lesions of this group arise near the commencement of the sigmoid sinus (sinudural angle).

10.1.2 Tentorial Meningiomas

The next most frequent subgroup is tentorial meningiomas, constituting up to about 30% [54]. Growth inferiorly into the posterior fossa alone or associated with a supratentorial extention is very frequent in these tumours. In the material of Sekhar et al. [252] 80% of tentorial meningiomas extended into the posterior fossa. These tumours are described in Chapter 9.

10.1.3 Clivus Meningiomas

The third most frequent subgroup is clivus meningiomas, constituting about 11% of posterior fossa meningiomas [54]. In Yasargil's highly selected material, 96% of clival meningiomas arose from the upper two thirds of the clivus. About 40% took their origin only from the sphenoid and most extended upwards out of the posterior fossa, and 60% were petrosphenoclival lesions. Meningiomas of the lower clivus and foramen magnum are rare and constitute less than 3% of all intracranial meningiomas [199, 304]. Usually they lie anterolaterally to the neuroaxis and extend downward into the spinal canal rather than upwards into the intracranial cavity.

10.1.4 Tumours of the Cerebellar Convexity

Some 10% of the posterior fossa meningiomas are tumours of the cerebellar convexity, arising from the dura over the cerebellar hemispheres. Many of these also encroach on the sinudural angle.

10.1.5 Meningiomas of the Fourth Ventricle

There are occasional report of meningiomas of the posterior fossa arising in or in the vicinity of the fourth ventricle which have no dural attachment.

10.1.6 Other Meningiomas

The posterior cranial fossa may be involved secondarily by extension from more distant origins, usually from the middle cranial fossa and tentorial hiatus (see Chaps. 8 and 9). Some meningiomas arise within the petrous bone itself and may extend medially into the posterior fossa (see Chap. 11).

10.2 Meningiomas of the Posterior Surface of the Petrous Bone

Computed tomography (CT), magnetic resonance imaging (MRI) and also angiography usually demonstrate these lesions well. By far the commonest lesion to present in the cerebellopontine angle is acoustic neurinoma, and it is from this lesion that meningioma needs to be distinguished. The mass effect and pattern of spread of all tumours in this region have much in common. They involve mainly the cerebellopontine angle and lateral cerebellomedullary cisterns and, when large, the lateral pontine and even the superior vermian cistern. They invaginate and rotate the brain stem; the medulla oblongata at the level of and just above the olives is commonly most severely distorted, but the middle cerebellar peduncle, cerebellar hemisphere and the posterolateral aspect of the midbrain may be compressed with larger lesions. The fourth ventricle is compressed and may be rotated and displaced from the midline; sometimes it is almost obliterated.

10.2.1 Computed Tomography

Meningiomas are relatively large at diagnosis. In a recent study by Catz and Reider-Groswasser [56] the mean diameter of meningiomas was about 4 cm, whereas that of acoustic neurinomas was 2.6 cm. About 80% of meningiomas are ovoid in shape with their long axis orientated along the posterior surface of the petrous bone, and lobulation is rare; neurinomas are more often spherical and large tumours are usually lobulated [201, 282, 283]. The margin is circumscribed and usually forms an obtuse angle with the posterior surface of the petrous bone. Neurinomas may occasionally show the same findings, and conversely some meningiomas are pedunculated, displaying a slender stalklike attachment to the dura, and these may appear very like an acoustic neurinoma [201]. Moreover, meningiomas less than 2.0 cm in size often are round in shape and can be impossible to distinguish from neurinomas if they arise in or near the internal auditory canal. Furthermore, meningiomas may extend into the internal auditory canal as may be demonstrated sometimes with CT, but much better with MRI (Figs. 10.1, 10.2).

Extension of a cerebellopontine angle tumour into the petroclival angle or above the tentorium suggests meningioma (Figs. 10.2, 10.3). Transcisternal supratentorial extension of the tumour gives rise to a characteristic comma-shaped appearance on CT and MRI [282, 283], due in part to the fact that such lesions are limited laterally by the straight edge of the tentorium (Figs. 10.2, 10.3). In rare cases the tumour has spread through the tentorium itself.

Typically, meningiomas appear hyperdense, hypodense examples being a rarity in the posterior fossa. Inhomogeneity and hypodensity are common in larger acoustic neurinomas; only 15% of neurinomas are hyperdense, and 22% are partially or totally hypodense, the rest being homogeneously isodense with normal brain [283].

Tumoral calcification is frequent in meningiomas of the posterior fossa (Fig. 10.3). It was recognizable in 53% of the cases of New et al. [207] and in 25% of those of Valavanis [282]. Calcification can be very

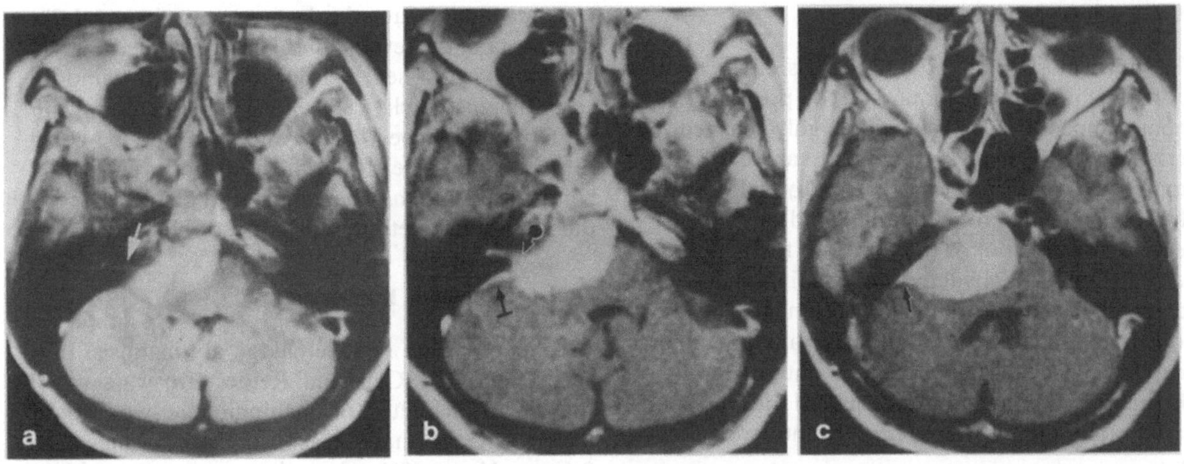

Fig. 10.1 a–c. Meningioma of the posterior surface of the petrous bone. **a** MRI, proton density-weighted image. The tumour is slightly hyperintense. Its border are poorly defined. There is no involvement of the acoustic nerve *(white arrow)*. **b, c** MRI, T1-weighted images after Gd-DTPA. **b** Rich and homogeneous enhancement of the tumour. There is a minimal en plaque portion of the tumour *(black arrow from line)* as well as a partial intracanalar extension *(black arrow from circle)*. **c** Note the obtuse angle between tumour and petrous bone *(black arrow)*

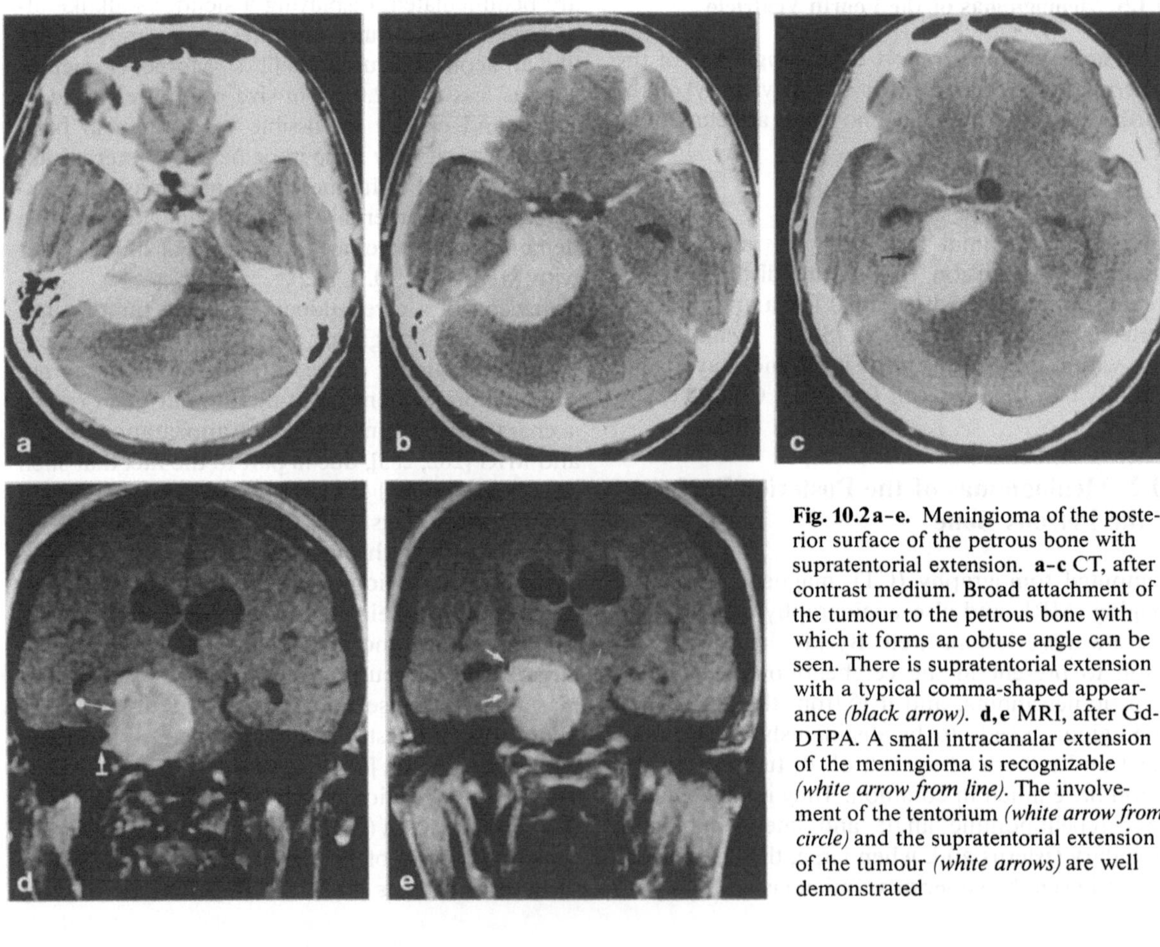

Fig. 10.2 a–e. Meningioma of the posterior surface of the petrous bone with supratentorial extension. **a–c** CT, after contrast medium. Broad attachment of the tumour to the petrous bone with which it forms an obtuse angle can be seen. There is supratentorial extension with a typical comma-shaped appearance *(black arrow)*. **d, e** MRI, after Gd-DTPA. A small intracanalar extension of the meningioma is recognizable *(white arrow from line)*. The involvement of the tentorium *(white arrow from circle)* and the supratentorial extension of the tumour *(white arrows)* are well demonstrated

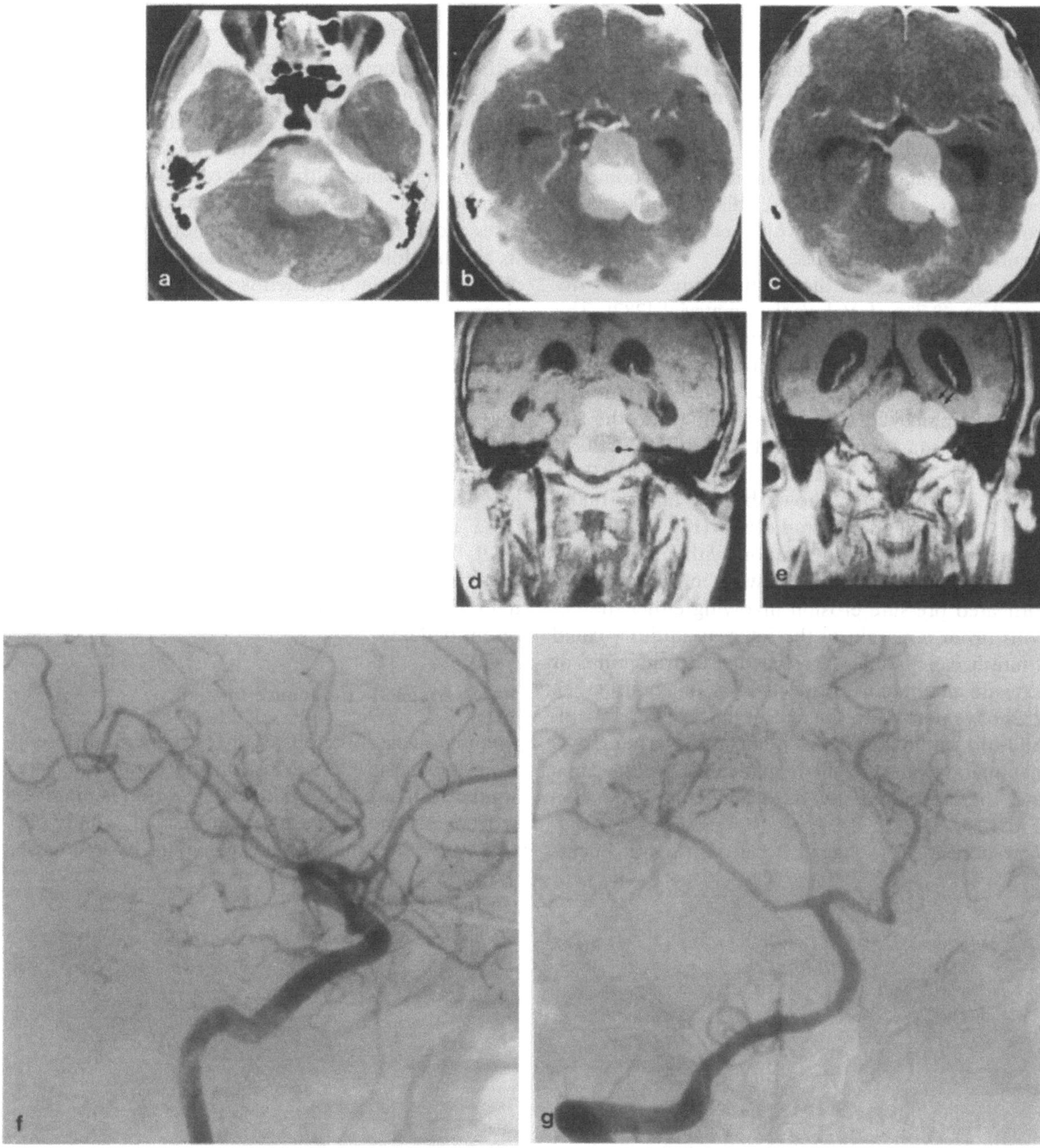

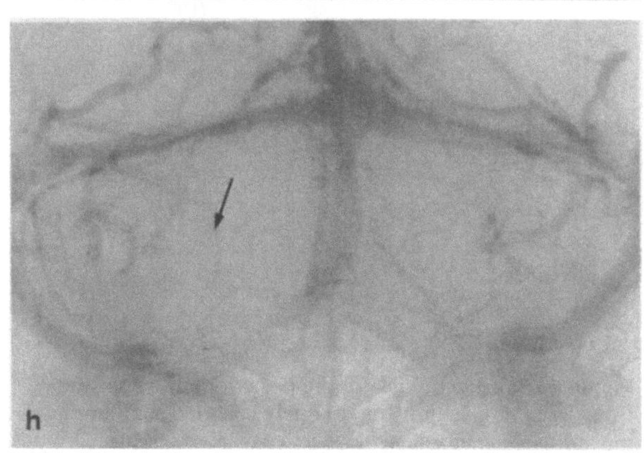

Fig. 10.3 a–h. Meningioma of the posterior surface of the petrous bone with secondary attachment to tentorium and supratentorial extension. **a–c** CT, shows broad attachment to the petrous bone. The tumour shows contrast enhancement, but it is largely calcified. Note the comma shape. **d, e** MRI, coronal plane, T1-weighted images after Gd-DTPA. The relationship of the tumour with the petrous bone (•→) and the tentorium *(parallel arrows)* are clearly recognizable. **f** Angiogram of ICA. There is some supply from meningeal branches of intracavernous portion of the ICA. **g, h** Angiogram of vertebral artery. There is no pathological vascularization. Dorsal shifting of posterior cerebral and particularly of superior cerebellar arteries. The petrosal *vein (→) is* not opacified, suggesting compression or infiltration by the tumour

extensive, and differentiation from chordomas and chondromas can be difficult. In contrast only 2% of acoustic neuromas show calcification on CT [282, 283].

Contrast enhancement is prominent and homogeneous even in large lesions; this is unlike large acoustic neurinomas, in which enhancement frequently is inhomogeneous.

Bony changes are of diagnostic value. These occurred in 43.7% of Valavanis's material [282]. The most characteristic osseous abnormalities seen with meningiomas of the petrous bone are hyperostosis and thickening of a diffuse, but variable extent and a focal, nipplelike exostosis extending into the site of primary tumour attachment (Fig. 10.4). Such an exostosis is usually identifiable at surgery [303] although it is not often shown by CT, and virtually never by conventional radiology [141, 282, 283]. Bone destruction is uncommon with meningioma and when present is almost always in the form of a corticated pressure erosion involving either the petrous tip or a margin of the internal auditory canal where it can simulate erosion due to trigeminal or acoustic neurinoma, respectively. Valavanis et al. [283] have noted also that entrapment of cerebrospinal fluid within the fundus of a canal overhung by a meningioma may result in widening of the canal and therefore simulate intracanalicular extension (Fig. 10.4).

Very occasionally, ragged bone destruction occurs with meningiomas, and exceptional cases have extended through the petrous bone into the middle ear or downwards into the neck (Fig. 10.5) [283, 303]. This type of bone destruction suggests malignant meningiomas, although it can also occur in benign lesions. The differential diagnosis in such cases includes chemodectoma, chordoma, metastasis and myeloma. Bone destruction around the middle ear or jugular foramen is also typical in meningiomas arising in the petrous bone itself (Fig. 11.8).

Hydrocephalus due to compression of the fourth ventricle or distortion of the cerebral aqueduct is present in about 60% of patients with meningioma [189, 201, 251, 283]; whereas it is seen in only about 15% of patients with acoustic neurinoma.

Peritumoral hypodensity is relatively frequent and has been observed in about 50% of the posterior fossa meningiomas recorded by Valavanis et al. [282]. The nature of the hypodensity is frequently doubtful. It usually appears as a peripheral rim or halo of variable thickness and may or may not represent oedema.

10.2.2 Magnetic Resonance Imaging

Meningiomas of the posterior fossa are no different from those elsewhere. Most display signal intensity similar to that of the brain. Calcification is relatively frequent and may appear as areas of signal void (Fig. 10.3). Neurinomas are generally hyperintense

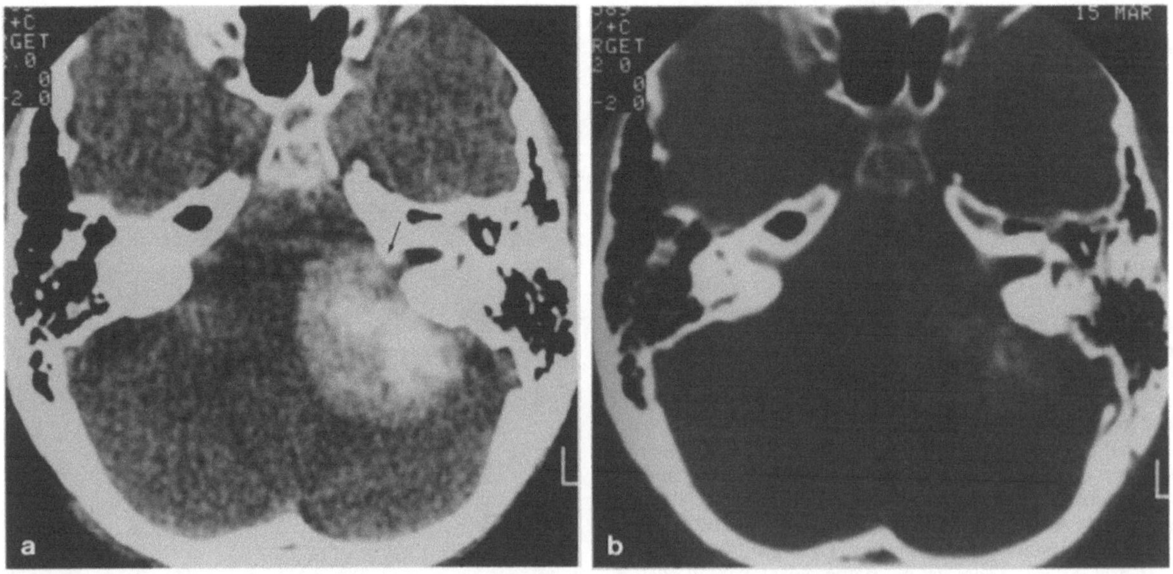

Fig. 10.4a, b. Meningioma of the posterior surface of the petrous bone. CT demonstrates largely calcified tumour showing diffuse enhancement. Hyperostosis *(arrow)*, probably at the primary point of attachment. Enlargement of the internal auditory canal is also evident

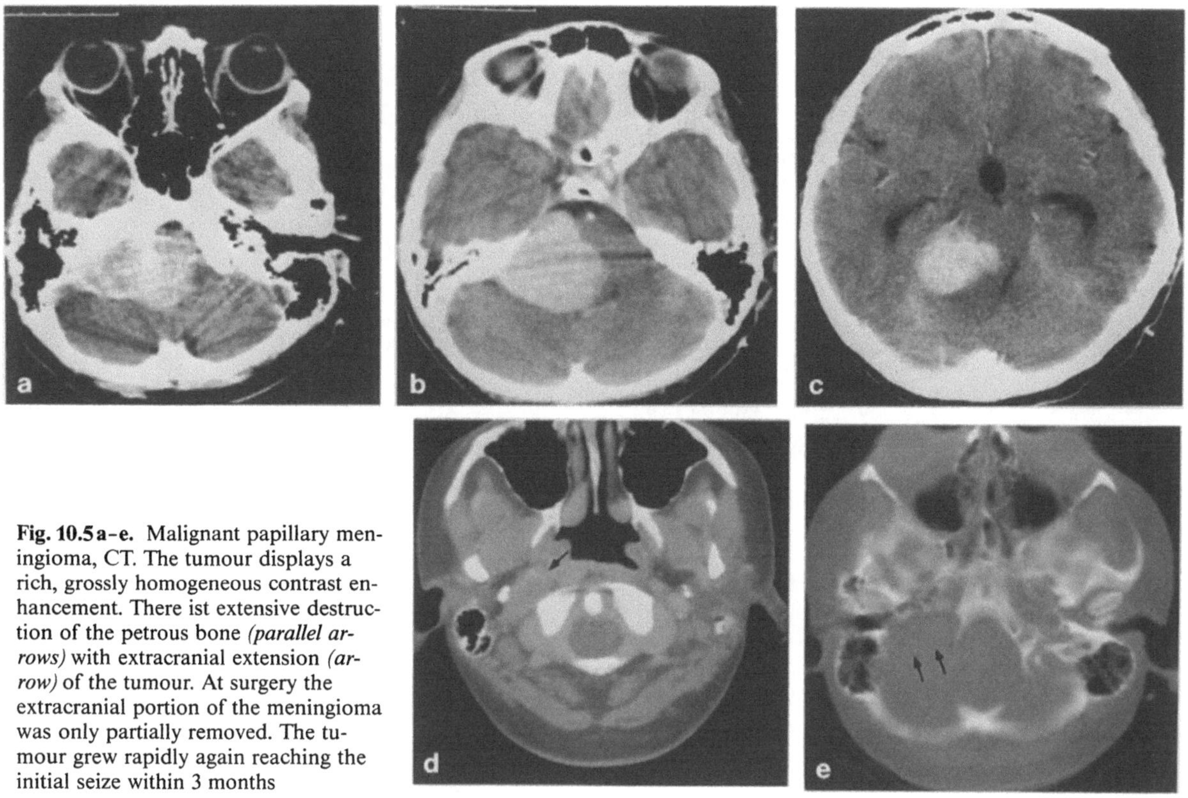

Fig. 10.5 a–e. Malignant papillary meningioma, CT. The tumour displays a rich, grossly homogeneous contrast enhancement. There ist extensive destruction of the petrous bone *(parallel arrows)* with extracranial extension *(arrow)* of the tumour. At surgery the extracranial portion of the meningioma was only partially removed. The tumour grew rapidly again reaching the initial seize within 3 months

on T2-weighted images, and large neurinomas are more often inhomogeneous due to necrotic and cystic areas. Involvement of the auditory canal is well demonstrated with MRI (Fig. 10.6), and in some cases it is possible to identify the seventh and eighth cranial nerve complex separate from the tumour which effectively excludes a neurinoma [197]. Sometimes a little intracanalar extension occurs in meningioma (Figs. 10.1, 10.2) [40, 41]. After intravenous Gd-DTPA, both meningiomas and neuromas are enhanced, but this is generally more homogeneous in meningiomas [40, 41].

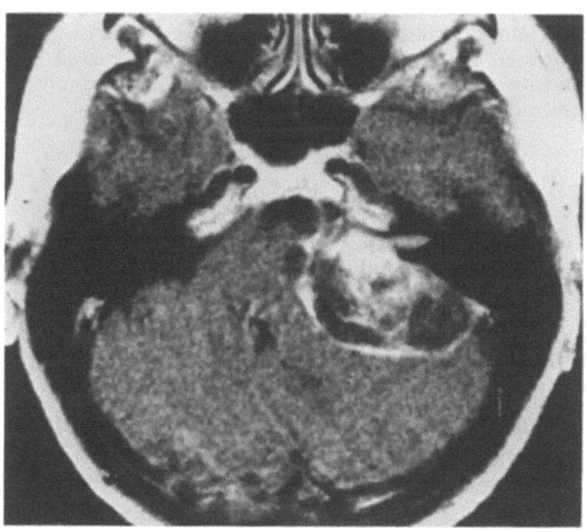

Fig. 10.6. Large acoustic neurinoma. MRI examination after Gd-DTPA. The intracanalar extension of the tumour is well demonstrated. The enhancement is inhomogenous

The great advantage of MRI is its ability to demonstrate the tumour in the three orthogonal planes so giving a better topographical demonstration of the lesion. The relationship to brain stem, and tentorium are particularly well demonstrated and displacement of large arteries is recognizable (Fig. 10.7).

10.2.3 Angiography

Tumours of the posterior fossa virtually always have some supply from the external carotid artery (ECA), typically from the petrosquamous branches of the middle meningeal, ascending pharyngeal and occipital arteries. Meningeal branches of the internal carotid artery (ICA) are also frequently involved, while supply from vertebral and basilar arteries is less common (Fig. 10.3) [73]. In the material reported by Sekhar and Jannetta [251] over 50% of

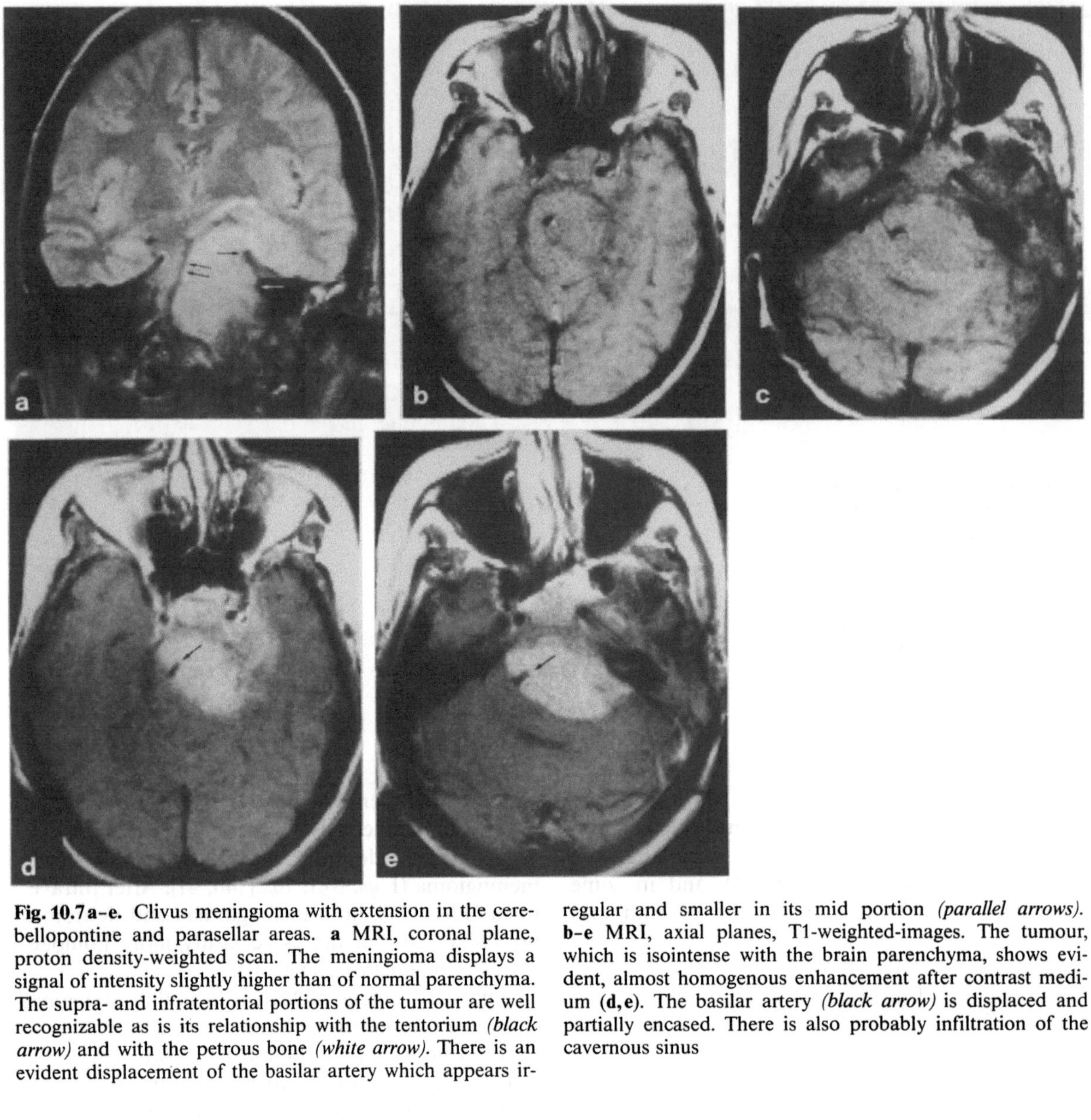

Fig. 10.7 a–e. Clivus meningioma with extension in the cerebellopontine and parasellar areas. **a** MRI, coronal plane, proton density-weighted scan. The meningioma displays a signal of intensity slightly higher than of normal parenchyma. The supra- and infratentorial portions of the tumour are well recognizable as is its relationship with the tentorium *(black arrow)* and with the petrous bone *(white arrow)*. There is an evident displacement of the basilar artery which appears irregular and smaller in its mid portion *(parallel arrows)*. **b–e** MRI, axial planes, T1-weighted-images. The tumour, which is isointense with the brain parenchyma, shows evident, almost homogenous enhancement after contrast medium (**d, e**). The basilar artery *(black arrow)* is displaced and partially encased. There is also probably infiltration of the cavernous sinus

meningiomas of the posterior surface of the petrous bone received the major blood supply from branches arising from C5–C4 portion of ICA and only about 12% specifically from the middle meningeal artery. Therefore, most meningiomas in this site receive their major blood supply from the carotid artery circulation, unlike acoustic neurinomas in which the blood supply is usually mainly from branches of the vertebral artery.

Vertebral angiography usually demonstrates a large extra-axial posterior fossa mass, which usually appears avascular. Depending on the precise location of the lesion, and its size, the basilar artery and anterior and posterior inferior cerebellar arteries will be displaced, usually away from the side of the lesion and from the posterior surface of the petrous bone (Fig. 10.3). Encasement is unusual in these lesions. The veins may be involved, the petrosal vein and its cerebellar tributaries often being elevated or occluded (Fig. 10.3). The superior petrosal and sigmoid sinuses also may be invaded by tumour. These anatomical relationships are of importance in the preoperative assessment. Also relevant is the vascular anatomy, especially whether the anterior inferior cerebellar or posterior inferior cerebellar arteries are dominant, and the position and na-

ture of vertebral artery loops and the location of the junction of the vertebral arteries with the basilar artery.
Moreover, depending on the surgical technique used, the venous anatomy may be relevant [3, 189, 252]. The drainage of a major part of one cerebral hemisphere can occur mainly through the vein of Labbé. The superior sagittal sinus usually drains mainly into one or other transverse sinus, and the vein of Labbé draining into the dominant transverse sinus may be particularly important and require planned preservation if the tentorium has to be divided during surgical exposure. Finally, if the sigmoid sinus is infiltrated, it can be resected with the tumour, provided that adequate drainage of the sagittal sinus occurs into the opposite transverse sinus.

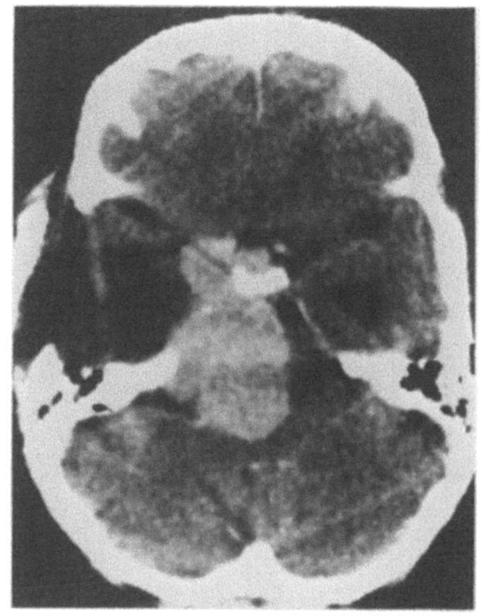

Fig. 10.8. Clivus meningioma with extension in the cerebellopontine and parasellar areas. CT after contrast medium

10.3 Clival Meningiomas

Clival meningiomas are less common than those of the posterior surface of the petrous bone [54, 303], and over 80% occur in women [303]. Clival meningiomas, like medial tentorial meningiomas, have a high morbidity and operative mortality [189, 251, 252, 303]. Earlier radiological diagnosis can help improve the surgical results.

10.3.1 CT and MRI

In the series of Mayberg and Symon [189] the correct diagnosis was made by CT in every case. By contrast, 20% of the cases of meningiomas of the posterior surface of the petrous bone reported by Sekhar and Jannetta [251] were diagnosed incorrectly as acoustic neurinomas. Clival meningiomas nearly always have a broad dural attachment, usually to the upper two thirds of the clivus and medial part of the petrous bone [303]. Between 17%-24% extend through the anterior part of the tentorial hiatus, and the supra- or parasellar extension is characterized in CT and MRI by the comma-shaped appearance (see 10.2.1). Extension into the cerebello-pontine angle is also frequent (Fig. 10.8).
The appearance of these lesions on CT and MRI is similar to meningiomas elsewhere. Osseous changes, in which erosion of the petrous apex is particularly frequent, are, however, slightly more common than in meningiomas in other parts of the posterior fossa, occurring in about 70% of Yasargil's [303] material compared with about 50% in cerebellopontine angle meningiomas. These bone changes can be demonstrated with high definition CT, but often they are only recognized at surgery [189, 251, 303].
MRI is very useful in demonstrating the full extent of the tumour and its relationship to the brain stem and important vessels such as the basilar artery (Fig. 10.7). Moreover, MRI is particularly helpful in diagnosing small lesions located near the foramen magnum (Fig. 10.9), a region often poorly shown by CT.
Peritumoral oedema is usually absent.

10.3.2 Angiography

Angiography may be useful for surgical planning, but generally is not required for diagnosis. A circumscribed hypervascular blush has been recognized in only about 35% of meningiomas of the clivus [303], far less than in meningiomas of the cerebellopontine angle. Blood supply is usually mainly from meningeal branches of the ICA, but meningeal branches of the ECA, particularly the petrosquamous branch of the middle meningeal artery, and branches from the ascending pharyngeal artery (Fig. 10.10) are often also involved, as are anterior meningeal branches of the vertebral artery which arise just below the skull base [72, 73]. Displacement of the arteries, particularly posteriorly and laterally (Fig. 10.10), is visible on the vertebral angiogram. Encasement of the basilar artery can occur. According to the surgical technique used, the angiogram may also be important in demonstrating the venous anatomy.

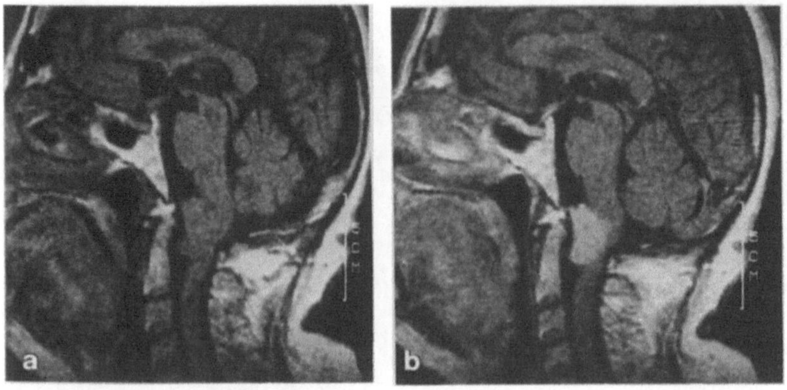

Fig. 10.9 a, b. Lower clival meningiomas extending into the cervical spinal canal. **a** MRI. The tumour is typically located rostrally to the spinal cord. On this T1-weighted image the tumour is isointense with brain parenchyma. **b** MRI. Shows rich contrast enhancement of the tumour after Gd-DTPA

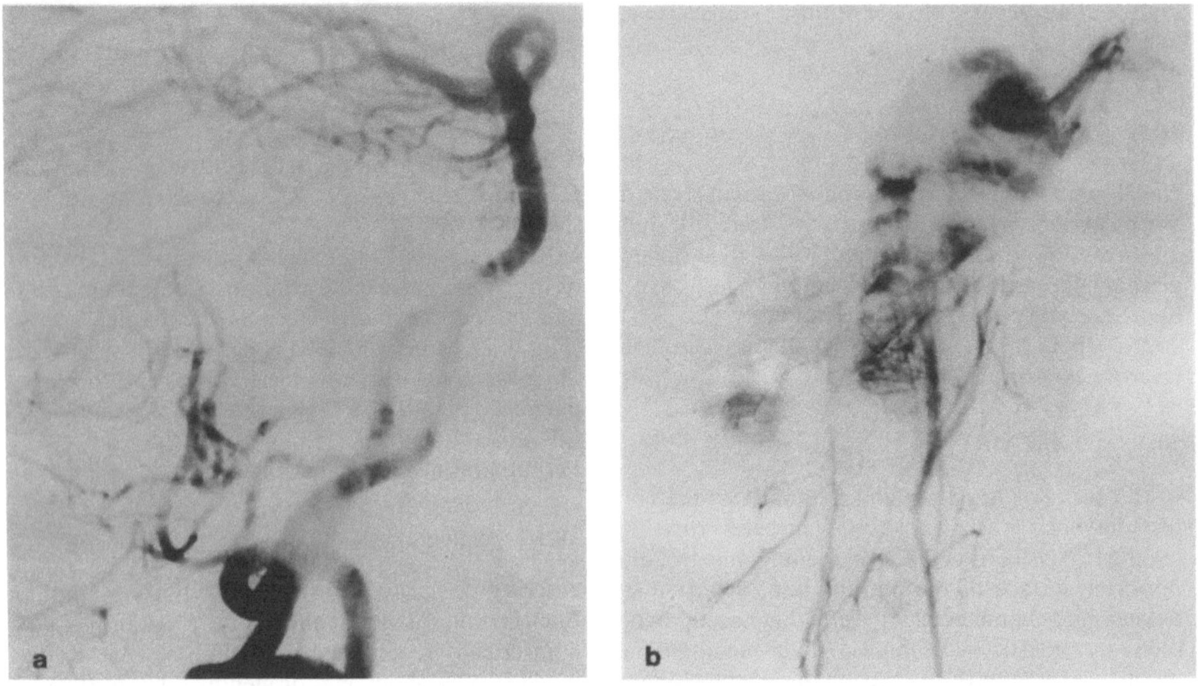

Fig. 10.10 a, b. Clivus meningiomas. **a** Angiographic study of the vertebrobasilar territory showing dorsal displacement of the vertebral artery. There is no abnormal vascularity. **b** Angiogram of the ascending pharingeal artery. There is a marked tumoral vascularization coming from the posterior branches of the ascending pharangeal artery

10.4 Meningiomas of the Cerebellar Convexity

Meningiomas of the cerebellar convexity arise from the dura over the cerebellar fossae of the occipital bone. Examples located laterally overlap with lesions of the posterior surface of the petrous bone, where they both may involve the sinudural angle. Medially located lesions arise near the falx cerebelli and may cross the midline. Rarely, they may encroach on the posterior margin of the foramen magnum. As they grow, they compress the convexity of the inferior surface of the cerebellar hemisphere or vallecula and posterior cerebellar notch. Diagnosis rests on similar principles to those enumerated for meningiomas in other locations in the posterior cranial fossa. Blood supply derives mainly from the petrosquamous branch of middle meningeal artery, from branches of the ascending pharyngeal artery and frequently from the meningeal-mastoid branch of the occipital artery (Figs. 10.12, 13.8)
Peritumoral oedema may occur.

10.5 Meningiomas of the Fourth Ventricle

Meningiomas of the fourth ventricle have no dural attachment. They arise from the choroid plexus or tela choroidea, and therefore may be found in the fourth ventricle itself, in the vallecula, or more laterally between the biventral lobule and medulla when the origin is in the tela of the posterolateral cerebellar fissue. They will be discussed further in Chap. 11.

10.6 Differential Diagnosis

Differential diagnosis is a lesser problem with clival than with cerebellopontine angle meningiomas. In the cerebellopontine angle the main differential diagnosis is with acoustic neurinoma which has already been discussed in detail.

10.6.1 Neurinomas

Neurinomas of cranial nerves other than the vestibuloacoustic are rare. Intradural components in the cerebellopontine or cerebellomedullary cisterns are not centered over the internal auditory meatus, and they may simulate meningioma closely. However, on CT and MRI these neurinomas are inhomogeneous (Fig. 8.21) even more frequently than acoustic tumours, especially those of the trigeminal nerve in which large low density components are common, and about 20% of these show mainly ring enhancement [101]. Neurinomas characteristically cause pressure erosion of adjacent osseous structures and widening of the basal foramina and canals for the affected nerves, in particular, the foramen ovale, Meckel's cave, jugular foramen and facial and hypoglossal canals. Meningiomas, on the other hand, may cause sclerosis around the margin of these canals and possibly even stenosis, but widening is rare.

10.6.2 Chordomas

Most chordomas resemble sphenopetroclival meningiomas, but some originate from the inferior part of the petrous bone and exocciput near the margins of the jugular foramen, and these constitute about 2% of lesions of the cerebellopontine angle [283]. Nodular calcification occurs in about 40%, but nodular calcification near the base of a lesion may be difficult to distinguish from the exostosis present in the base of a meningioma [139, 283]. Bone destruction is usually a salient feature and was demonstrable in over 90% of the cases in the material of Meyer et al. [194]; however, diffuse sclerosis of the skull base has also been recorded [139]. Low density regions representing gelatinous areas in the tumour matrix are present in about 50% of these lesions [194], whereas similar appearances in mainly posterior fossa meningiomas occur in less than 10%. Enhancement after intravenous contrast medium is generally poor and inhomogeneous. On MRI, parts of the matrix are often isointense

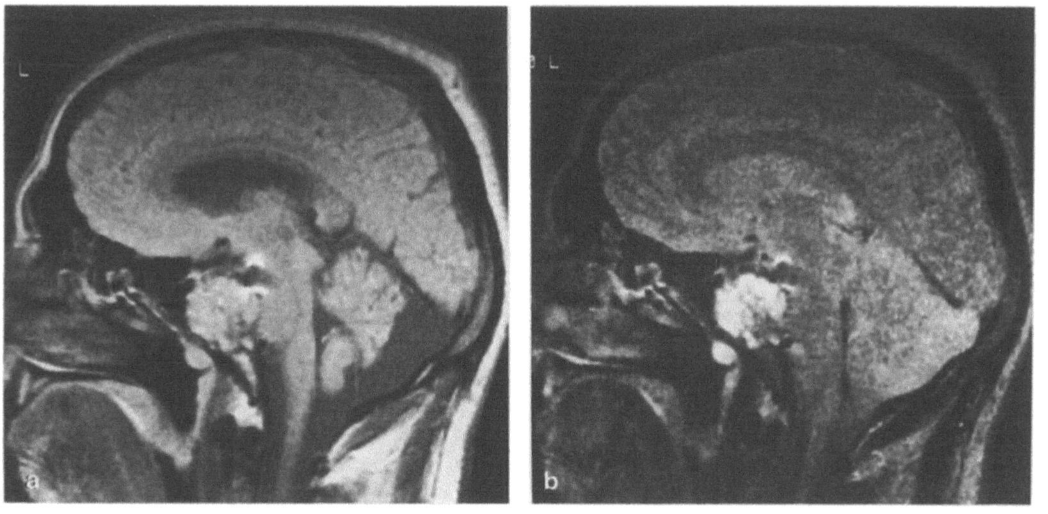

Fig. 10.11. Clivus chordoma, MRI. **a** Proton-density and **b** T2-weighted images. The tumour appears inhomogeneous and displays a high signal intensity on T2-weighted image. There is extensive destruction of clivus with the tumour also extending into the sphenoid sinus

with brain, but calcified areas and gelatinous cyst-like regions give rise to typical signal changes and render the mass inhomogeneous in appearance (Fig. 10.11).

10.6.3 Chemodectomas

Chemodectomas arising in the region of a jugular foramen comprise 4% of the cerebellopontine angle lesions [282], and intracranial extensions may resemble some meningiomas. Chemodectomas are often minimally hyperdense on CT and exhibit homogeneous contrast enhancement, however, the hallmark of these lesions is ragged destruction of the inferior surface of the petrous bone around the jugular foramen, usually well demonstrated by high definition CT. Involvement of the middle ear cavity results in opacity due to tumour or accumulated secretions. On MRI, chemodectomas commonly have a characteristic mottled appearance due to high flow in tumoral vessels with signal void contrasting strongly against the rest of the tumour tissue.

10.6.4 Chondromas

Chondromas are rare intracranial lesions. Most of the material collected by Bingas [24] came from lesions which occurred in the skull base. Many have arisen in the region of the petroclival synchondrosis. Such lesions may be of large size when diagnosed.

They are heavily calcified or ossified masses on CT which cause pressure erosion rather than widespread bone destruction. They can be indistinguishable from meningioma.

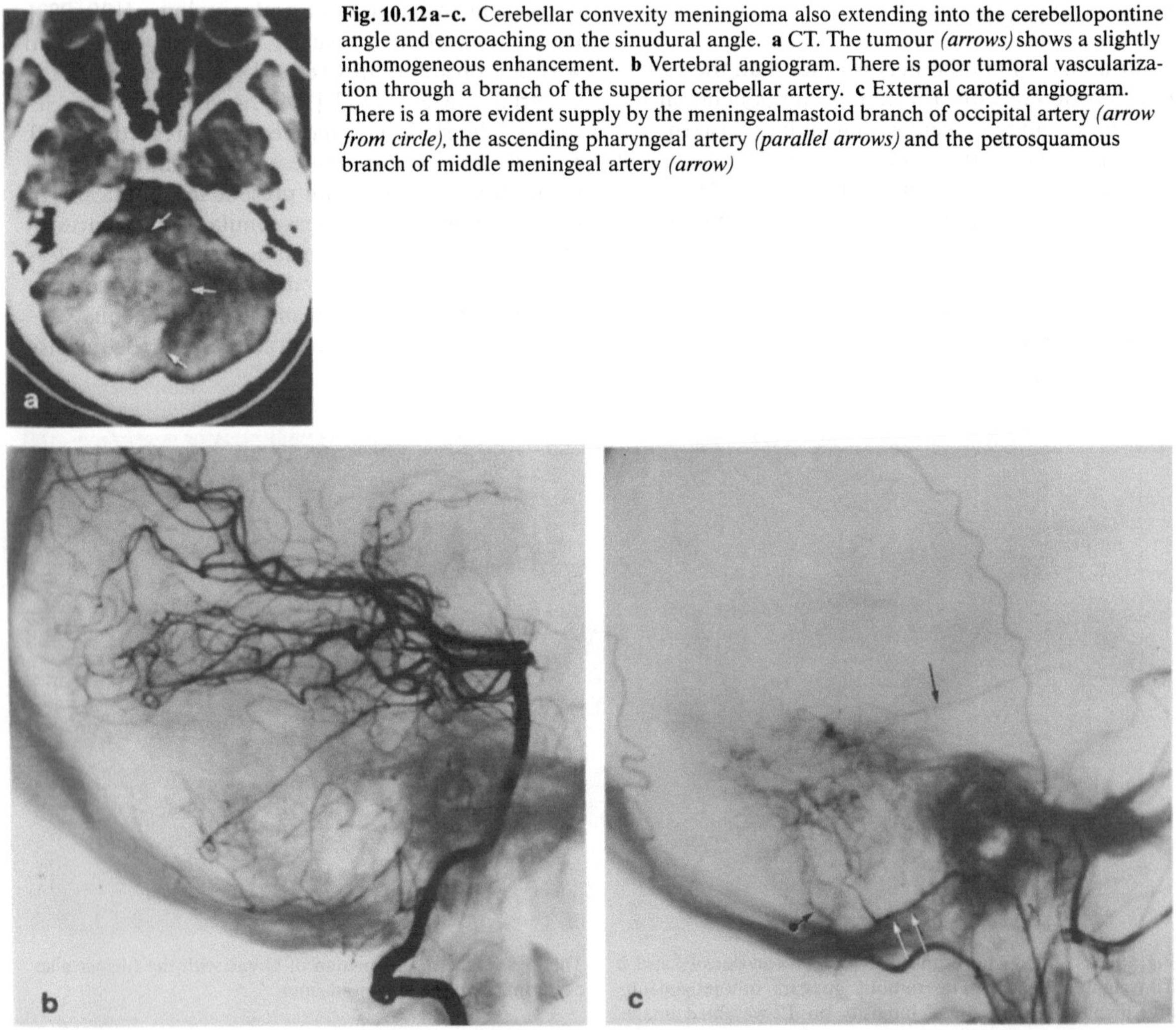

Fig. 10.12 a–c. Cerebellar convexity meningioma also extending into the cerebellopontine angle and encroaching on the sinudural angle. **a** CT. The tumour *(arrows)* shows a slightly inhomogeneous enhancement. **b** Vertebral angiogram. There is poor tumoral vascularization through a branch of the superior cerebellar artery. **c** External carotid angiogram. There is a more evident supply by the meningealmastoid branch of occipital artery *(arrow from circle)*, the ascending pharyngeal artery *(parallel arrows)* and the petrosquamous branch of middle meningeal artery *(arrow)*

10.6.5. Aneurysm and angiomas

Aneurysm and angiomas may occur in the cerebello pontine angle. They may appear on CT as hyperdense, diffusely enhancing lesions, which sometimes require MRI or angiography to establish the correct diagnosis.

10.6.6 Haemangioblastomas

Haemangioblastomas can extend into the cerebello pontine angle and be difficult to differentiate from meningiomas especially if their typical cystic component is absent and they abutt against the dura (Fig. 3.4).

10.6.7 Low density lesions

Low density lesions on CT, such as cisternal epidermoid tumours, cystic acoustic neuromas, arachnoid cysts and brainstem gliomas with exophytic growth should virtually never be confused with meningiomas, although a small meningioma associated with large intracerebellar cyst has been described pathologically [236]. Very occasionally epidermoid cysts are hyperdense, but they are not enhanced after intravenous contrast medium [42].

10.6.8 Metastasis, Lymphoma and Myeloma

Metastases and lymphoma can be identical in appearance to meningiomas since they do not always cause bone destruction. Myeloma, lacking calcification, is centred on bone causing extensive destruction and should not be confused with meningioma.

10.6.9 Other Tumours in the Cerebello pontine Angle

The cerebello pontine angle may be invaded by local extension of nasopharyngeal carcinoma; lymphoma or metastasis and many other lesions arising from the petrous bone may invade or encroach on it: these include histiocytosis, rhabdomysarcoma, malignant ceruminoma, Paget's disease or its complications and brown tumour.

11 Particular Conditions

11.1 Cystic Meningiomas

The pathology of cystic structures in and around meningiomas is discussed in Chaps. 1 and 3. Cystic meningiomas are often misdiagnosed on computed tomography (CT) and magnetic resonance imaging (MRI), particularly as gliomas (Figs. 11.1, 11.2, 4.5, 4.14, 6.8). Helpful CT features are: contrast enhancement of the solid part, clear separation between this portion and the cystic part and demonstration of dural attachment. These are demonstrated particularly well with the multiplanar facility of MRI (Fig. 4.14). Angiography may be helpful by demonstrating the extra-axial location of the lesion and predominantly meningeal blood supply [167, 216, 225, 298]. Nevertheless a biopsy is usually mandatory for final diagnosis.

It is important to completely resect the cystic as well as the solid portion of the tumour. Incomplete resection of the cyst wall can lead to a recurrence [81, 110]. The possibility that a meningioma may be associated with an adjacent cystic glioma should also be kept in mind [196].

11.2 Intraventricular Meningiomas

11.2.1 Incidence and Localization

Cushing and Eisenhardt [67] estimated that intraventricular meningiomas comprise 2%–3% of all intracranial meningiomas. In more recent studies [90, 107, 182] the frequency has been between 1% and 2%. The tumours most often occur in a lateral ventricle near the trigone with a clear proponderance on the left side [90, 107, 156, 182, 285]. Intraventricular meningiomas are encountered only rarely in the third and fourth ventricles. In some series [162, 182] intraventricular meningiomas occurred more frequently in children, but this has not been found in others [68]. It is probable that most of these tumours arise from the stromal cells of the choroid plexus, but occasionally may arise from the tela choroidea. They are most commonly of the fibromatous type.

11.2.2 Lateral Ventricles

CT usually shows a globular, slightly hyperdense mass within the ventricle in the region of the trigone, often associated with hydrocephalus or dilatation of an entrapped temporal horn. If the lesion is small origin from the choroid plexus is demonstrable. Calcification is frequent. Commonly, homogeneous enhancement occurs after intravenous contrast medium, as in meningiomas elsewhere. Bilateral intraventricular meningiomas, sometimes involving the whole of both choroid plexuses, have been described in patients with neurofibromatosis [236].

MRI shows an intraventricular mass having the previously described characteristics of a meningioma. The advantage of MRI is the ability to demonstrate the tumour in three orthogonal planes and so to establish its relationship to the ventricle and surrounding structures.

There is no peritumoral oedema in small intraventricular meningiomas. Sometimes large tumours adhere to the underlying tissue, and these often induce oedema (see Chap. 12).

Angiography often indicates and can diagnose intraventricular meningiomas. According to one group, angiography established the diagnosis in 16 of 18 cases [90], the most characteristic feature being vascularization predominantly from the choroidal arteries. The anterior choroidal (Fig. 11.3) artery is consistently enlarged, and the tortuous plexal segment is displaced usually laterally. In many cases the posterolateral choroidal arteries on the affected side are also enlarged.

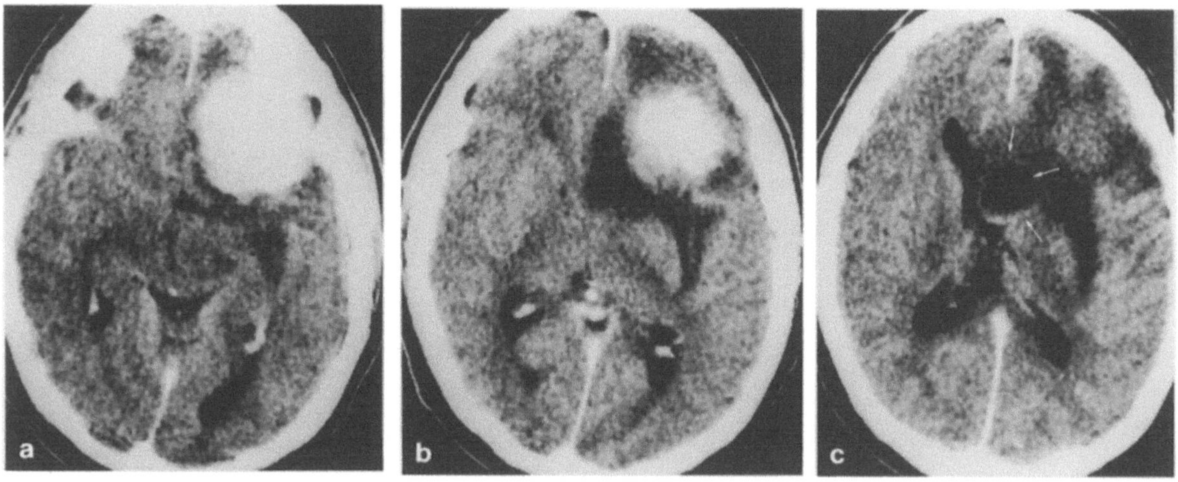

Fig. 11.1 a–c. Lateral sphenoid wing endotheliomatous meningioma with a cystic component. CT after contrast medium. The cyst is located peripherally to the solid tumour mass. There is contrast enhancement of the solid portion and of the capsule of the cyst *(arrows)*. There is evident oedema also involving the external capsule

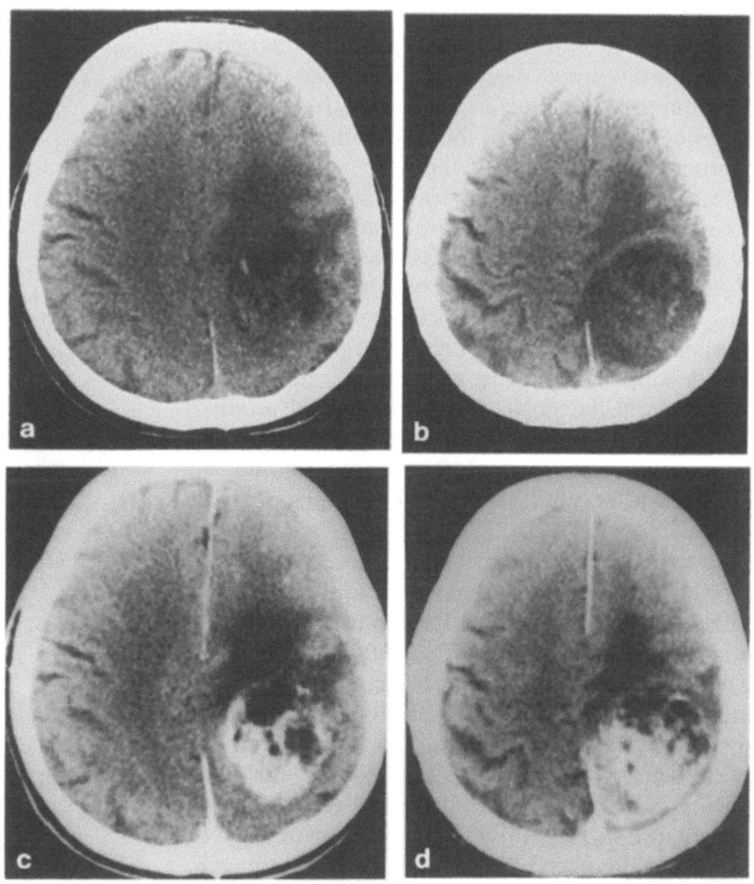

Fig. 11.2 a–d. Parasagittal endotheliomatous meningioma with fatty and cystic components. **a, b** CT. The tumour mass appears almost totally hypodense. **c, d** CT. After contrast medium there is enhancement involving also some of the areas appearing hypodense on the routine scan

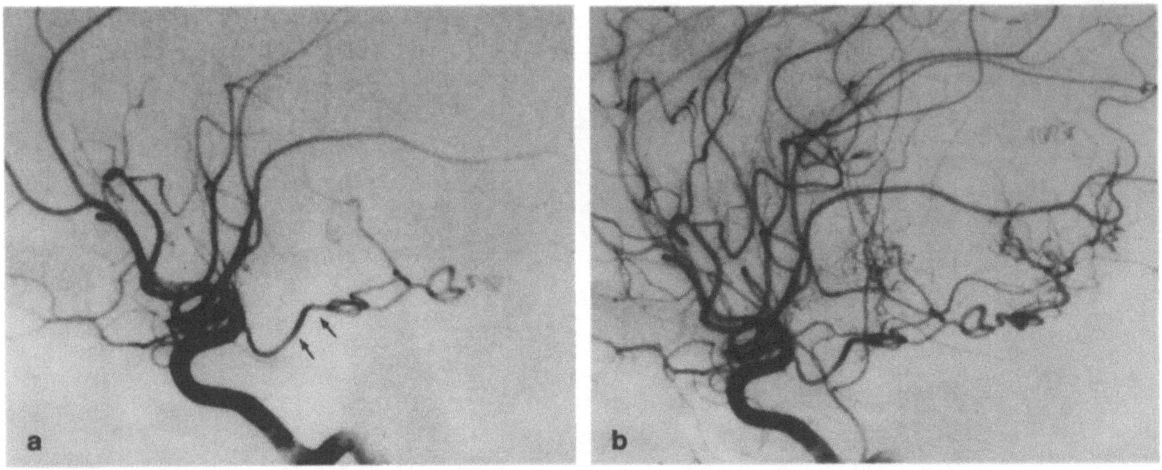

Fig. 11.3 a, b. Angiogram in intraventricular meningioma located in the trigone and temporal horn. Hypertrophic anterior choroidal artery *(arrows)*

11.2.3 Meningiomas of the Third and Fourth Ventricles

Russell and Rubinstein [236] regard meningiomas of the third ventricle as considerably more common than those of the fourth. They arise from the tela choroidea where it forms the velum interposition, a component of the roof of the third ventricle lying within the transverse cerebral fissure. They can arise posteriorly near the pineal gland [8, 115, 233], or more anteriorly near the foramen of Monro [1, 50, 55, 162, 184]; 75% have occurred in children. On CT the lesions have been dense, appearing like meningiomas elsewhere. On angiography, blood supply would be expected to be derived mainly from the posteromedial choroidal arteries, and vascular displacement to follow those of a third ventricular mass. MRI findings would be expected to be similar to those of meningiomas in general.

Cantore et al. [51] have recently reviewed meningiomas arising from the region of the fourth ventricle. The lesions were divided into three types: those arising from the choroid plexus and confined to the cavity of the fourth ventricle, those arising from the attachment of the tela choroidea to the velar lip of the peduncle of the flocculus and growing into the posterolateral fissure of the cerebellum, and those arising from the tela choroidea attached to the nodular part of the inferior medullary velum and growing down into the vallecula and cisterna magna. Their approximate frequencies were 68%, 18% and 14%, respectively. The reported cases appeared on CT like partly calcified meningiomas in other sites, often incorrectly diagnosed because of the predominantly intraventricular location and lack of dural attachment. Angiography has revealed only a faint tumour blush in less than half the reported meningiomas. However, careful analysis of the retromedullary branches especially of the posterior inferior cerebellar artery on magnification or tomographic angiography, may reveal choroidal arterial supply in a higher proportion; in practice, this finding is only of limited differential diagnostic values. Experience with MRI is very limited. In one patient examined by us, the tumour displayed the characteristics of meningioma, and its intraventricular location was clearly demonstrated (Fig. 11.4).

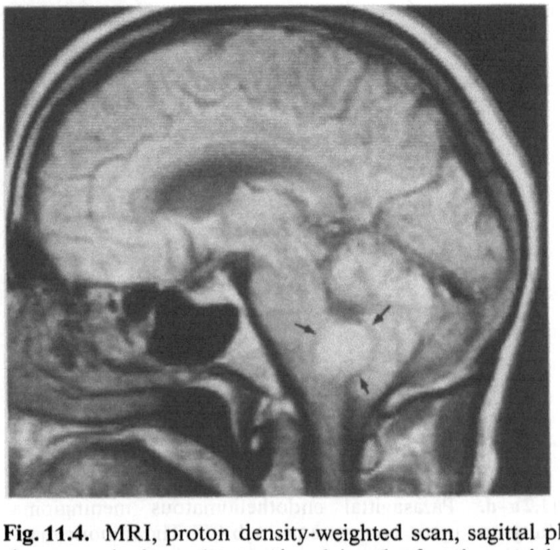

Fig. 11.4. MRI, proton density-weighted scan, sagittal plane shows meningioma *(arrows)* involving the fourth ventricle

11.2.4 Differential Diagnosis

Numerous tumours present as primarily intraventricular masses, and not all are neoplastic. It is necessary to differentiate tumours which extend into the ventricle from the surrounding brain and those which arise actually within the ventricle itself; there is a distinct propensity for the former to show changes in the underlying or adjacent brain [143, 266].

Medulloblastoma of the fourth ventricle appears in CT as a hyperdense mass showing rich homogeneous enhancement, difficult to distinguish from meningiomas, which is, however, rare in this localization. Furthermore, medulloblastoma usually occurs in the first decade of life.

Plexus papilloma and ependymoma are slightly hyperdense lesions with borders which appear more irregular than in meningioma. In both tumours cystic components, particularly in ependymoma, calcifications as well as inhomogenous enhancement are frequent. They are found in young patients. Very rare are subependymomas which appear as hypodense tumours with poor and irregular enhancement. Haemangioblastomas of the fourth ventricle are rare tumours, showing usually a richly enhanced solid part associate to a cystic component. There is a rich vascularisation of the solid portion on the vertebral angiogram.

Epidermoid and teratomas can arise from the choroid plexuses, or their vicinity, teratomas either in the fourth ventricle or near the pineal gland. Calcifications, solid and cystic elements without uniform enhancement should distinguish teratomas. Low density meningiomas occurring in the choroid to our knowledge have not been reported in this location, this eliminating confusion with typical epidermoids.

Other rare lesions such as colloid cyst of the third ventricle and xanthogranuloma of the choroid plexus should be easily distinguished from meningioma. Usually the colloid cyst is a hyperdense mass with well-defined borders showing no enhancement. Xanthogranulomas of the lateral ventricles are usually bilateral lesions displaying marked marginal enhancement sparing the central part of the tumour.

11.3 Primary Orbital Meningiomas

11.3.1 Incidence and Localization

The prevalence of primary orbital meningiomas, that is, those occuring within the orbit and excluding those extending into it from the orbital walls, is about 1% of all cranial meningiomas [67, 170]. They have been estimated to account for about 10% of all intraorbital neoplasms [136, 193, 269]. In a more recent study [138], they were the fourth most frequent group of intraorbital lesions following malignant tumours (carcinomas, sarcomas and metastases), cavernous angiomas and gliomas of the optic nerve. The tumour is predominant in women in whom it is more frequently found in the left orbit, while the right side tends to be more affected in men [269]. There is a comparatively high rate of intraorbital meningiomas in young children and infants [136], usually those suffering from neurofibromatosis [68]. Primary orbital meningiomas occurring in children and infants seem clinically more aggressive than those occurring in older patients [136], although histology generally gives no indication of malignancy.

11.3.1.1 Optic Nerve Sheath Meningiomas

According to their site of origin, optic nerve sheath meningiomas can be divided into those arising from that part of the optic nerve between the end of the optic canal and the eyeball and those arising from the optic nerve within the optic canal, the so-called foraminal meningiomas, which are extremely rare. These meningiomas are thought to arise from arachnoid cells lying in clusters within the connective tissue sheath surrounding the optic nerve.

11.3.1.2 Other Rare Meningiomas

Other rare meningiomas occurring in the orbit have no connection to the optic nerve sheath and are presumed to originate from embryonic rests of arachnoid cells located here.

11.3.2 Radiological Diagnosis

Meningiomas of the optic nerve sheath usually are shown well by CT. They may appear either as more or less diffuse thickening of the optic nerve or as a rounded mass. There is strong enhancement after contrast medium (Figs. 11.5, 11.6). Often the thickened sheath of the optic nerve is visible, distinct from the slightly lower density of the optic nerve; this appearance is highly characteristic of optic nerve sheath meningioma. Calcification in the optic nerve sheath also strongly suggests meningioma.

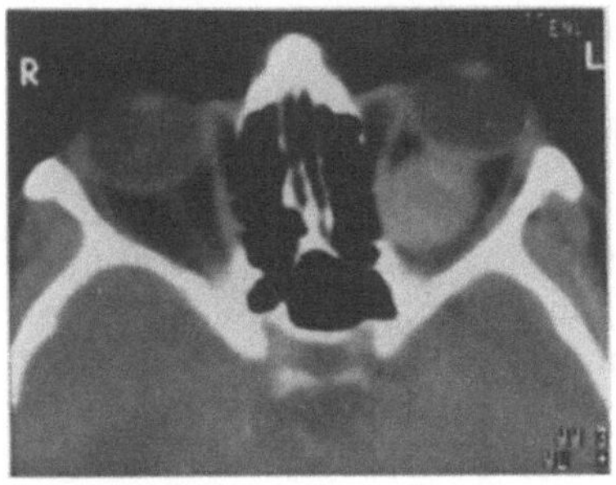

Fig. 11.5. Meningioma of the optic nerve, on CT a defined mass showing good enhancement

The meningioma can appear as a rounded mass with well-defined borders which occasionally may be irregular [92]. Foraminal lesions are sometimes difficult to diagnose. These grow in the optic canal and may have only a small intracranial or intraorbital extension. The anatomy and modifications induced by pathology can be most accurately assessed when CT is performed in the axis of the optic canal, which is orientated in a plane inclined downward and forward forming an angle of minus 40° with the orbitomeatal plane [19]. A widening of the optic canal can occur, most particularly in foraminal meningiomas. This used to be demonstrated with conventional tomography, but is now more easily and reliably shown with high definition CT.

In angiography capillary blush persisting in the venous phase is frequently present (Fig. 11.6). In general, however, angiography is no longer essential in the evaluation of orbital pathology except when an angiomatous malformation is suspected.

High resolution MRI may also demonstrate thickening of the optic nerve sheath in meningiomas, although distinction of sheath from optic nerve is not always possible.

11.3.3 Differential Diagnosis

The specific diagnosis of intraorbital lesions is often difficult if not impossible. We summarize some criteria which can be helpful in differentiating meningiomas, from the other frequent pathological processes [138].

Cavernous angiomas are the most common autochthonus orbital tumours [138]. They appear in CT as well-defined masses with clear enhancement similar to meningiomas. They are, however, frequently located in the lateral or medial portion of the orbit and usually can be well demarcated from the optic nerve. Bone changes are in general absent. Unlike cavernous angiomas, arteriovenous malformations present frequently with poorly demarcated borders. These lesions are very rare.

Fig. 11.6 a, b. Meningioma of the optic nerve, CT and angiogram. There is a faint pathological vascularization *(arrows)* visible in the capillary-venous phase

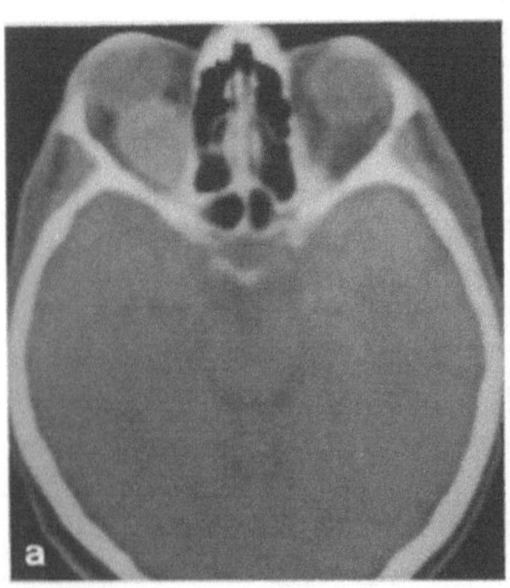

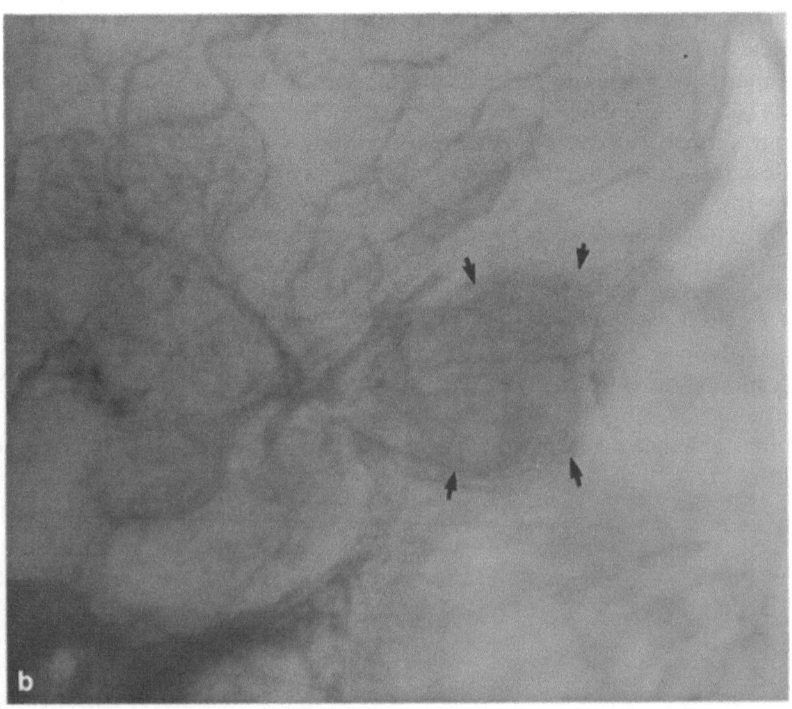

In the material of Kazner et al. [138] optic nerve gliomas represented 5%, while meningiomas accounted for 3% of all intraorbital tumours. The optic nerve gliomas may resemble meningiomas in CT, but are virtually confined to childhood, while meningiomas occur almost exlusively in adults, apart from cases of neurofibromatosis. The optic canal may be enlarged as in meningiomas, but intracranial extension of the glioma occurs into the chiasma, where meningioma spreads along the meninges.

Malignant tumours such carcinomas, metastases, and lymphomas are very frequent intraorbital lesions. They do not have a uniform appearance. Some are well outlined with strong enhancement, similar to meningiomas; others are not demarcated from surrounding structures. There is frequent bone destruction, which will help in the diagnosis. Rhabdomyosarcoma, which is the most common orbital tumour in children, belongs to this group of highly malignant tumours. Its appearance is like that of other malignant tumours.

Pseudotumours are also relatively frequent. They represent, in general, either a chronic inflammation or a reactive hyperplasia. They are irregularly shaped masses which may fill the entire orbit. Orbital enlargement as well as local bone erosion may occur. In mucoceles there is a soft tissue lesion originating in the paranasal sinuses, causing displacement or bone destruction.

Though rare, neurinomas may be found. They can simulate meningiomas; bone changes are unusual, and these lesions are usually associated with neurofibromatosis.

Other pathological processes which involve intraorbital structures are epidermoid and dermoid cysts. The former are characterized by density values similar to those of CSF, in the latter areas of a very low density due to fatty tissue are characteristic.

In Grave's disease spindle-shaped enlargement of one or more intraorbital muscles is very typical, and the diagnosis of this disease usually poses no problems.

11.4 Ectopic Meningiomas

11.4.1 Incidence and Localization

Ectopic meningiomas make up less than 1% of all meningiomas [96, 271]. The most frequently described sites are the paranasal sinuses, particularly the maxillary sinus and the nasal-oral cavity [11, 20, 100, 218, 232, 241, 287, 296]. The second most frequent localization is the parapharyngeal region [15, 112, 122, 195, 234, 254, 271, 295]. More rare localizations are the petrous bone [74, 103, 109, 183, 204, 242], the diploë and the outer table of the calvarium [9, 58, 106, 308]. Finally, ectopic meningiomas may occur in the orbits [169] and in the skin [132].

According to Hoye et al. [122] and to Geoffray et al. [96], the origin of ectopic meningiomas are arach-

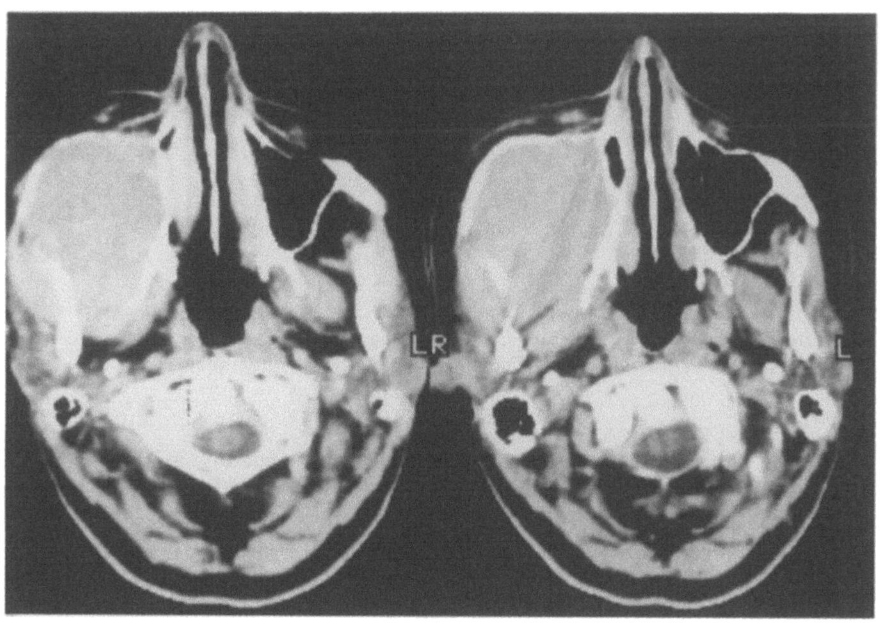

Fig. 11.7. Ectopic meningioma of the right maxillary sinus. CT, the richly enhanced tumour has completely filled the sinus which also appears enlarged. There is erosion of the lateral and medial wall of the sinus with extension of the tumour into the infratemporal fossa and the parapharyngeal area

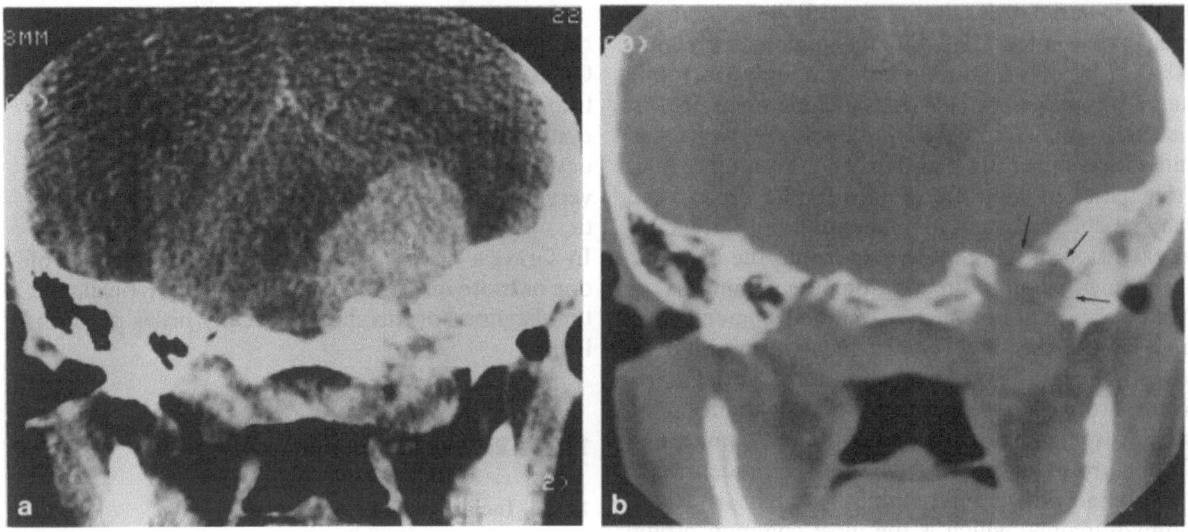

Fig. 11.8 a, b. Intrapetrous meningioma with intra- and extracranial growth. There is extensive destruction of the petrous bone *(arrows)*

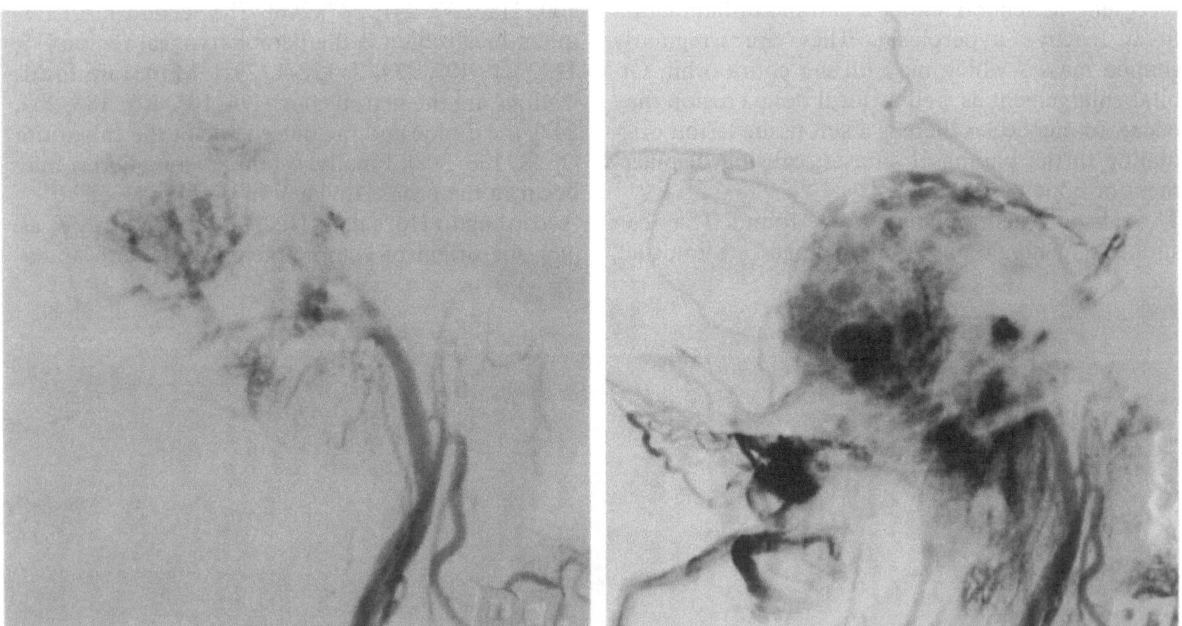

Fig. 11.9 a, b. Meningioma of the epipharynx extending intracranially. Angiogram of the hypertrophied ascending pharyngeal artery shows a very richly vascularized tumour. The angiographic appearance is similar to that of a chemodectoma

noid cells within the sheaths of the cranial nerves close to their foramina in the skull base, especially of the facial, hypoglossal and nerves of jugular foramen. This is probably the case in parapharyngeal meningiomas taking their origin from cranial nerves VII, IX, X, XI and XII and in some petrous bone lesions arising from arachnoid cells within the sheaths of lesser and greater petrosal nerves [204]. In other cases, extracranial growth of such a tumour is thought to occur from nests of embryonic cells of arachnoid differentiation which are not connected with cranial nerves. The tumours of the paranasal sinuses and the oral-nasal cavity as well as tumours of the calvarium, some orbital and some petrous bone tumours and those of the skin probably belong to this group. Sometimes meningiomas are found near the cranial sutures, and it has been suggested that the origin are arachnoidal cells disseminated during the formation of the skull [9].

11.4.2 Radiological Diagnosis

We have already treated ectopic lesions of the calvarium in Chap. 6. Here we will briefly consider the diagnosis of ectopic meningiomas located in the nasal, paranasal, oral cavities, those in the parapharyngeal regions and in the petrous bone.

Radiological findings commonly fail to deliver a specific diagnosis. They are, however, very useful in demonstrating the lesion which generally appears in CT as a well-defined mass showing rich enhancement (Fig. 11.7). Destruction of the skull base and intracranial extension is frequent (Fig. 11.8). This accounted for 47% of the cases in the report of Geoffray et al. [96]. MRI can be helpful in giving a better topographical demonstration of the tumour [15, 271].

Angiography shows a moderate capillary blush supplied by related branches of the exernal carotid artery. Intracranial and intraorbital components may be supplied by branches of the internal carotid artery. Angiography in general does not contribute to the specific diagnosis. It can be useful in differential diagnosis with chemodectomas, which always show a very rich vascularization. Occasionally, however, a similar angiographic appearance is present in meningiomas which makes a differential diagnosis impossible (Fig. 11.9).

12 Peritumoral Oedema in Meningiomas

12.1 Introductory Comments

A regional increase in the water content of the brain adjacent to meningiomas, termed oedema, is common. It is a paradox that a slow-growing tumour arising outside the brain should frequently induce oedema, especially when other extracerebral masses such as neurinomas, epidermoids and giant aneurysm seldom do so. Although oedema contributes to mass its role in causing cerebral dysfunction and determining false localizing signs is doubtful [95, 220]. Oedema surrounding meningiomas is difficult to study microscopically because fragments of brain tissue attached to operative specimens usually are traumatized, and in necropsy cases the brain is affected by terminal and post-mortem processes. Nevertheless, swelling of peritumoral brain tissue, mainly of the white matter, is easily recognized macroscopically. Animal models of brain oedema have been extensively studied, and many observations on propagation, distribution and resorption of vasogenic oedema suggest a close similarity to the oedema seen near meningiomas.

12.2 Peritumoral Oedema in Computed Tomography - Magnetic Resonance Imaging

12.2.1 Incidence

The precise incidence of oedema with meningiomas is not known because not all changes shown by computed tomography (CT) and magnetic resonance imaging (MRI) in peritumoral brain represent oedema. In one report [37] oedema was recorded on CT in 73% of patients examined but in 25% of these it was confined to within 2.5 cm of the tumour margin. In another report [264] low attenuation in surrounding brain was seen in 67% of patients examined, but only that which showed a fingerlike pattern in cerebral white matter was definitely ascribed to oedema, and this occurred in 46%. In the posterior fossa where brain substance around meningiomas is less well shown by CT, incidences of oedema of between 33% and 66% have been reported [56, 207, 282], suggesting a slightly lower frequency than with supratentorial lesions.

12.2.2 Distribution

On CT a near linear relationship between tissue water content (specific gravity) and attenuation has been demonstrated by Rieth et al. [226] although specific gravity may be a significantly less satisfactory measure of water content when oedema fluid is protein rich [84]. With MRI not only protein content, but also compartmentalization of tissue water has a profound effect on relaxation times, especially on T2 - weighted scans [16].
Experience with CT and MRI suggests that the distribution of oedema depends on its amount and site

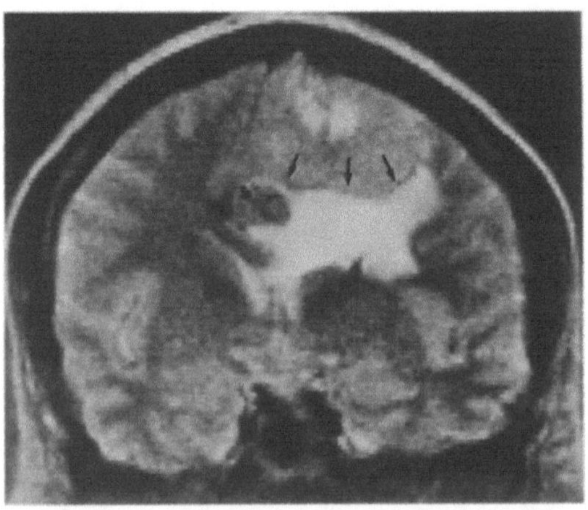

Fig. 12.1. Parasagittal meningioma. MRI. T2-weighted scan, coronal plane. The meningioma is isointense with the cortex. Inside of the tumour one can recognize an area with high signal intensity corresponding to a small cyst. The tumour is separated by the oedema by a small ring of hypointensity *(arrows)*. The oedema involves largely the corona radiata, but does not extend caudally into the capsule

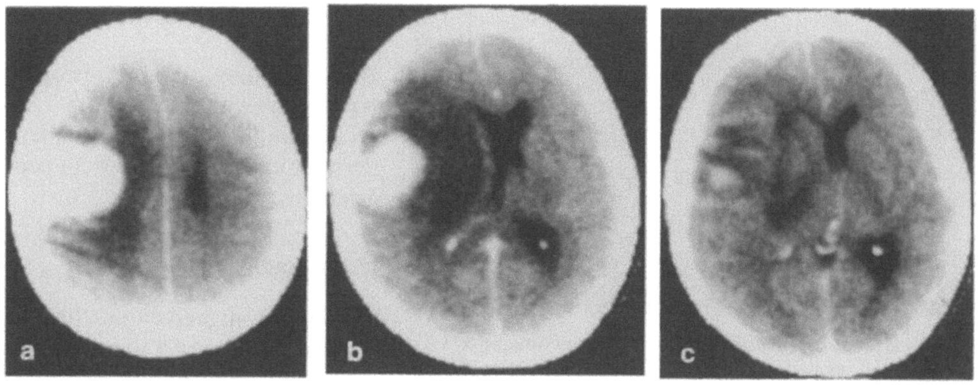

Fig. 12.2 a–c. Convexity Haemangiopericytic meningioma with large oedema involving the corona radiata, the external and posterior limb of the internal capsules

of origin [159, 264], and it is always most prominent near the tumour. The characteristic appearance is of a fingerlike or flame-shaped, homogeneous abnormality extending into the external capsule and posterior limb of the internal capsule, and having a scalloped or lobulated lateral margin where it extends into the white matter of the cerebral gyri. These features are usually only visible when oedema extends more than 2.5 cm beyond the tumour margin [264]. The centrum semiovale and the external capsule are most often involved (Fig. 12.1). The corpus callosum and the internal capsule are involved only when edema is severe or the meningioma is nearby (Fig. 12.2); involvement of the posterior limb of the internal capsule is particularly characteristic of tumours of the middle cranial fossa [264] (Figs. 12.3, 12.7, 8.18).

This distribution strongly suggests that oedema propagates by centrifugal spread from an origin lying at or near some part of the surface of the tumour [75, 202, 264]. Moreover, it conforms closely to vasogenic or extracellular oedema in experimental animals produced by superficial cold injury or microdrip infusion [83, 84, 151, 187, 228]. The dynamics of these types of experimentally produced oedema are well known. As fluid is added to the interstitium of brain tissue, there is a near linear rise in tissue pressure, until it reaches a certain level, referred to as the critical opening pressure. Large volumes of fluid may then be added with only minimal increase in tissue pressure; in other words, an abrupt change in tissue compliance occurs. It is hypothesized that fluid enters and spreads preferentially in the regions of greatest compliance and that the neuropil in the less compact regions of the white matter, such as the centrum semiovale and external capsule, have a lower critical opening pressure than more compact areas, such as grey matter, the corpus callosum and internal capsule. When there is a continuous source of fluid production, as is probably the case in peritumoral oedema, it is suggested that a steady state is reached in which the increased tissue pressure initially determining oedema propagation has dissipated sufficiently at the oedema margin to be below the critical opening pressure of adjacent tissue. In the cerebral hemispheres it is common for the oedema to involve an ependymal surface; oedema fluid has been shown to enter the ventricles, and there is evidence that this is an important physiological route for the removal of extracellular fluid [228, 229].

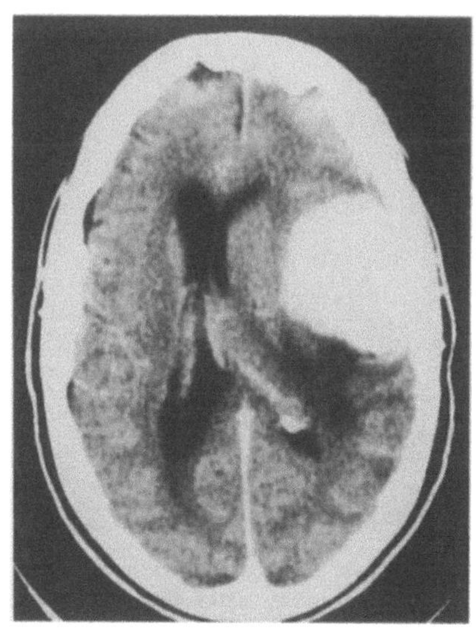

Fig. 12.3. Endotheliomatous lateral sphenoid wing meningioma. There is oedema in the corona radiata, extending also into the external and the posterior limb of the internal capsule

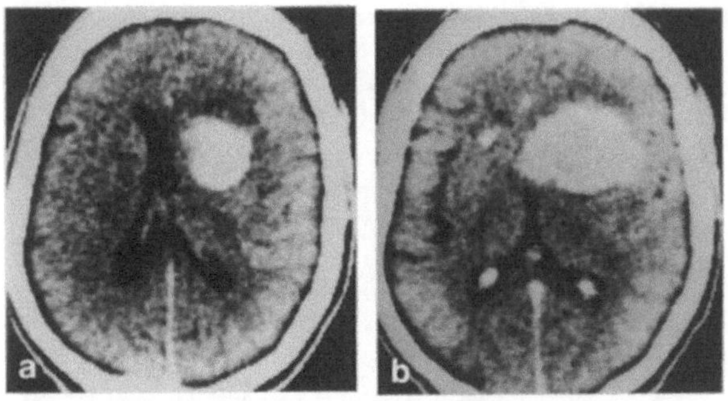

Fig. 12.4 a, b. Large medial sphenoid wing meningioma, CT. There is only negligeble oedema. The histological study revealed a poorly vascularized tumour without signs of perivascular exudation

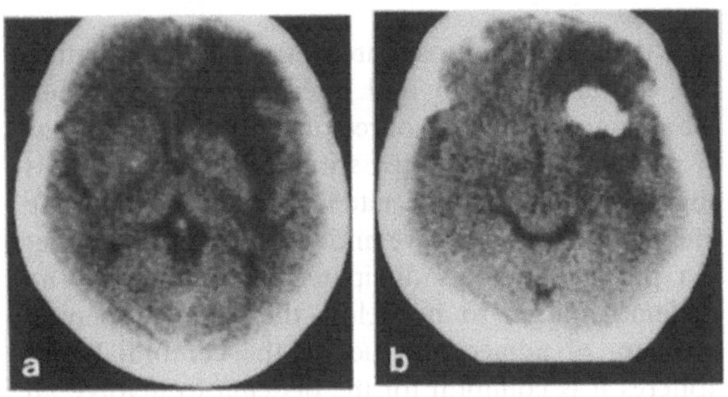

Fig. 12.5 a, b. Small calcified sphenoid wing meningioma, CT. There is extensive peritumoral oedema involving the corona radiata and the external capsule. The histological examination showed a richly vascularized tumour, particularly near the capsule. There was also evident perivascular protein accumulation

12.3 Factors Involved in Oedema production

Many radiological and histopathological features associated with peritumoral oedema have been studied in humans with specific reference to meningioma, but the available data contains many inconsistencies.

12.3.1 Radiological Features

Experience suggests that there is little correlation between the size of a meningioma and the degree of oedema. Large tumours without any and small tumours with marked oedema are seen frequently (Figs. 12.4, 12.5, 12.6, 7.11). Nevertheless, in a review of 160 supratentorial meningiomas it was shown statistically that oedema was more frequent with large lesions [264], and also that lobulation of the cerebral surface of the tumour was related to the presence of oedema [264]. These observations suggest that the surface area of tumour in contact with the brain is relevant in some way to the genesis of oedema.

Meningiomas appearing richly vascularized on angiography have been associated with oedema more frequently than those appearing poorly vascularized [37], although this has not been evident in all studies [264]. The demonstration of a blocked dural venous sinus was proposed as an important cause of oedema in meningioma [86], but subsequent observations have consistently denied this [37, 264].

The site of a meningioma may have relevance.

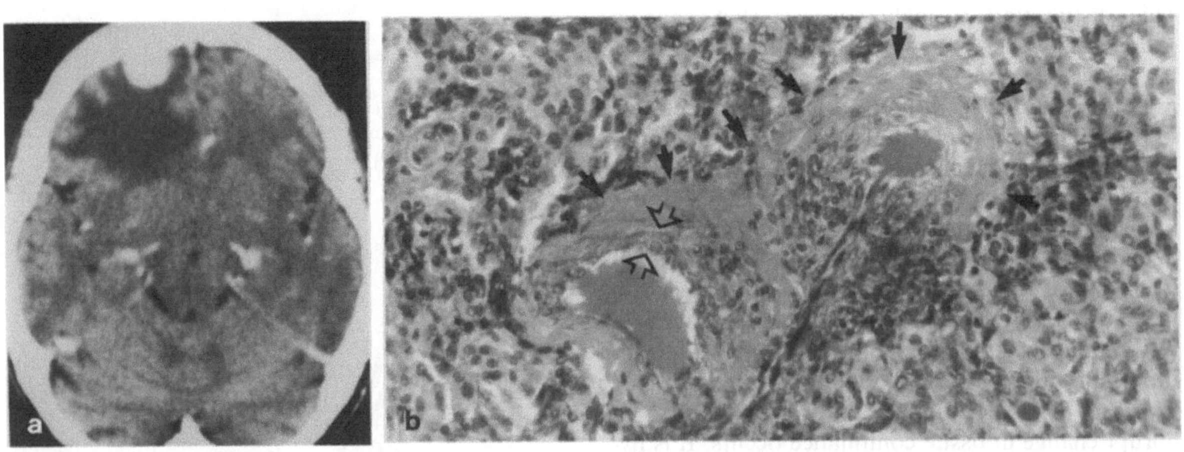

Fig. 12.6 a, b. Small meningioma of the frontal convexity. **a** CT. There is very extensive peritumoral oedema. **b** Histological study with PAS stain, magnification, ×450. Highly vascularized endotheliomatous meningioma. The figure shows two small veins. Both vessels contain grey homogeneous PAS-positive material in their lumen. The vessel wall is demarcated by the *two light arrows*. Beyond the wall, similar PAS-positive material is seen penetrating the tumour tissue and coalescing with exudate from the neighbouring blood vessel. The *black arrows* show the border of the resulting lack of protein-rich fluid

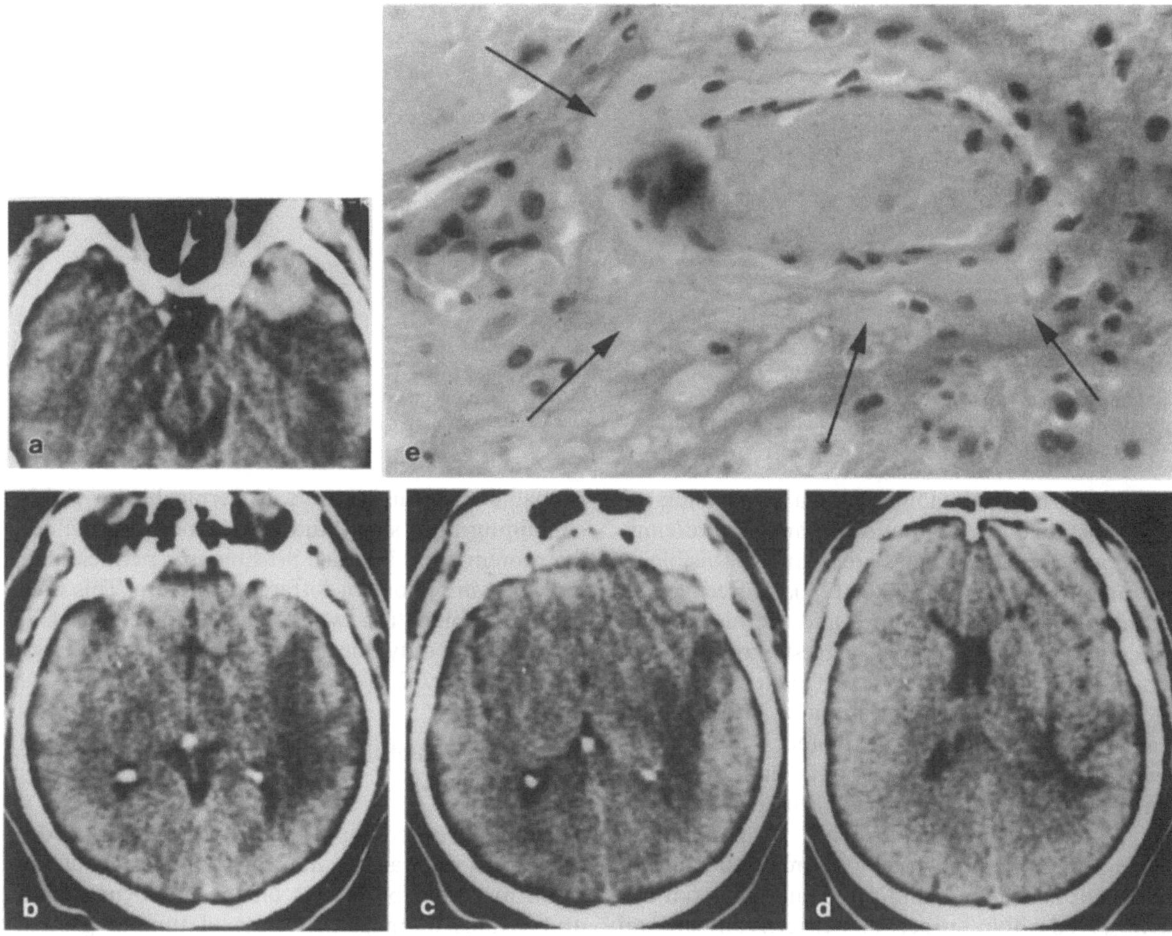

Fig. 12.7 a–e. Temporobasal meningioma. **a–d** CT. The tumour is well recognizable after contrast medium. There is evident peritumoral oedema, also involving the external and the posterior limb of the internal capsules. **e** Histological examination. The tumour appears richly vascularized, particularly in the areas near the capsule where perivascular exudation *(arrows)* can also be demonstrated (H. E., ×650)

Oedema is significantly less common with meningiomas of the tuberculum sellae and free margin of tentorium than with tumours in contact with the medial or superolateral surface of the hemispheres, particularly of the frontal lobe. However, parafalcine and high convexity meningiomas tend to be larger lesions, and experience dictates that tumours of similar size in the same location may or may not be surrounded by oedema (Figs. 12.7, 12.8).

12.3.2 Histological Features

Most meningiomas classified as malignant are associated with oedema. When the peritumoral tissue is examined in these cases, astroglial proliferation, perivenular haemorrhages and proteinaceous perivascular exudates may be seen, which are histological features suggesting microcirculatory failure. Oedema is also found in the great majority of hemangiopericytomas. It is also more frequent in the angioblastic (Fig. 12.2) and endotheliomatous types than in fibromatous lesions. Smith et al. [259] demonstrated an unusually rich capillary and venular network in four small meningiomas, all of which were associated with extensive brain oedema; Bradac et al. [37] and Ferszt and Bradac [82] subsequently showed a statistically significant relationship in a larger number of cases and also demonstrated that this histological appearance did not correlate with the degree of vascularization indicated by angiography. Indeed, this seems to represent a true independent variable influencing oedema production, but the fact that it is not found in all indicates that it also is not the crucial determinant.

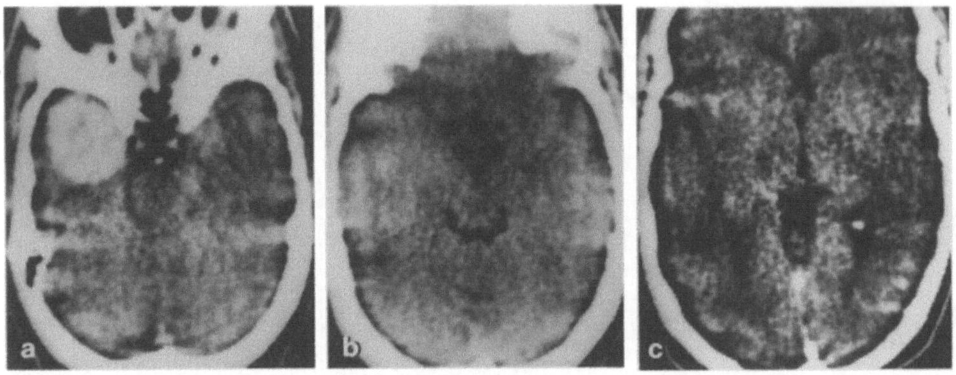

Fig. 12.8a-c. Temporobasal meningioma, CT. The tumour is well visible after contrast medium. There is no oedema. Histologically the tumour appreared poorly vascularized without perivascular exudation

The vessels in meningiomas lack a morphological and functional blood-tumour barrier. Proteinaceous perivascular exudates are frequently visible in the tumour matrix (Figs. 12.6, 12.7). Moreover, the texture of meningiomas varies and the histological appearance in some cases suggests intratumoral oedema [37, 82]. However, exact data are lacking and correlation between intratumoral and adjacent brain oedema has not been explored.

Secretory activity is demonstrable in the cells of some meningiomas, and it has been suggested that this correlates with the presence of peritumoral oedema [221]. The rough endoplasmic reticulum of these cells is enlarged, and proteinlike material can be observed within intracellular cisterns and around a proliferated golgi apparatus, resulting in vesicles which open into the extracellular space. It is possible that this represents the secretion of oedema-producing factors, possibly polypeptide vasoactive substances which could determine oedema production by migrating into surrounding brain. Further studies on a larger number of patients have not confirmed a relationship between secretory phenomena and oedema [37, 82]. Nevertheless, it is possible that secretory activity is important in some cases and capillary hypervascularity in others. For example, in one patient [37] with a large parasagittal tumour and marked oedema, conventional histological examination showed poor vascularization and the tumour was classified as fibrous in type; however, retrospective electron microscopic analysis revealed abundant secretory activity of the tumour cells (Fig. 12.9).

Capsulelike structures (Fig. 12.10) often form around meningiomas. Such structures vary considerably with regard to the density of the collagen fibres and the number of blood vessels embedded within them, even around the same tumour. It is probable that this capsule is permeable to fluids containing both small and large molecules including proteins, and it is also possible that permeability may vary in regions of different structure. This may be one explanation why oedema sometimes [37] spreads from only one sector of the surface of large tumours (Figs. 12.11-12.13, 7.2, 7.5).

12.3.3 Theories of the Pathogenesis of Oedema in Meningioma

The long-favoured hypothesis for peritumoral oedema formation was mechanical compression of the brain mediated by effects on the microcirculation and venous drainage. The rate of tumour growth was considered important. However, the cases in which serial CT or MRI studies have been available indicate that rapid tumour growth is not crucial for development of brain oedema (Fig. 12.14), and the accumulated radiological data indicate strongly that factors other than compression are involved.

A new hypothesis was propounded recently by Stevens et al. [264, 265] based mainly on radiological observations, but grounded in the hydromechanical concepts of vasogenic oedema developed by others [151, 152, 228, 229]. The hypothesis states that the oedema fluid is derived from vessels within the tumour. This fluid leaks from the capillary bed of the tumour and determines the interstitial pressure within the tumour; when the pressure exceeds the critical opening pressure of contiguous brain tissue, brain oedema may develop. The interstitial pressure in the majority of meningiomas is probably lower than the critical opening pressure of the normal cerebral cortex, but higher than that of most cerebral white matter. Focal thinning of parts of the cortex contiguous with even small meningiomas is well known pathologically, progressing in some cases to

Fig. 12.9 a–e. Large parasagittal fibrous meningioma which evolved within 4 months to a meningosarcoma. The tumour was poorly vascularized on the angiogram, where a partial infiltration of the sinus was demonstrated. **a** CT. There is a large area of oedema around the inhomogeneously enhanced tumour. **b** Angiogram. Infiltration of the sinus *(arrows)*. **c–e** Electron micrograph. **c** Note the large number of vesicular structures and the rich Golgi apparatus. Original magnification, × 8000. **d** Tumour cell processes with a typical interdigitating pattern of membranes. The rectangular process contains cytoplasm with many vesicular structures and, at two sites at least *(arrows)* these vesicles fuse with the cell membrane, indicating perhaps secretory activity. Magnification, × 5000. **e** Two tumour cells with some vesicular activity in the cytoplasm. The *dark arrows* depict two vesicles fusing with the cell membrane, the *light arrow* shows the Golgi apparatus. Magnification, × 8000

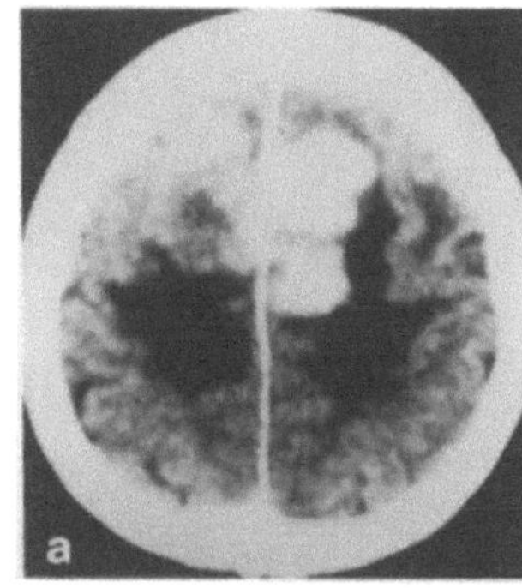

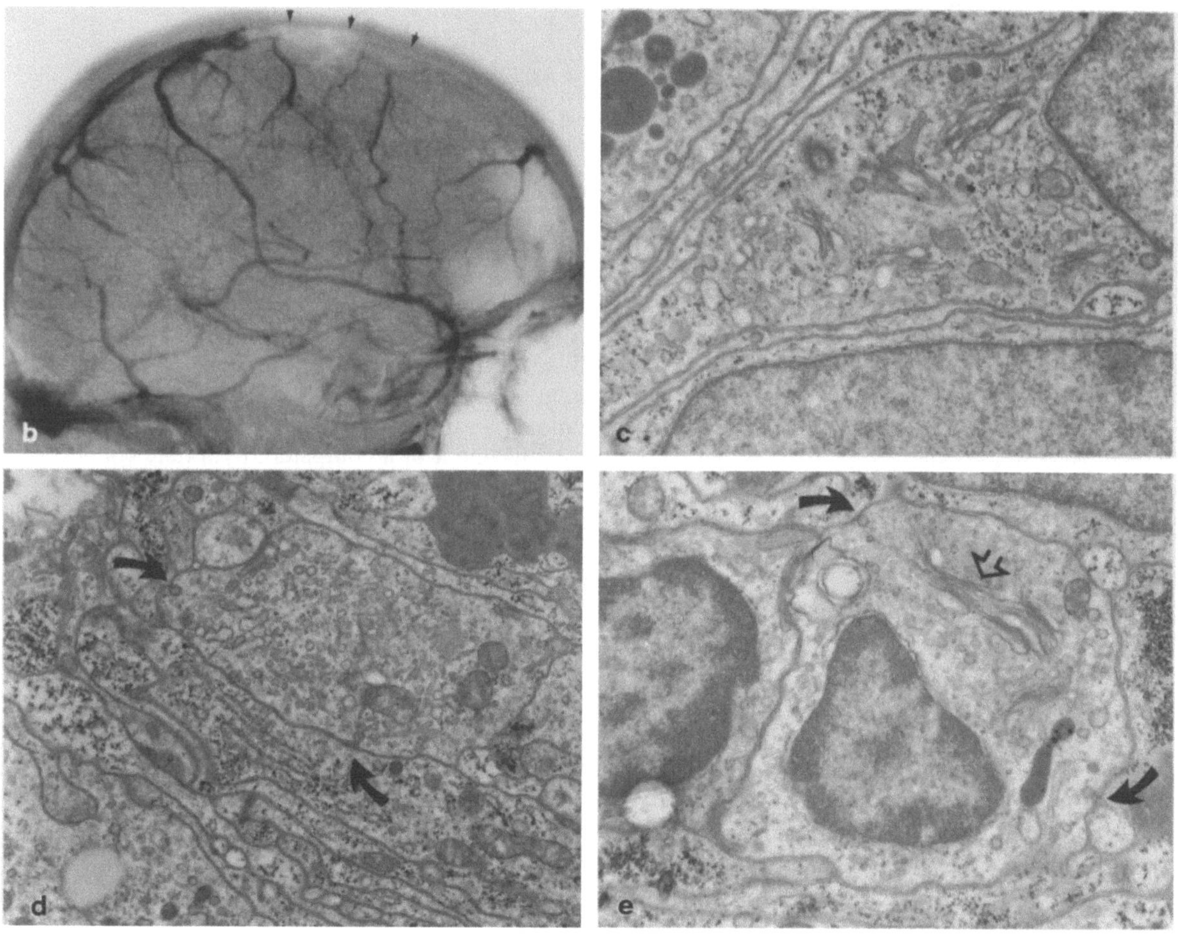

destruction of the cortex and its replacement by a thin gliomesodermal scar [99, 264]. The hypothesis holds that at some stage in this degenerative process the hydraulic resistance of cortical grey matter falls sufficiently for it not to constitute a barrier between the interstitial fluid pressure of the tumour and the more compliant white matter, and oedema results. Experimental work on ultraviolet-induced lesions of the cerebral cortex of cats has shown that vasogenic oedema spreads very slowly through normal cortex in spite of its higher vascular density, and it is further inhibited by subcortical U fibres [84, 244].

Intraventricular meningiomas come into contact with ependyma and the subedendymal white matter which, observation suggests, have a high compliance and in which oedema easily develops. That not all intraventricular meningiomas are associated with brain oedema suggests that another important factor in the production of oedema is the establish-

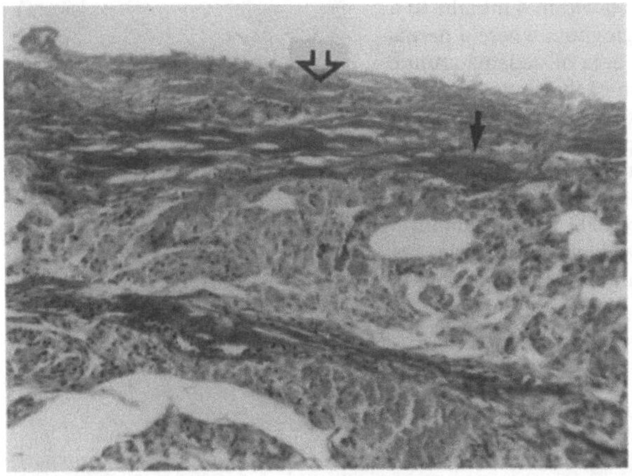

Fig. 12.10. "Capsule" of a meningiotheliomatous meningioma. Comparatively loose tumour tissue is shown in the *lower half* of the picture. The *light arrow* shows a few strands of neighbouring gliotic brain tissue adhering to the tumour surface. The *dark arrow* shows a dense feltwork of interlacing collagen fibres tapering out into the tumour tissue and forming a highly variable capsulelike structure. Elastica van Gieson stain, × 250

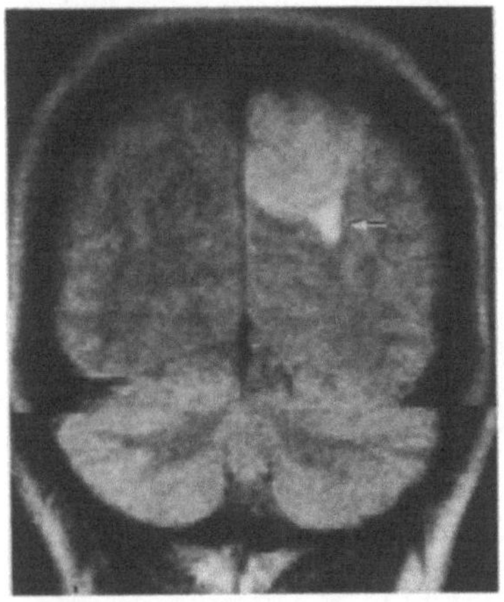

Fig. 12.11. Parasagittal meningioma. MRI, T2-weighted scan. The meningioma displays a slight increase of signal intensity. The oedematous reaction *(arrow)* characterized by a high signal intensity is present only in a limited sector of the tumour's surface

ment of a competent hydraulic connection between the interstitium of tumour and brain, and that for many intraventricular lesions the available path of least resistance for fluid excaping from the tumour surface remains the ventricular cavity. Similarly, lesions contacting the brain stem, which also lacks a cortical mantle, do not always produce brain stem oedema since the fluid escaping from tumour finds direct access to CSF; but also the compliance of the neuropil is known to be very different from that of

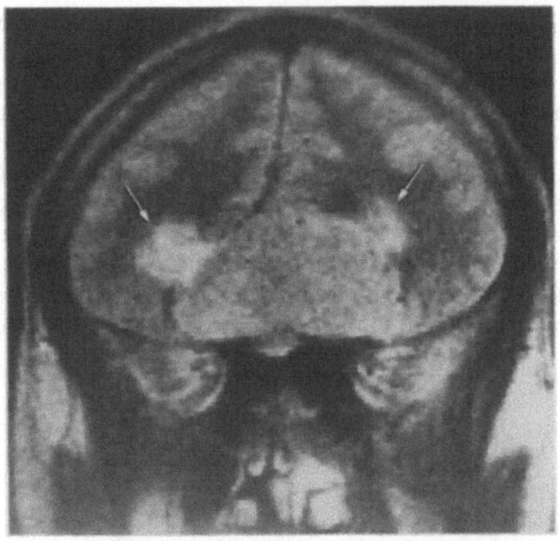

Fig. 12.12. Large frontobasal meningioma. MRI, T2-weighted scan, coronal plane. The peritumoral oedema characterized by a signal of high intensity is not recognizable on the whole surface of the meningioma, but only in two limited sectors (→)

the centrum semiovale, as was shown experimentally [111]. The role of the permeability of the capsulelike structure of some meningiomas in this process is unclear, but it seems likely to be of less importance than the compliance of contiguous brain and establishment of a competent hydraulic connection between the interstitium of tumour and brain.

It is possible that oedema fluid arises from cerebral vessels rather than from those of the tumour. Indeed, the abnormal fluid in the brain usually appears less proteinaceous than the perivenular exudates seen in some meningiomas, and therefore may have a different origin. Secretion of oedema factors by the tumour is a hypothesis favoured by many, and a number of possible substances have been studied [10]. The density of capillaries, arterioles and venules in the cerebral cortex is considerably greater than in white matter, and these vessels could constitute the source of oedema fluid under the influence of oedema factors, produced by meningioma. The extravasated fluid would be contained initially by the perivascular glial sheaths and the dense cortical neuropil. Once the texture of the cortex had been altered by the presence of the tumour only the subcortical U fibre layer would remain as a barrier to separate the oedema forming in the grey matter from the more compliant white matter. In animal experiments focal oedema usually takes about 24 h to develop, and this may represent the time required for the rising interstitial fluid pressure to exceed the critical opening pressure of the underlying white matter.

The relevance of the secretory phenomena first re-

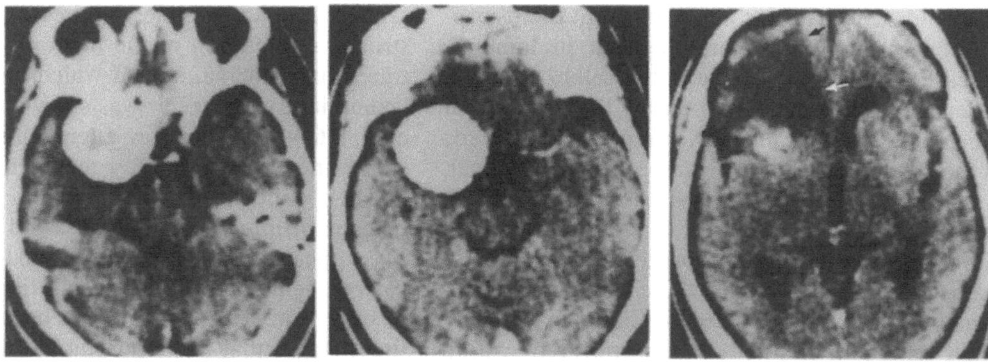

Fig. 12.13. calcified large medial sphenoid wing meningioma, CT. The oedema spreads only in the frontal region *(arrows)*

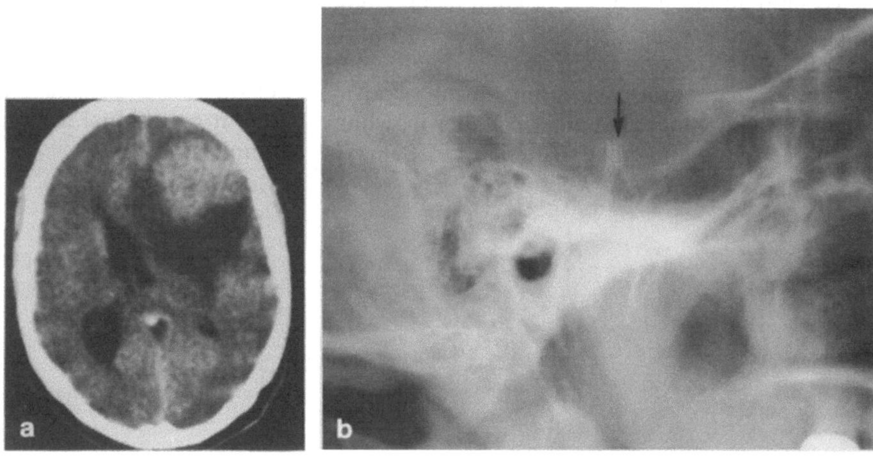

Fig. 12.14a, b. Large frontal convexity meningioma in a patient with a long clinical history. **a** CT showed a large area of peritumoral oedema. **b** On the plain skull erosion *(arrow)* of dorsum sellae, a sign of long-lasting compression, was visible. The tumour appeared richly vascularized on the angiogram and in histological studies. Nevertheless, there was only little evidence of perivascular exudation and no sign of secretory activity of tumour cells

ported by Philippon and his group [221] is obscure, but it is at least possible that it represents secretion of substances which promote vascular permeability outside the tumour. Also, mast cells are occasionally seen in meningiomas, and frequently they have a perivascular arrangement; it is conceivable that these, too, may promote increased vascular permeability.

In summary, many mechanisms may be at work in producing oedema around meningiomas. It is clear that the tumour is not an inert space-occupying lesion, but actively involved in the process.

The nature of this involvement is a matter of controversy. Vasogenic oedema produced in experiments is essentially an acute phenomenon elicited by tissue breakdown, whereas oedema around meningiomas may take months or years to develop, and necrosis of adjacent brain is not a prerequisite. Pressure atrophy and chronic mild distension of the interstitial spaces of the cortex are seen with meningiomas, but are not encountered in experimentally induced oedema; however, neither has been shown to be associated with oedema production. Nevertheless, it is highly probable that the tumour and perhaps the surrounding brain produce fluid which eventually accumulates in the extracellular spaces of the cerebral white matter and constitutes peritumoral oedema.

12.4 Peritumoral changes after Meningioma Excision

Oedema fluid may be removed from brain tissue by at least three processes, all of which have been demonstrated in acute experimental oedema in animals: (1) absorption into the ventricular cerebrospinal fluid, (2) removal of osmotically active solids (particularly proteins) from the oedema fluid by astrocytes and (3) endothelial reasorption of fluid and solids by the capillaries themselves, which seems linked to astrocyte function [152]. It seems likely that similar mechanisms are involved in the resorption of chronic peritumoral oedema in humans. When a cold lesion is made in the cerebral cortex, oedema rises to a maximum during the few days in which the blood-brain barrier remains disrupted; as the barrier recovers oedema begins to disappear, a process which usually takes about 1 week [229]. Stevens et al. [264] showed that in humans peritumoral oedema usually disappeared after meningioma excision inside 8 weeks; there was some dependence on the amount of oedema initially present - small amounts of oedema disappeared within 1 week and larger amounts took up to 8 weeks. In many cases, however, some residual low attenuation persists indefinitely in brain substance, but it is related more to the size of the original meningioma rather than the severity of oedema [264], suggesting that usually it represents brain damage due to compression by the tumour or occuring during removal. Notwithstanding, there are also patients in whom the characteristic fingerlike pattern of oedema is retained, which probably represents a permanent structural alteration of the neuropil due to the extracellular oedema, a state which has been termed "compliant wetness". It was shown also by Stevens et al. [264] that when low attenuation in brain substance increased soon after meningioma excision it invariably indicated a complication such as haemorrhage or infection. In no case did the postoperative appearances suggest further extension of typical vasogenic oedema into brain tissue in response to operation. This is significant because it is sometimes stated that an important cause of perioperative morbidity is the occurrence of brain oedema, caused by liberation of oedema factors from the tumour during operative manipulation. The observations of Stevens et al. [264] suggest that such a conception is fallacious. When a fingerlike pattern of white matter oedema is shown to be extending on postoperative CT, this strongly suggests either recurrent or residual tumour or a surgically induced complication.

13 Meningioma Embolization

13.1 General Considerations

Meningiomas are frequently highly vacularized and can cause heavy bleeding during surgery. Reduction of tumour vascularity by embolization decreases the blood loss during surgery and can facilitate removal of the tumour.
The first reports of embolization of meningiomas appeared in the early 1970s [114, 179, 210] and were followed by studies from several groups [36, 72, 80, 116, 180, 181, 230, 238, 275]. Today embolization is considered a useful complementary method to surgery and is regularly employed in selected patients in many neuroradiological centres.

13.2 Meningioma Vascularization

13.2.1 Role of Meningeal Supply

The central part of the tumour is supplied by meningeal branches entering the meningioma at the site of dural attachment.
The peripheral portion is often supplied by cortical arteries whose leptomeningeal branches enter the surface of the tumour laying adjacent to the brain.
In our experience about 25% of meningiomas are supplied almost exclusively by the external carotid artery. In these patients the advantages of embolization are most evident, but in tumours with mixed supply, embolization of the territory of the external carotid artery (ECA) can be useful since emboli in the central part of the tumour cause partial necrosis (Figs. 13.6, 13.7), resulting not only in reduced bleeding but also facilitating extirpation of the meningioma [116, 181].

13.2.2 Anastomosis of External Carotid with Internal Carotid and/or Vertebral Arteries

In embolization of the ECA it is important to be aware of the possibility of anastomosis with internal carotid (ICA) or vertebral arteries. A careful study of the external carotid angiogram before and during the embolization is mandatory because anastomoses may open up during embolization. We described these potential anastomoses in Chap. 5.
The most frequent dangerous anastomoses are between:

1. Middle meningeal and ophthalmic arteries
2. Accessory meningeal artery and C_4-C_5 portion of the carotid siphon
3. Foramen rotundum artery and C_4-C_5 portion of the carotid siphon
4. Ascending pharyngeal artery and C_4-C_5 portion of the carotid siphon
5. Ascending pharyngeal artery and vertebral artery
6. Occipital artery and vertebral artery

13.2.3 Cranial Nerves

It is important to be aware of the blood supply of some cranial nerves from the meningeal branches of the ECA:

1. The middle meningeal and/or accessory meningeal arteries are responsible for some of the blood supply of the nerves III, V, VI and peripheral part of nerve VII.
2. The occipital and/or posterior auricular arteries also supply the vertical part of nerve VII.
3. The ascending pharangeal artery supplies, via its jugular branch, nerves IX, X, XI and partially XII.

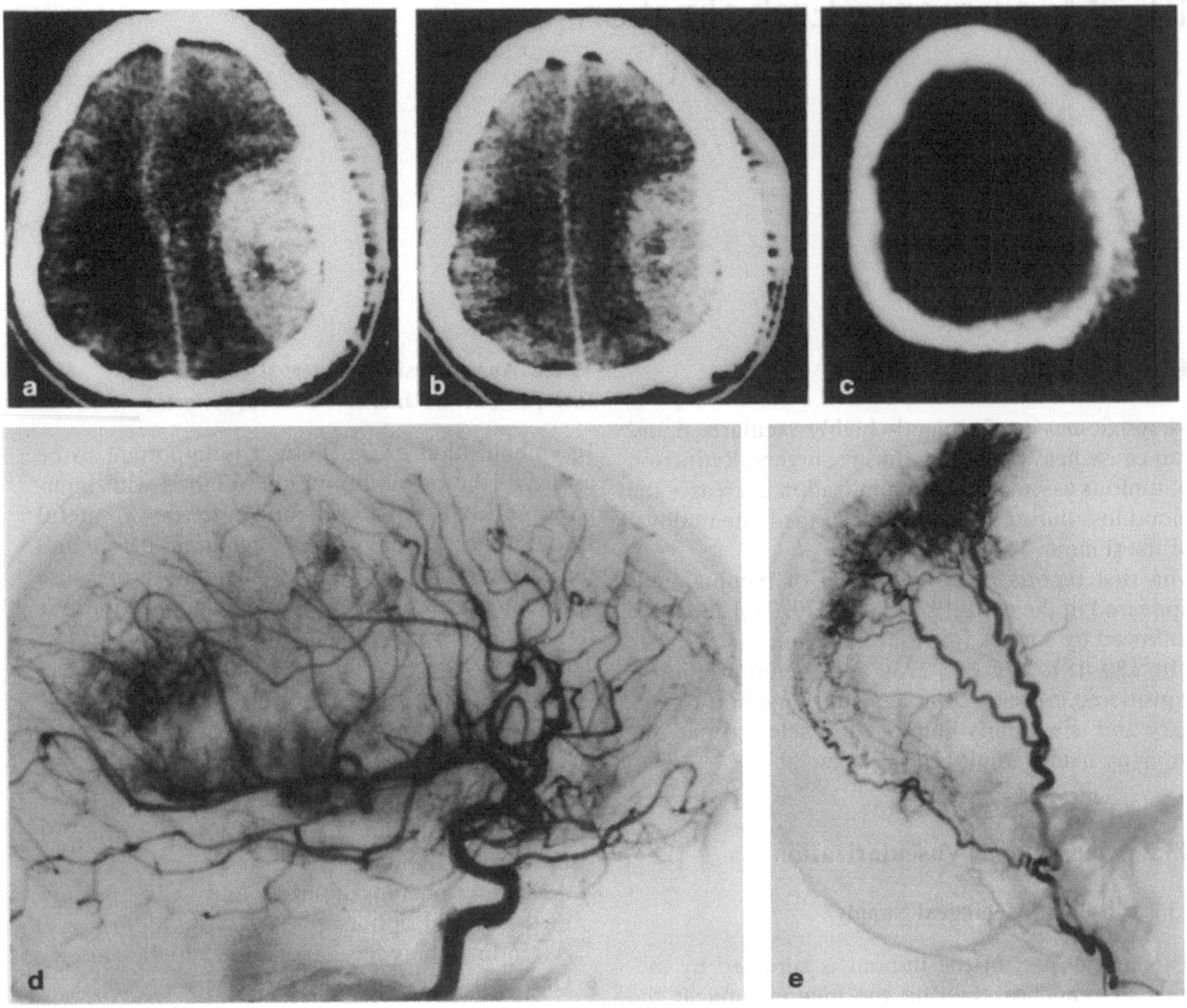

Fig. 13.1 a–e

13.3 Technical Aspects

Angiography is usually carried out through the femoral artery under mild sedation, using nonionic contrast medium. Discomfort for the patient is minimal and the angiographer can monitor the patient's neurological status throughout the procedure. It is preferable to perform the embolization during the same session as diagnostic angiography, so that the possibility of embolization should have been discussed with the clinician and with the patient and full consent obtained before angiography is performed.

Superselective catheterization of different branches of the ECA can generally be performed without damage or spasm of the arteries. The internal maxillary artery (IMA) is the most sensitive vessel, and spastic reactions are not infrequent. If catheterization of the middle meningeal artery and other peripheral branches of IMA is too difficult, the tip of the catheter may have to be left near the origin of IMA. When particulate emboli are injected slowly, they mainly enter the large tumoral feeders; partial embolization of other branches of IMA may not be avoidable, but this does not usually cause any significant complications [275]. If dangerous external to internal carotid or vertebral anastomoses are present, there are two options: (1) advance the tip of the catheter beyond the origin of the anastomosic branch, which often is not difficult to do, but embolization should not be attempted if the catheter tip cannot be advanced far enough; (2) since these anastomoses are often vary small, it may be safe to use larger particles which will not pass through the anastomoses. Fluid embolic material for this kind of embolization is best avoided.

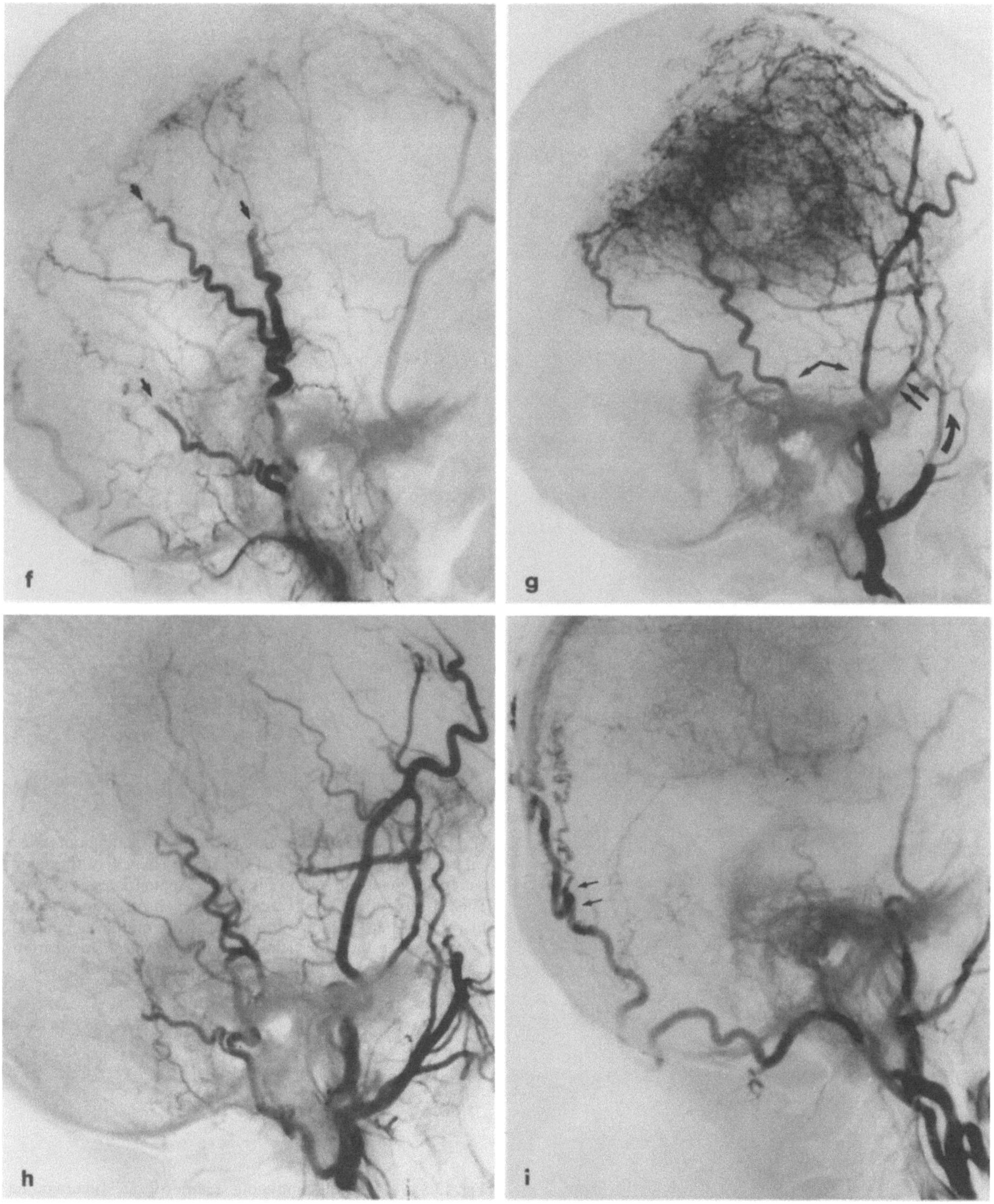

Fig. 13.1 a–i. Endotheliomatous convexity meningioma involving also the vault and extending extracranially. **a–c** CT. There is evident thickening of the calvarium with formation of spiculae. **d–i** Angiogram. There is rich vascularization by branches of the ICA and, particularly, ECA. **d** ICA. **e, f** Posterior auricular artery before and after embolization. **g, h** Middle meningeal *(parallel arrows)*, accessory meningeal *(curved arrow)* and superficial *(double arrow)* temporal arteries before and after embolization. **i** External carotid angiogram after embolization of the above demonstrated branches. There is still a small supply through the occipital artery *(parallel arrows)* which was embolized too

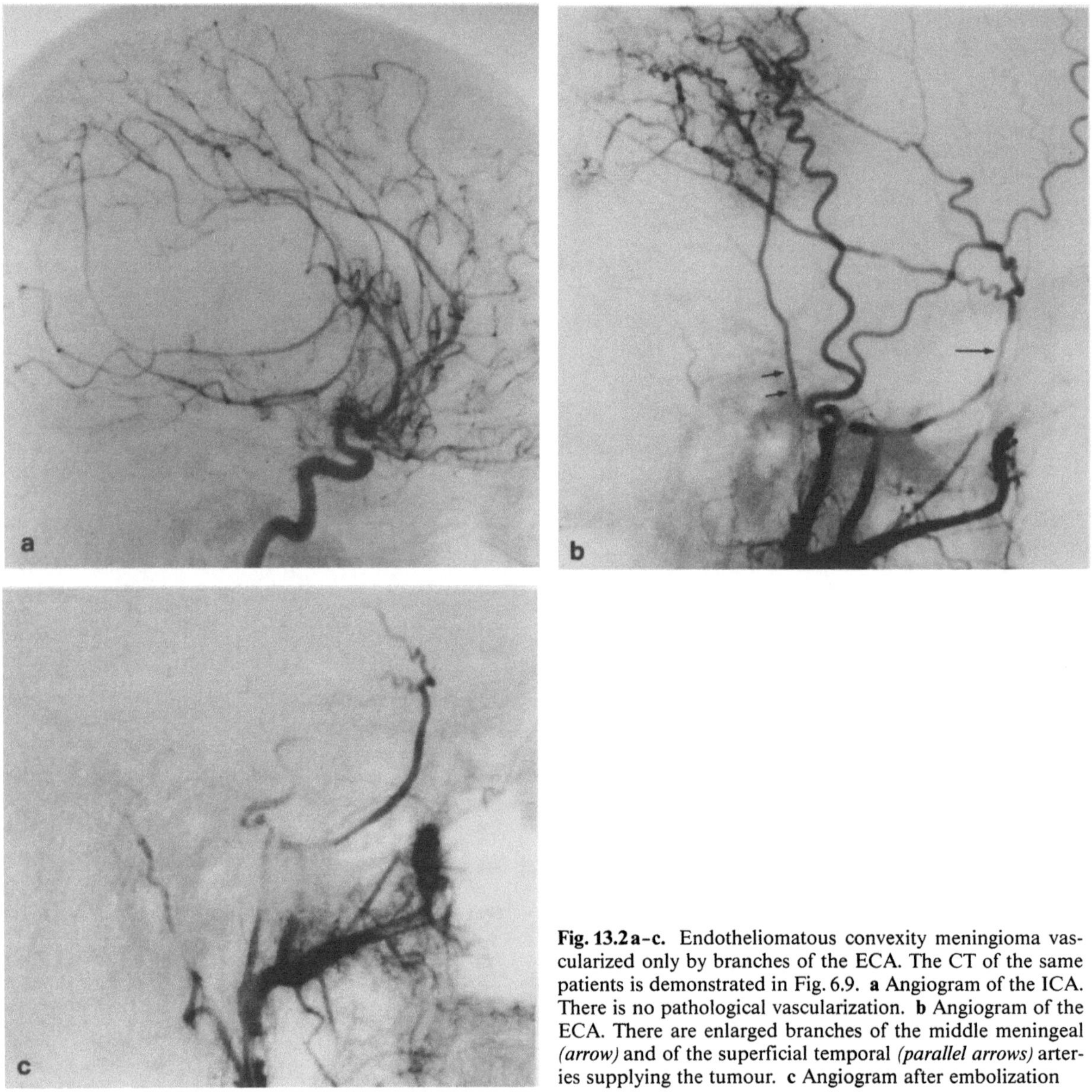

Fig. 13.2 a–c. Endotheliomatous convexity meningioma vascularized only by branches of the ECA. The CT of the same patients is demonstrated in Fig. 6.9. **a** Angiogram of the ICA. There is no pathological vascularization. **b** Angiogram of the ECA. There are enlarged branches of the middle meningeal *(arrow)* and of the superficial temporal *(parallel arrows)* arteries supplying the tumour. **c** Angiogram after embolization

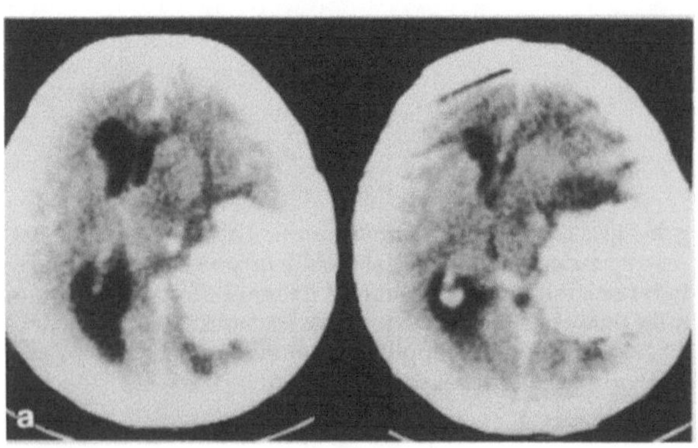

Fig. 13.3 a–c. Endotheliomatous temporobasal meningioma with attachment also to tentorium. The tumour is vascularized only by branches of the ECA. **a** CT study with contrast medium. **b** Angiogram of the common carotid artery. The tumour is supplied by the petrosquamous branch *(three parallel arrows)* of the middle meningeal artery and by the posterior auricular artery *(parallel arrows)*. **c** Angiogram after embolization of these two branches. The tumour appears now poorly vascularized

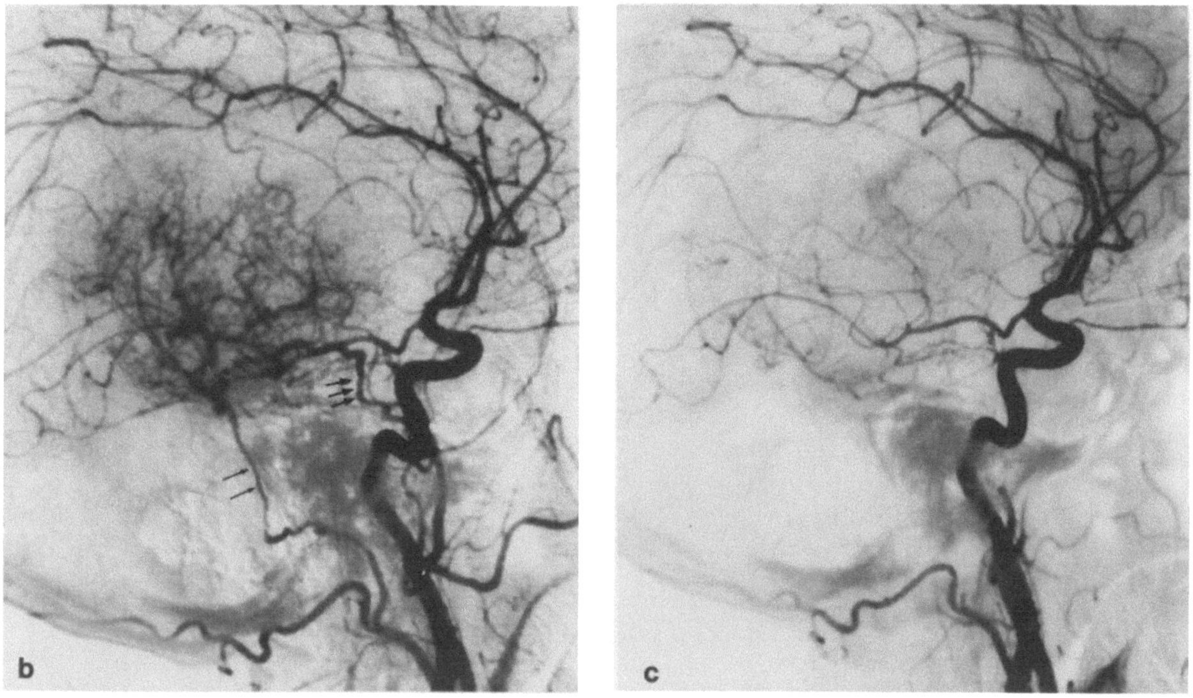

Fig. 13.3 b, c

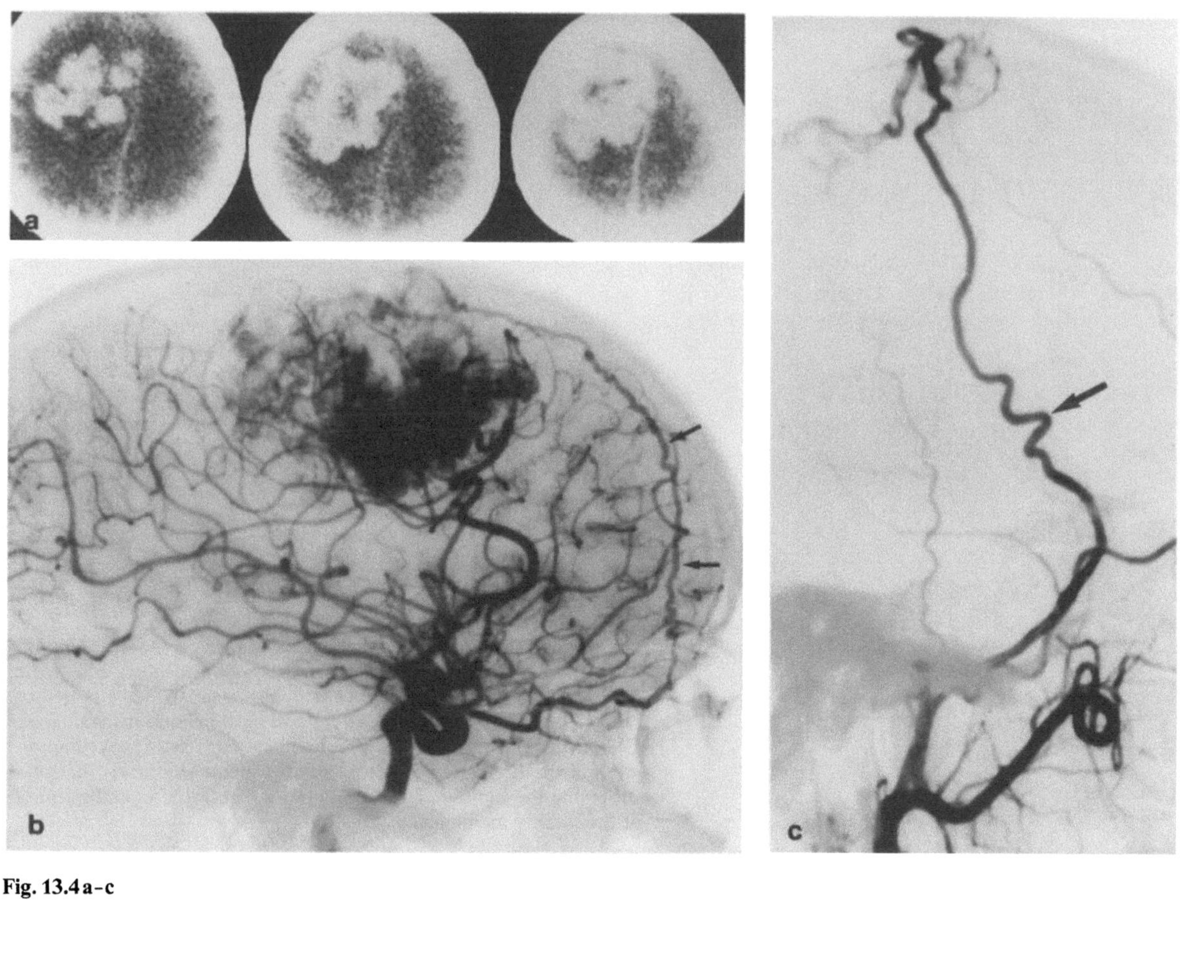

Fig. 13.4 a–c

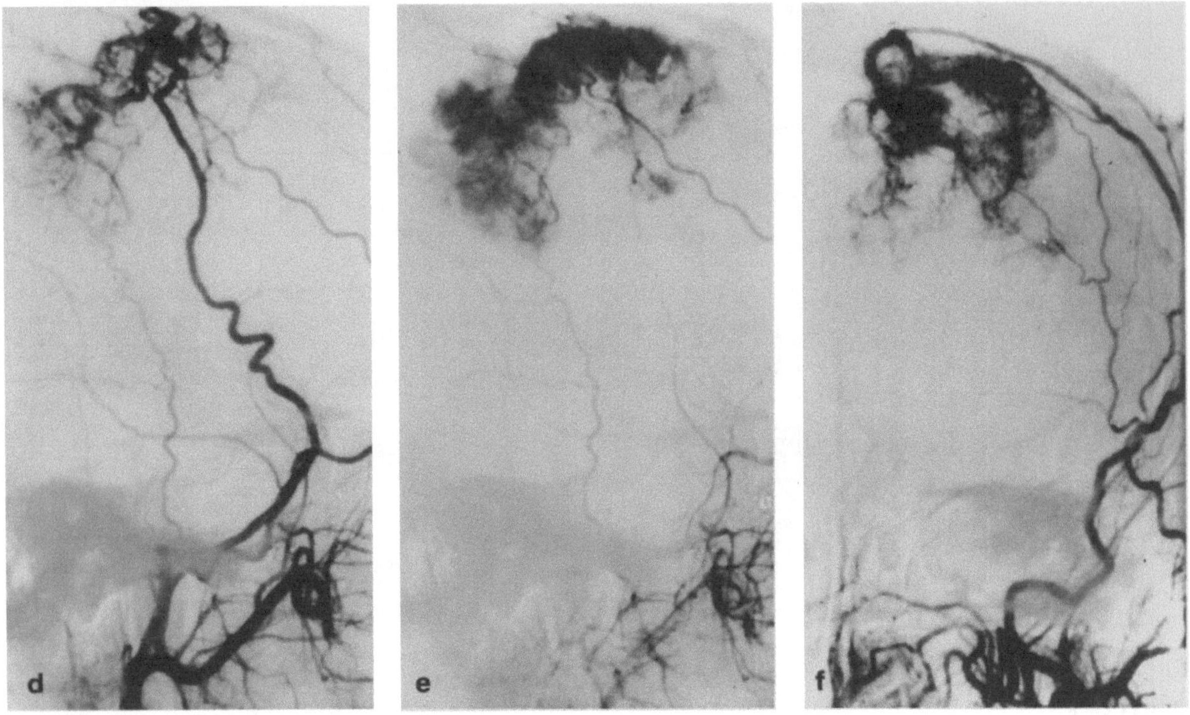

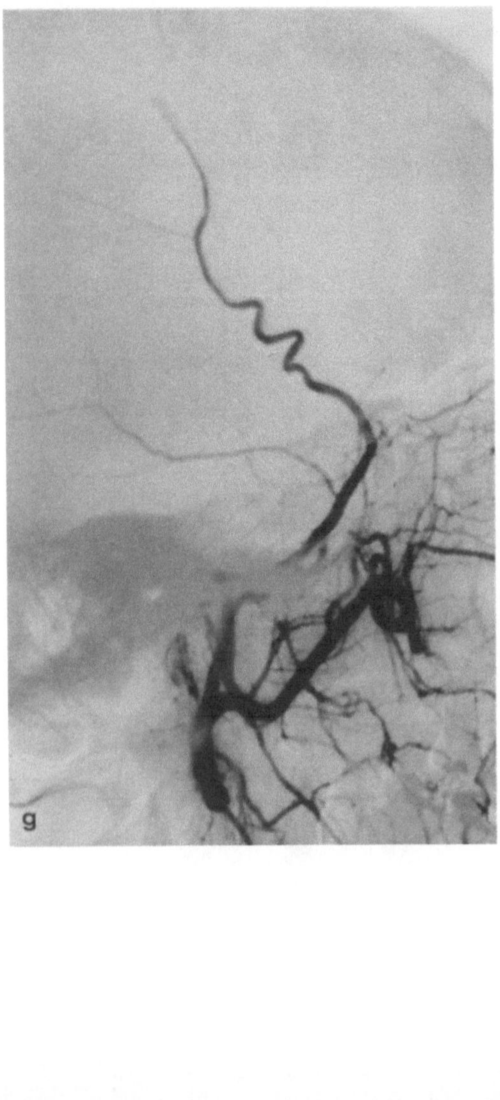

Fig. 13.4 a–g. Haemangiopericytic meningioma. **a** CT examination with contrast medium. Irregularly shaped tumour shows enhancement. **b** Angiogram. The tumour is richly vascularized, supplied by branches of anterior cerebral artery and by the anterior meningeal artery *(arrows)* branch of the ophthalmic artery. **c–f** On the angiogram of the ECA there is a large middle meningeal artery *(arrow)* supplying the tumour. **f** Frontal view. **g** Control after embolization of the middle meningeal artery

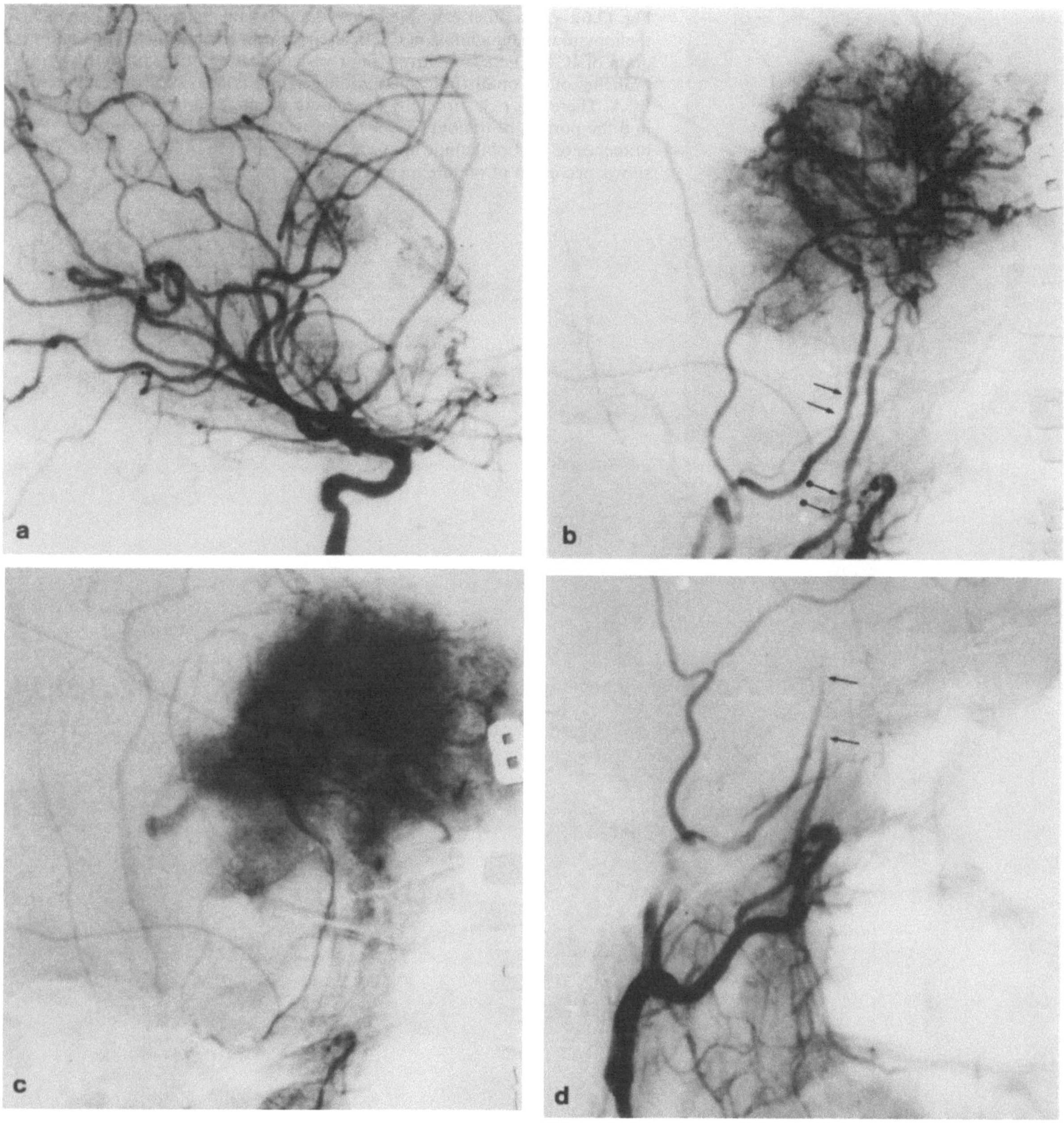

Fig. 13.5a-d. Endotheliomatous lateral sphenoid wing meningioma. **a** Angiogram of ICA. There is a poor pathological vascularization by branches of the ophthalmic and middle cerebral arteries. **b,c** Angiogram of ECA. The middle meningeal *(parallel arrows)* and deep temporal *(parallel arrows from circles)* arteries extensively supply the tumour. **d** Angiogram of ECA after embolization. Occlusion of the feeding arteries *(arrows)*

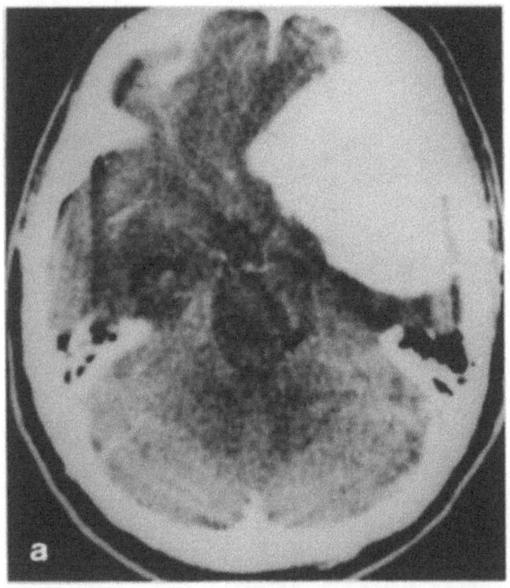

Fig. 13.6 a–e. Another example of very large lateral sphenoid wing endotheliomatous meningioma. **a** CT. There is strong enhancement. **b** Angiogram of ICA. There is relatively poor vascularization of the tumour by branches of the ophthalmic and middle cerebral arteries. **c, d** Angiogram of ECA. There is a rich supply by the middle meningeal artery *(arrows)*. Note in **d** the portion of tumour *(arrow from circle)* supplied by meningeal branches of the ophthalmic artery. **e** Angiogram of ECA after embolization shows occlusion of middle meningeal artery *(arrow)*

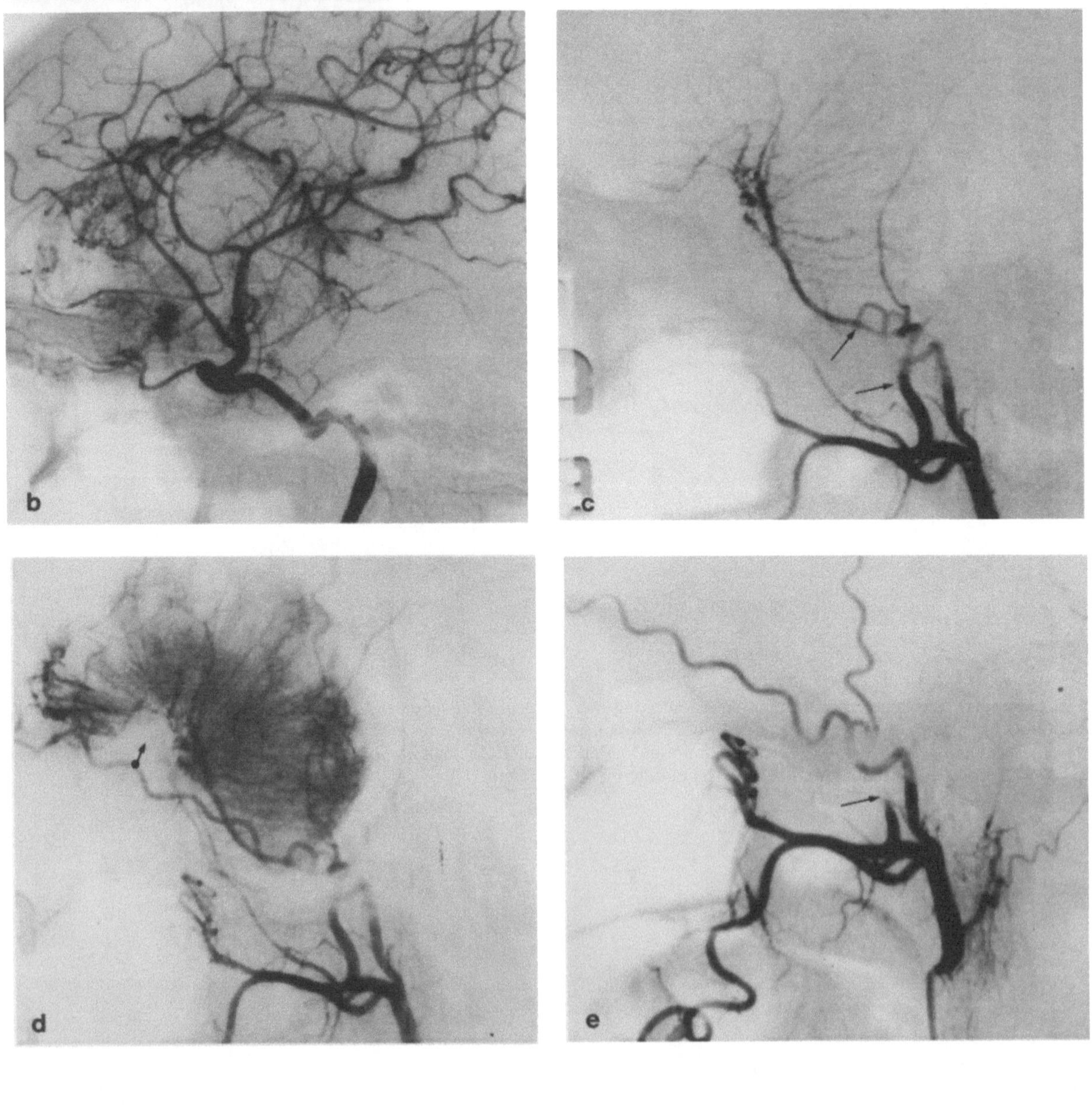

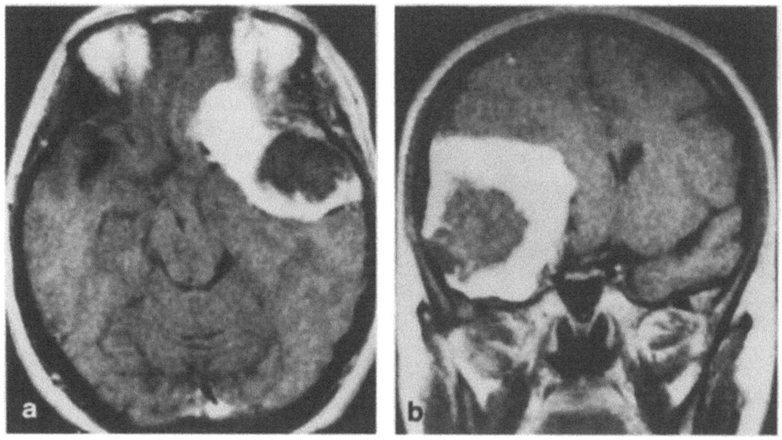

Fig. 13.7 a, b. Same patient demonstrated in Fig. 13.6. MRI with Gd-DTPA performed 24 h after the embolization. There is no longer enhancement in the central part of the tumour supplied by the middle meningeal artery

We use polyvinyl alcohol foam (Ivalon) microparticles (150-200; 300-500 mm). The emboli are not radio-opaque and so flow must be monitored during injection using contrast medium. The injection is made slowly to allow the blood flow to carry the particles distally and avoid reflux.

A few short angiographic series are performed during the procedure to stage the embolization in a controlled manner and to check for reflux and opening up any dangerous anastomoses which may preclude injection of further emboli. Ideally the procedure is terminated when the tumoral blush is no longer recognizable, which is normally associated with marked slowing of blood flow through or peripheral occlusion of the arteries feeding the tumours. However, flow conditions often make it wise to terminate earlier when a substantial reduction in vascularity has been achieved since further thrombosis often occurs in the embolized vessels. Surgery should be performed within a week of the embolization.

In meningiomas of the skull base, particularly cavernous sinus and medial sphenoid meningiomas, encasement of Internal carotid artery (ICA) can occur. This can make a total removal of the tumour very difficult or impossible. In such cases test of occlusion of the proximal intracavernous portion of ICA using a non-detachable balloon may be useful to assess tolerance [181]. Extraintracranial anastomosis should be considered prior to surgery if occlusion is not tolerated.

13.4 Results

The usefulness of embolization has been recently reported in a large series of meningiomas [181]. We have employed embolization in 55 meningiomas.

Table 1. Site of embolized meningiomas

Site	No. embolized
Falx	5
Parasagittal	7
Convexity	15
Sphenoid wing and middle cranial fossa	25
Petrous ridge-tentorial	1
Falx-tentorial	1
Cerebellar convexity	1

Of these, 47 were endotheliomatous, 3 were haemangiopericytic and the remaining 5 were of the haemangioblastic type. In most cases the supply was predominately from the ECA. The localization of tumours in our material is shown in Table 1 and examples are demonstrated in Figs. 13.1-13.8, 6.1, 6.3, 6.6, 8.1, 8.2.

13.4.1 Findings in Embolized Meningiomas

Low density areas indicating necrosis and reduction up to almost complete disappearance of the tumoral contrast enhancement have been described in about 50% of meningiomas examined by CT after embolization [181, 230, 238, 275]. In our series the frequency of changes on computed tomography (CT) and/or magnetic resonance imaging (MRI) after embolization was similar (Fig. 13.7). However, in some patients there was discrepancy between the postembolization angiogram showing a complete disappearance of the tumoral blush and CT in which little or no changes were recognizable. In such patients embolizations were still regarded as successful by the neurosurgeon because there was mild to minimal bleeding in the majority of them. The lack of change in postembolization CT can be

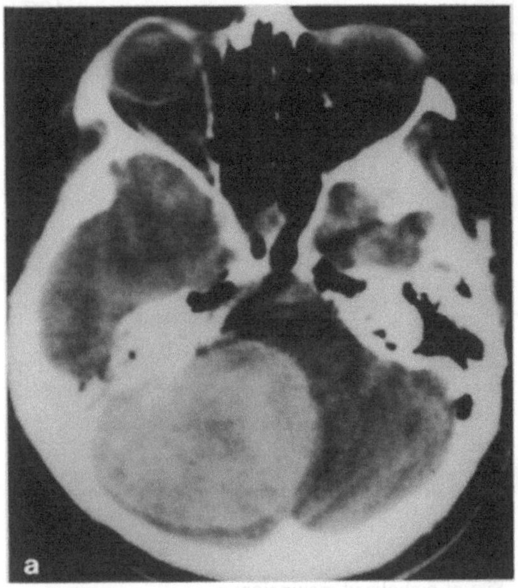

Fig. 13.8a–e. Very large endotheliomatous meningioma of the cerebellar convexity with extension in the cerebellopontine angle and encroaching on the sinudural angle. **a** CT shows richly enhanced tumour. **b–d** Angiogram. Selective study of the occipital artery, which gives off an enlarged meningeal-mastoid branch *(arrow)* supplying the tumour. **d** Drainage of the tumour mainly in the mastoid vein *(arrows)*. There was no additional supply of the tumour recognizable on the carotid and vertebral angiograms. **e** Angiogram. Postembolization study

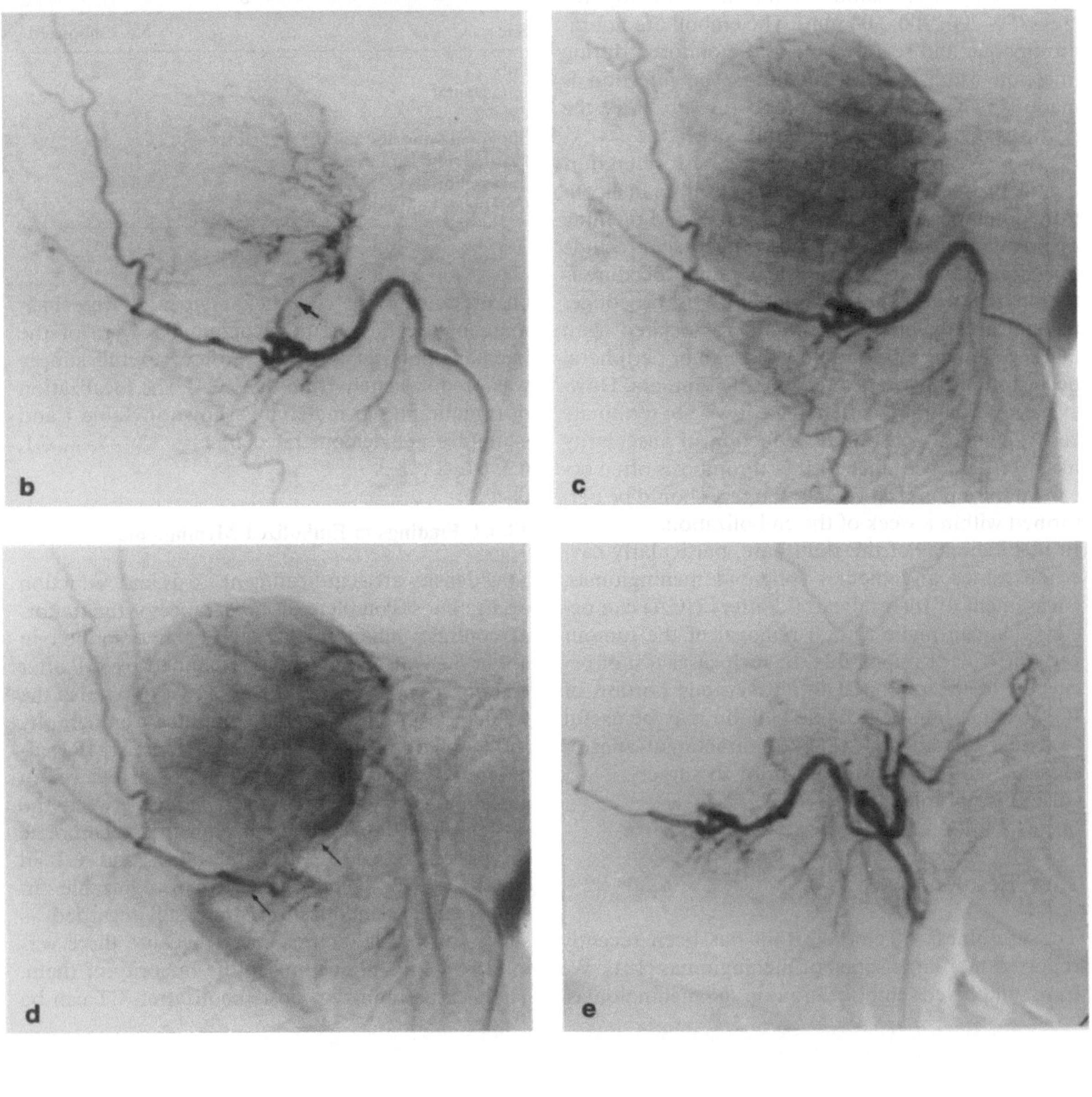

due in some patients to a presence of internal carotid supply [181, 275], and in others intratumoral necrosis may not have been visualized by CT though present at subsequent pathology [181]. Some authors [116] have described a decrease in the tumour mass, but this was not found by others [181] or in our material.

In all our patients the procedure was valuable in terms of the diminished intraoperative bleeding and ease of removal of the meningioma, particularly in tumours with a predominant supply from the ECA, which corroborates also the results of other authors [181, 275].

13.4.2 Recurrence of Embolized Meningiomas

It has been stated that embolization may be helpful in diminishing the rate of recurrence. This may occur through two mechanism; the first is the facilitated total removal of the tumour, the second is the occlusion of the nourishing meningeal branches entering the meningioma at the site of its dural attachment [181]. This latter hypothesis needs more confirmation.

13.4.3 Complications

Minor complications such as transient temporal or facial pain and trismus due to embolization of branches of IMA can occur. This was present in about 20% of our patients, which is in accordance also with other authors [140, 181].

Serious neurological complications due to passage of emboli into the carotid and vertebral circulation through reflux or anastomosis rarely occur [46, 73]. Cranial nerve palsy has been described [181]: it usually occurred when fluid embolic material was used, and this is not advised.

Finally, neurological complications may be linked to intratumoral changes occurring during or after embolization. A case of peri- and intratumoral haemorrhage has been reported during embolization of a haemangiopericytoma which was performed using Gelfoam [267]. This was attributed to the rupture of tumoral vessels proximal to the occlusion as a result of increased pressure. A similar event may have occurred in one of our patients (Fig. 13.4) with a richly vascularized haemangiopericytoma in whom a slight increase of paresis was recorded at the end of the embolization.

13.5 Conclusions

Embolization of highly vascular meningiomas may facilitate surgical treatment of these lesions. It is complementary to surgery, and the decision to perform preoperative embolization depends upon local facilities and on the requirements of the neurosurgeon in each individual case.

14 Surgical Perspective of Meningiomas

14.1 Historical Background

The first reliable description of a meningioma is that of Louis [173] although many descriptions of cranial hyperostosis predate that. Richard Bright [45] in his celebrated *Reports of Medical Cases* illustrates the post-mortem findings of a parasagittal meningioma, commenting "the tumour was a growth from the dura mater or rather perhaps from the arachnoid lining the dura mater".

The first successful removal of a tumour that may have been a meningioma was performed by Professor Pecchioli of Siena [cf. 98] in 1835: the tumour was described as a fungating tumour of the sinciput, and at operation the tumour, which involved skull and dura, was completely excised.

Harvey Cushing first operated on a cranial meningioma in 1908, however, his most celebrated case was the successful removal of a parasagittal meningioma in Major General Leonard Wood, the US Army Chief of Staff, in 1910. Wood was discharged from hospital 1 month later and led a vigorous public and political life thereafter. He developed signs of recurrence with occasional epilepsy in 1921 and finally died in 1927 following a further tumour removal by Cushing [cf. 168].

Cushing [66] first coined the term meningioma in his Cavendish Lecture of 1922 to avoid the confusing term endothelioma, which had been applied to a number of different tumours. In 1938 Cushing and Louise Eisenhardt in their classic book reported their experience with 313 cranial and spinal meningiomas [67].

14.2 Clinical Presentation and Individual Sites

Meningiomas present clinically by compressing adjacent brain or cranial nerves, causing focal neurological deficits or epilepsy, or by causing raised intracranial pressure either by their size and associated cerebral oedema or, in the case of posterior fossa meningiomas, obstructive hydrocephalus. Tumours adjacent to the sensory motor cortex present either with epilepsy or focal neurological deficit. Occasionally the deficit can occur in a stepwise manner mimicking vascular transient ischaemia attacks. Cranial nerve palsies are seen most commonly in suprasellar meningiomas (optic chiasm/nerve) and in posterior fossa meningiomas (cranial nerves V–XII).

Meningiomas are conventionally classified according to their site of origin into: convexity, parasagittal, falx, basal, posterior fossa and intraventricular. Within all the major divisions are subdivisions, again based on the anatomical origin of the tumour (see Chap. 1). The majority of the large series of meningiomas were reported in the pre-CT scan era when the clinical syndromes are likely to be much more advanced that is seen today. However, even today meningiomas still attain considerable size, compressing silent areas of the brain before they present, and the clinical syndromes presented in these early papers still have relevance today.

14.2.1 Convexity Meningiomas

Cushing and Eisenhardt [67] subdivided the group of convexity meningiomas into seven anatomical subdivisions according to the site of origin of the

Table 1. Symptoms at presentation from 54 convexity meningiomas [67]

Site of origin No.	Headaches (%)	Visual failure (%)	Epilepsy (%)	Focal limb motor deficit (%)
Precoronal (5)	60	40	40	40
Coronal (17)	59	65	29	47
Postcoronal (7)	43	29	43	70
Paracentral (9)	56	22	100	89
Parietal (12)	33	42	100	33
Temporosylvian (4)	75	25	100	25

tumour: (1) precoronal, (2) coronal, (3) postcoronal, (4) paracentral, (5) parietal, (6) occipital (of which he had no examples) and (7) temporosylvian. They noted that in their series 30% of the convexity meningiomas were of coronal origin. As can be seen from Table 1 the incidence of epilepsy increases to 100% and the occurrence of focal motor deficit to 89% in tumours close to the sensory motor cortex; concurrently, the incidence of visual failure secondary to raised intracranial pressure falls. Although in more current series the incidence of raised intracranial pressure is likely to be much lower due to the earlier investigation and treatment of these tumours, the underlying trend is the same.

14.2.2 Parasagittal and Falx Meningiomas

Olivecrona [211] subdivided parasagittal and falx meningiomas into anterior, central and posterior according to the site of attachment to the sagittal sinus or falx. He felt the division justified because of the different presentation at the different sites as well as the different surgical approach required: subsequent authors have followed the logic of this subdivision. Parasagittal meningiomas are defined as those tumours with any attachment to the superior sagittal sinus, whereas falx meningiomas arise from the falx only. Cushing and Eisenhardt [67] reported a relative incidence of 90% parasagittal to 10% falx, whereas the report by Hoessly and Olivecrona [119] as well as that of Gautier-Smith [95] recorded a relative incidence of approximately 70% parasagittal tumours to 30% falx tumours. The difference in the relative incidence reported almost certainly reflects judgments by the authors as to whether or not the attachment involves the sagittal sinus rather than any true variation between the series. In Gautier-Smith's [95] series headache was a very frequent presenting symptom in all lesions. The commonest clinical sign was dementia for the anterior and poterior parasagittal tumours (71%), occurring slightly less in the anterior and posterior falx tumours. Epilepsy was commonest presenting symptom for central tumours: 44% in the parasagittal tumours and 27% in the falx lesions. Pyramidal weakness was present in 77% of the central parasagittal and in 96% of central falx meningiomas. Papilloedema was also very frequent in all the lesions.

14.2.3 Basal Meningiomas

Basal meningiomas may be subdivided into (1) anterior frontobasal meningiomas (crista galli, olfactory groove, orbital roof), (2) posterior frontobasal (tuberculum sellae, planum sphenoidale, dorsum sellae), (3) medial sphenoid wing, (4) lateral sphenoid wing, (5) cavernous sinus and Meckel's cave and (6) superior surface of tentorium. Clearly the last group will overlap with the posterior fossa tumours, but this is unavoidable. Many surgeons would include a subgroup arising from the floor of the middle fossa, however, we feel that this group overlaps other adjacent subgroups.

14.2.3.1 Anterior Frontobasal Meningiomas

Anterior frontobasal tumours usually remain clinically silent, as do other frontal tumours, until they attain a considerable size. They usually arise from the junction of the cribriform plate and the planum sphenoidale, according to Cushing and Eisenhardt [67]. Epilepsy, visual failure and psychological change are the dominant clinical features of the presentation [268], of which visual failure is the commonest. Loss of olfaction is not a symptom frequently noted by patients; in only three patients was loss of olfaction the presenting symptom in Cushing's series of 29 meningiomas of this type, although it was affected unilaterally in 20% and bilaterally in 66% of patients on clinical testing.
Symon [268] noted the sense of smell was recorded as being present in four of eight patients of massive bilateral tumours at initial presentation in his series. As Symon comments, the reason for this is most likely to be the difficulty in testing pure smell clinically, especially in patients with clinical dementia. The commonest symptom is asymmetrical visual loss, usually reported as blurred vision in one eye due to a central scotoma. The classical Foster Kennedy [144] syndrome is uncommon today, occurring in 25% of patients in Cushing's series, but only 1 out of 40 patients in Symon's more recent series. Some 30% of patients present with epilepsy, which is almost always grand mal. Minor psychological symptoms of frontal lobe dysfunction occur commonly; major psychological disturbance occurs rarely, although even today patients present from psychiatric institutions.

14.2.3.2 Posterior Frontobasal Meningiomas

Posterior frontobasal tumours commonly arise from the planum sphenoidale. In contradistinction to the olfactory groove meningiomas, these tumours commonly present when much smaller because of their close proximity to the optic nerves. The commonest presenting symptom is visual failure, usually associated with headache; epilepsy and psychological changes are uncommon. Gregorus et al. [104] analysed the visual loss in 23 suprasellar meningiomas. They noted that associated headache was a feature in 65% of patients. The presenting subjective visual failure consisted of gradual or fluctuating visual loss in one eye, followed later by loss of central acuity in the other eye. In the 16 patients from whom information was available, the time between onset of unilateral visual loss to subjective bilateral loss was 1 year or less in seven patients, 3 years or more in seven patients and 8 years in one: in the other patient the time could not be determined. On assessing the patients' vision objectively, 20 of 23 had signs of visual impairment in both eyes. Three patients had unilateral field defects: the commonest field defect was an asymmetrical, bitemporal field loss, and classical symmetrical bitemporal haemianopsia was seen in only three patients. Four patients had a central or paracentral scotoma in one eye associated with a temporal or nasal field defect in the other. Optic atrophy was the commonest finding on funduscopical examination. Following surgery, the three eyes that were completely blind preoperatively showed no improvement. Of the 35 eyes in which postoperative results could be assessed, 22 of the 35 fields were improved and five patients had full return of a field in at least one eye. Visual acuity improved in 21 of the 35 eyes, was unchanged in 9 and worse in 5.

14.2.3.3 Medial Sphenoid Ridge Meningioma

Tumours of the medial sphenoid ridge arise from the medial sphenoid ridge or the anterior clinoid process. They can be broadly divided into two main groups. In one group they present as masses compressing or encircling the internal carotid artery (ICA) and middle cerebral artery and branches and compressing the optic nerve. These usually present with unilateral visual failure or epilepsy. In the second group the tumours grow diffusely, en plaque meningioma, in the region of the anterior clinoid process medial sphenoid wing and cavernous sinus and can present with optic nerve compression, third nerve palsy, superior orbital fissure syndrome or proptosis due to extension into the orbit and/or hyperostosis. This second group accounts for ca. 30% of all medial sphenoid ridge meningioma [62]. In both types of tumour, radical excision is usually impossible.

14.2.3.4 Lateral Sphenoid Ridge Meningioma

The lateral sphenoid ridge meningiomas overlap with the convexity tumours and differ from the medial sphenoid wing tumours in that they usually do not involve the ICA of proximal middle cerebral artery or the optic nerve, but may, of course, involve the peripheral branches of the middle cerebral artery. Proptosis due to extension into the orbit and/or hyperostosis can occur. They usually present with epilepsy or limb weakness due to compression of the adjacent motor cortex.

14.2.3.5 Cavernous Sinus and Meckel's Cave Meningiomas

The typical clinical symptom of lesions in the cavernous sinus or Meckel's cave is a varying early involvement of cranial nerves (III, IV, V, VI) present in the cavernous space. Progressive impairment of visual acuity may occur. This is due either to anterior extension of the tumour with involvement of the optic nerve or to progressive stenosis of the cavernous portion of internal carotid and ophthalmic arteries. High definition computed tomography (CT) and, particularly well, magnetic resonance imaging (MRI) [38] are very useful diagnostic methods to discover these lesions early and to improve their management.

Total surgical removal of these meningiomas is impossible.

The treatment of these lesions has been considered recently in a review by Lesoin et al. [166]. According to the extension and grading of the tumour, surgery associated with radiotherapy, radiotherapy alone or no therapy has been proposed.

14.2.3.6 Superior Surface of Tentorium

Guidetti et al. [108] reviewing their series of 61 tentorial meningiomas, of which 23 were purely supratentorial and 13 were both supra- and infratentorial, found the commonest presenting symptom to be headache (40%), with 20% of the patients with supratentorial meningioma presenting with epilepsy and 16% of all patients presenting with a psychiatric disturbance. Papilloedema was present in 63% of their patients and fifth to twelfth nerve plasies were also reported, presumably associated with posterior fossa extensions of the tumours.

14.2.4 Posterior Fossa Meningiomas

Lesions of the posterior fossa can be subdivided into (1) posterior surface of petrous bone, (2) tentorium, (3) clivus and (4) cerebellar convexity. In Yasargil et al.'s series [303] of basal posterior fossa meningiomas the average length of history before presentation was 4 years, ranging from 4 months to 16 years. Meningiomas arising from the petrous bone and the clivus as well as medial tentorial meningiomas can cause a wide range of cranial nerve palsies. Involvement of cranial nerve V occurs in more than half of the patients, nerve VIII involvement in about half and nerve VII involvement (usually only mild) in just less than half of the patients. The distinction between a cerebellopontine angle (CPA) meningioma and the more common acoustic neuroma is not possible on clinical grounds alone. However, CPA meningiomas tend to involve cranial nerves V and VII more than acoustic neuromas and less often involve cranial nerve VIII. In particular, preservation of the caloric responses in the presence of CPA tumours increase the likelihood of a meningioma. As pointed out by Yasargil et al. [303] and recently confirmed by Mayberg and Symon [189] cranial nerves III, IV and VI were rarely affected symptomatically in spite of their frequent involvement by tumour mass. Involvement of the lower cranial nerves is unusual. Other frequent symptoms in meningioma of posterior fossa are ataxia due to compression of brain stem and/or cerebellum and signs of increased intracranial pressure due to obstructive hydrocephalus.

Meningiomas encroaching into the foramen mangum are very rare. There are no symptoms pathognomonic of a tumour in this area. Pain in the cervical and occipital regions which may be exacerbated by flexion of the neck, coughing and straining is frequent. Sensory and motor symptoms as well as involvement of lower cranial nerves follow [199, 303].

14.2.5 Intraventricular Meningiomas

Intraventricular meningiomas are very rare lesions. Tumours located in the third and fourth ventricles usually present with symptoms of increased intracranial pressure due to hydrocephalus, without localizing neurological deficit. In meningiomas of the lateral ventricle a controlateral hemiparesis is also frequent.

14.2.6 Intraorbital Meningiomas

Progressive decrease of visual acuity associated with a varying degree of proptosis and impairment of ocular motility are the typical symptomas of intraorbital meningiomas. Today they can easily be well investigated with high definition CT and/or MRI.

14.3 Surgical Technique

Surgical removal is the principal, and in most cases the only form of treatment of a meningioma. The aim of surgery is to excise the tumour in its entirety along with its dural attachment and any overlying infiltrated bone. If this can be achieved, then the risk of recurrence of most meningiomas is very low (see Sect. 14.4). Where excision of the dural attachment is impossible, then coagulation with diathermy is undertaken. The ideal treatment is nearly always possible with convexity tumours, but it is often impossible for tumours arising at other sites. In addition to CT scanning, angiography is important in the preoperative surgical assessment of most meningiomas. It indicates the source of the primary blood supply of the tumour as well as an assessment of its vascularity so that preoperative embolization (Chap. 13) can be undertaken if appropriate. In addition the venous phase is important in assessing the patency of major venous sinuses and the proximity of large cortical veins whose preservation will minimize postoperative brain swelling.

The poor positioning of a bone flap can change an operation for removal of a meningioma from a relatively easy technical exercise into an extremely difficult or impossible one. CT scans with external markers can minimize this risk and in some cases are a valuable additional investigation.

14.3.1 New Surgical Techniques

The underlying principle of meningioma surgical excision is to debulk the centre of the tumour before developing a plane between the tumour and the surrounding brain so that total excision can be achieved. If the meningioma is soft and avascular, the debulking can be readily achieved using conventional suction. If, however, the tumour is fibrous, then this is more difficult, and cutting diathermy is often necessary with an increased risk of damage to surrounding structures. Over the last 10 years two particularly useful additional surgical tools have become available, the ultrasonic surgical aspirator and the laser. The ultrasonic surgical aspirator, of which the CUSA is the most widely used example in the UK, is a suction device with a tip that vibrates at 23 kHz. This causes fragmentation of tissue within 1-2 mm of the vibrating tip, which can then be aspirated by irrigation and suction in the same instrument. In practice meningiomas can be excised by the ultrasonic surgical aspirator with less brain manipulation, and tumours that are too fibrous to be removed by simple suction can be removed. However, its use is limited, and some meningiomas are too fibrous even for this instrument. The CO_2 laser is the commonest laser in clinical neurosurgery. This produces light in the infrared range at 10.6 μ. At this wavelength there is total absorption of the light by the surface cellular layer, leading to intracellular water vaporization, and thus removal of tissue without touch or manipulation [245]. This has led a number of surgeons to advocate use of this in the removal of meningiomas, especially basal and posterior fossa meningiomas [279]. Unfortunately, the rate of tissue vaporization is slow, and the laser fails to coagulate all but the smallest vessels, significantly limiting its value so that only relatively few surgeons use it today. More powerful lasers are becoming available that may increase the rate of tissue vaporization.

The Nd: YAG laser is far less generally available. This produces light in the near-infrared range, principally at 1060 nm. Light at this wavelength significantly penetrates tissues, causing an area of coagulative damage up to aproximately 0.5-1 cm below the surface [289]. This laser is a much better blood vessel coagulator and has been used by a number of neurosurgeons in the surgical excision of arterio-venous malformations (AVM's) [290], but has not gained widespread use in tumour neurosurgery because of the potential associated damage to normal brain.

14.3.2 Adjuvant Therapy

14.3.2.1 Radiotherapy

The commonest, and in the majority of centres the only form of adjuvant therapy used for meningiomas, is radiotherapy. There is still doubt as to the efficacy of this form of treatment among some neurosurgeons. The best support for its use comes from a paper by Wara et al. [286], who reviewed retrospectively 213 meningiomas treated at University of California, San Francisco. Of the 104 patients that had subtotal removal of the tumour 58 did not receive postoperative irradiation: the recurrence rate in these patients was 74%. 34 patients underwent subtotal resection of tumour followed as soon as the wound has healed by post-operative radiotherapy. There was a 29% recurrence rate with over half the recurrences appearing within the first 5 years. Yamashita et al. [302] reviewed the effect of radiotherapy on meningiomas that had multiple recurrences. In four of the seven patients in this group radiotherapy did not prolong the time to further recurrence: in two patients the effect of radiotherapy was regarded as equivocal and in one it appeared to significantly slow down the rate of recurrence. They concluded that radiotherapy for recurrent meningiomas was generally of little value.

In contrast, positive results have been reported by Carella et al. [52] in the treatment of subtotal excised and inoperable meningiomas. Lesoin et al. [166] in a study on cavernous meningiomas also showed positive results obtained with radiotherapy in the treatment of these lesions. Finally, Barbaro et al. [14] in a recent work about the efficacy of radiation therapy on partially resected meningiomas report 32% of recurrence in irradiated and 60% in nonirradiated tumours. These results confirm previous studies and seem to provide convincing evidence that radiation therapy is beneficial in the treatment of subtotally resected meningiomas. Radiotherapy has also been advocated as preoperative adjuvant treatment to reduce the size and vascularity of some meningiomas. Fukui et al. [91] concluded on the basis of their results and a review of the literature that preoperative radiotherapy may be helpful in the treatment of haemangiopericytomas only. This is further supported by the case report of Takase and Watanabe [270] of a dramatic response of a parasagittal haemangiopericytoma to radiotherapy; one of the authors has seen a similarly dramatic response to radiotherapy in a recurrent parasagittal haemangiopericytoma.

14.3.2.2 Hormonal Therapy

Only a limited number of reports are available on the use of hormonal therapy in the treatment of meningiomas. From our knowledge (Chap. 1., Sect. 1.8.4) of the receptor status of most meningiomas, an antiprogestagen would be likely to be most effective. Unfortunately, pure antiprogestagens that can be administered clinically are not available. Up to now reports on the use of hormonal therapy in a clinical setting [127, 185, 186] have failed to demonstrate any benefit.

14.4 Prognosis

The problem of recurrence of meningioma has been already discussed in Chap. 1 (Sect. 1.5). We briefly describe in this section a few other aspects which influence recurrence such the grade of removal, follow-up analysis and location of the tumour.

14.4.1 Degree of Surgical Removal

Simpson [257] in his classic paper, was the first to address the problem of recurrence in a systematic

Table 2. Recurrence-free percentage of patients from Simpson [257], Adegbite et al. [2] and Gautier-Smith [95]

Surgical grade	Simpson [257]	Adegbite et al. [2]		Gautier-Smith [95]
		5 years	10 years	
1	91%	86%	78%	83%
2	81%	82%	72%	83%
3	71%	-	-	-
4	56%	48%	32%	-

way. He concluded that the degree of surgical removal of the tumour which frequently corresponds to its site was the most important determinant of recurrence.

Simpson [257] classified the degree of surgical removal into five groups:

Grade 1: complete macroscopic removal of tumour and dural attachment with any abnormal bone

Grade 2: complete macroscopic removal of tumour with diathermy coagulation of its dural attachment

Grade 3: complete macroscopic removal of intradural tumour without resection or coagulation of its dural attachment or of any extradural extensions

Grade 4: partial removal leaving intradural tumour in site

Grade 5: simple decompression with or without biopsy

Tabulation of these results along with those of Gautier-Smith [95] and Adegbite et al. [2] is shown in Table 2. It can be seen here, especially from Adegbite's results, that there was a significant difference between the combined recurrence-free percentage of grades 1 and 2 and grade 4, but no statistical difference between grades 1 and 2.

More recently Mirimanoff et al. [200] studied recurrence, taking into consideration the type of tumoral removal and varying follow-up times. He found an actuarial recurrence-free rate of 93%, 80% and 68%, respectively, at 5, 10 and 15 years following total excision of the meningioma and a progression-free rate following incomplete removal of 63%, 45% and 9% over similar time periods: the difference rates of recurrence of totally excised tumours and of progression of subtotally excised lesions were statistically significant ($P < 0.0001$).

14.4.2 Site of Meningioma

Site indirectly affects the likelihood of recurrence; sites with a higher incidence of complete excision, for example cortical meningiomas, have a lower incidence of tumour recurrence. This is due both to a higher incidence of total excision and also a higher degree of certainty that a total excision has been achieved. Mirimanoff et al. [200] found 96% of convexity meningiomas were removed in toto and the recurrence/progression rate at 5 years was only 3%. In contrast, in meningiomas of the sphenoid ridge total removal was possible in 28% of patients and at 5 years the probability of recurrence/progression was 34%. Between these two extreme groups, intermediate risk was found in parasagittal, parasellar, posterior fossa meningioma with a recurrence/progression rate, respectively, of 18%, 19%, 22% at 5 years.

Conclusion

1. Meningiomas are extra-axial intracranial and/or intraspinal tumours. Less than 1% grow outside the central nervous system. Meningiomas originate from arachnoid cells and occur considerably more frequently in middle-aged women. They are generally benign, but malignant forms occur with a preponderance in men. In the uncommon childhood meningiomas, the sexes are equally affected.
2. Most meningiomas have typical computed tomography (CT) and histopathological features and present no difficulty in diagnosis. Further diagnostic precision has come with magnetic resonance imaging (MRI), in which the anatomical relations of the tumour can be even better evaluated than on CT, and en plaque meningiomas as well as en plaque portions of globoid tumours are usually shown; highly vascularized tumours and the relationships of major vessels including the dural sinuses are often recognizable. Nevertheless, angiography is often performed to show these features and can help establish the correct preoperative diagnosis when CT and MRI are atypical.
3. Hyperostosis and peritumoral oedema are the most conspicuous effect of meningiomas on adjacent structures. The pathogenesis of oedema is not completely clear, but it seems certain that the tumour participates actively in its production.
4. Recurrence after surgery and sometimes metastases occur. Recurrence probably is due to incomplete surgical removal of the tumour, though it does occur after apparent total macroscopic excision. Radiological, cytohistological and metabolic features which suggest malignancy are present in some of these patients, but not in all.
5. In spite of recent progress in radiology, cytohistology, cytochemistry and biological behaviour, knowledge about meningiomas remains incomplete. The basic treatment of these tumours is surgical excision: mortality and morbidity is still relatively frequent, and excision is partial in many cases. Adjuvant therapies include preoperative embolization for highly vascular tumours and radiation therapy for inoperable and malignant lesions; endocrine therapy based on discovery of sex steroid receptors in meningiomas has also been used, although clear evidence of clinical benefit has not yet been demonstrated.

References

1. Abbott KH, Courville CB (1942) Intraventricular meningiomas. A review of the literature and report of two cases. Bull Los Angeles Neurol Soc 7: 12
2. Adegbite AB, Khan MI, Paine KWE, Tan LK (1983) The recurrence of intracranial meningiomas after surgical treatment. J Neurosurg 58: 51
3. Al-Mefty O, Fox JL, Smith RR (1988) Petrosal approach for petroclival meningiomas. Neurosurgery 22: 510
4. Alp H, Ceviker N, Baykaner K, Orbay T (1985) Giant meningioma in a fourteen-month-old infant. Surg Neurol 24: 77
5. Amano K, Miura N, Yasuhito T, et al. (1980) Cystic meningioma in a 10 month-old infant. J Neurosurg 52: 829
6. Andrews BT, Wilson CT (1988) Suprasellar meningiomas: the effect of tumor location on postoperative visual outcome. J Neurosurg 69: 523
7. Aron-Rosa D, Laloi M, Man HX, et al. (1977) Tumeur double méningiome et melanome malin de la choroide associés (à propos d'un cas). Bull Soc Ophthalmol Fr 77: 895
8. Auman N, Dincer C (1978) Meningiomas of the third ventricle. Acta Neurochir (Wien) 41: 217
9. Azar-Kia B, Sarwar M, Marc JA, Schechter MN (1974) Intraosseous meningioma. Neuroradiology 6: 246
10. Baethmann A, Oettinger W, Rothenfuber W, et al. (1980) Brain edema factors: current state with particular reference to plasma constituents and glutamate. Adv Neurol 28: 171-196
11. Bagchi AK, Sen Gupta KP (1969) Primary nasal meningioma. J Indian Med Assoc 523: 286
12. Bailey P, Bucy PC (1931) The origin and nature of meningeal tumors. Am J Cancer 15: 15
13. Baker HL, Houser OW, Campbell JK (1980) National Cancer Institute study evaluation of computed tomography in diagnosis of intracranial neoplasms. I. Overall results. Radiology 136: 91
14. Barbaro NM, Gutin PH, Wilson CB, Sheline GE, Boldrey EB, Wara WM (1987) Radiation therapy in the treatment of partially resected meningiomas. Neurosurgery 20: 525
15. Barloon TJ, Yuh WTC, de Marino DP, Maves MD, Godersky JC, Dolan KD (1987) Infratemporal fossa meningiomas: CT and MR findings. Case report. J Comput Assist Tomogr 11: 1050
16. Barnes D, McDonald WI, Tofts PS, et al. (1986) Magnetic resonance imaging of experimental cerebral oedema. J Neurol Neurosurg Psychiatry 49: 1341-1347
17. Barrows HS, Harter DH (1962) Tentorial meningiomas. J Neurol Neurosurg Psychiatry 25: 40
18. Bar-Sella P, Front D, Peyser E, Talmon A, Israel O, Nir I (1981) Correlation between radionuclides uptake and ultrastructural features of tight junctions in the capillary wall of meningiomas. J Neurol Neurosurg Psychiatry 44: 1024
19. Bazin A, Scherpereel B, Rousseaux P, Bernard MH, Peruzzi P, Baudrillard JC, Delattre JF (1988) Méningiomes du canal optique. Réflexions diagnostiques à propos de trois cas opérés. Neurochirurgie 34: 164
20. Belal A (1955) Meningioma infiltrating the nasal cavity, nasal sinuses and the orbit. J Laryngol 69: 59
21. Bellon G, Caulet T, Cam Y, et al. (1985) Immunohistochemical localisation of macromolecules of the basement membrane and extracellular matrix of human gliomas and meningiomas. Acta Neuropathol (Berl) 66: 245
22. Berry J, Brant-Zawadsky M, Osaki L, et al. (1986) Gd-DTPA in clinical MR of the brain. II. Extraaxial lesions and normal structures. AJNR 7: 789
23. Bickerstaff ER, Small JM, Guest IA (1958) The relasping course of certain meningiomas in relation to pregnancy an menstruation. J Neurol Neurosurg Psychiatry 21: 89
24. Bingas B (1974) Tumours of the skull base. In: Vinken PO, Bruyn N (eds) Handbook of clinical neurology, vol 17. North-Holland, Amsterdam, p 136
25. Blankenstein MA, Blaasnw G, Lamberts SWJ, et al. (1983) Presence of progesterone receptors and absence of estrogen receptors in human intracranial meningioma cytosols. Eur J Cancer Clin Oncol 19: 365
26. Bloomgarden GM, Byrne TN, Spencer DD, Heafner MD (1987) Meningioma associated with aneurysm and subarachnoid Hemorrhage: Case Report and review of the literature. Neurosurgery 20: 24
27. Bogdanowicz WM, Sachs E Jr (1974) The possible role of radiation in oncogenesis of meningioma. Surg Neurol 2: 379
28. Bonnal J, Thibaut A, Brotchi J, Born J (1980) Invading meningiomas of the sphenoid ridge. J Neurosurg 53: 587
29. Bonneville JF, Cattin F, Bouchareb M (1987) Dynamic CT scanning of the caverous sinus. In: Dolenc V (ed) The cavernous sinus. Springer, Berlin Heidelberg New York
30. Borovich B, Doron Y (1986) Recurrence of intracranial meningiomas: The role played by regional multicentricity. J Neurosurg 64: 58
31. Borovich B, Doron Y, Braun Y, et al. (1986) Recurrence of intracranial meningiomas: The role played by regional multicentricity. II. Clinical and radiological aspects. J Neurosurg 65: 168
32. Boylan SE, McCunniff AJ (1988) Recurrent meningioma. Cancer 61: 1447
33. Bradac GB (1976) Some aspects of the venous drainage dynamics with tumors at the base of the skull in the anterior and middle fossae. Neuroradiology 12: 115

34. Bradac GB, Schramm J (1981) Principles in the computed tomography study of pathologic changes of the skull base. In: Félix R, Kerzner E, Wegener OH (eds) Contrast media in computed tomography. Exerpta Medica, Amsterdam
35. Bradac GB, Schramm J, Kaernbach A (1981) Traumatic exophthalmos due to an uncommon arteriovenous fistula without involvement of the cavernous sinus. Case report. J Neurosurg 55: 993
36. Bradac GB, Stojanovic J (1985) Die selektive-superselektive Angiographie und die therapeutische Embolisation der Arteria carotid externa. Radiol Jugosl 19: 15
37. Bradac GB, Ferszt R, Bender A, Schörner W (1986) Peritumoral edema in meningiomas. A radiological and histological study. Neuroradiology 28: 304
38. Bradac GB, Riva A, Schörner W, Stura G (1987) Cavernous sinus meningiomas: An MRI study. Neuroradiology 29: 578
39. Bradac GB, Riva A, Schörner W, Berger T, Duca S, Liboni W (1987) MRI in the study of intracranial meningiomas. In: Calabrò A, Leonardi M (eds) Computer aided neuroradiology. CIC, Rome
40. Bradac GB, Riva A, Berger T, Stura G, Duca S (1988) Il gadolinium-DTPA nella risonanza magnetica. Esperienze cliniche nella patologia intracranica. Radiol Med (Torino) 76: 33
41. Bradac GB, Riva A, Stura G (1988) Il gadolinium-DTPA in risonanza magnetica. Studio della patologia tumorale intracranica e spinale. Riv Neuroradiol [Suppl] 1: 101
42. Brain IF, Naidich TP, Leeds NE, et al. (1977) Dense intracranial epidermoid tumours. Radiology 122: 717
43. Brant-Zawadzki M, Berry J, Osaki L, Brasch R, Murovic J, Norman D (1986) Gd-DTPA in clinical MR of the brain. I. Intraaxial lesions. AJNR 7: 781
44. Brennan TG Jr, Krishna Rao CVG, Robinson W, Itani A (1977) Tandem lesions. Chromofobe adenoma and meningioma. J Comput Assist Tomogr 1: 517
45. Bright R (1831) Diseases of the brain and nervous system. Longman, London, pp 342-347 (Reports of medical cases, vol 2/1)
46. Brismar J, Cronquist S (1978) Therapeutic embolization in the external carotid artery region. Acta Radiol [Diagn] (Stockh) 19: 715
47. Burns PR, Naresh JHA, Bain GO (1986) Association of breast cancer with meningioma: A report of five cases. Cancer 58: 1537
48. Burrows EH, Leeds NE (1981) Neuroradiology, vol 1. Livingstone, New York, pp 1-74
49. Bydder GM, Kingsley DPE, Brown J, Niendorf HP, Young IR (1985) MR imaging of meningiomas including studies with and without gadolinium-DTPA. J Comput Assist Tomogr 9: 690
50. Cabezudo JM, Vaquero J, Garcia di Sola B (1981) Meningioma of the anterior part of the third ventricle. Acta Neurochir (Wien) 56: 219
51. Cantore G, Ciappetta P, Delfini R, Raco A (1986) Meningiomas of the posterior cranial fossa without dural attachment. Surg Neurol 25: 127
52. Carella RJ, Ransohoff J, Newall J (1982) Role of radiation therapy in the management of meningioma. Neurosurgery 10: 332
53. Carr DH, Brown J, Bydder GM, Steiner RE, Weinmann HJ, Speck U, Hall AS, Young IR (1984) Gadolinium-DTPA as a contrast agent in MRI: Initial clinical experience in 20 patients. AJR 143: 215
54. Castellano F, Ruggiero G (1953) Meningiomas of the posterior fossa. Acta Radiol [Suppl] (Stockh) 104: 164
55. Castillo RG, Geise AW (1985) Meningioma of the third ventricle. Surg Neurol 24: 525
56. Catz A, Reider-Grosswasser I (1986) Acoustic neurinoma and posterior fossa meningioma. Clinical and CT radiologic findings. Neuroradiology 28: 47
57. Chen WYK, Kepes JJ, Teglbjaerg PS (1985) Intracellular mucoid changes in tumor cells of meningiomas: a manifestation of polyvinyl pyrrolidone (PVP) effect on tissues with mesenchymal characteristics. J Neuropathol Exp Neurol 44: 606
58. Choux R, Chan M, Hassoun J (1975) Meningiome intraosseux chez un enfant. Neurochirurgia (Stuttg) 21: 89
59. Chronwall BM, McKeeves PE, Kornblith PL (1983) Glial and monglial neoplasms evaluated on frozen section by double immunofluorescence for fibronectin and glial fibrillary acidic proteins. Acta Neuropathol (Berl) 59: 283
60. Chui M, Tucker W, Hudson A, Bayer N (1985) High resolution CT of Meckel's cave. Neuroradiology 27: 403
61. Claveria LF, Sutton D, Tress BM (1977) The radiological diagnosis of meningiomas, the impact of EMI scanning. Br J Radiol 50: 15
61a. Codd MB, Kurland LT (1985) Descriptive epidemiology of primary intracranial neoplasms. Progress in Exp. Tumor Research 29: 1
62. Cophignon J, Lucena J, Clay C, Marchac D (1979) Limits to radical treatment of spheno-orbital meningiomas. Acta Neurochir [Suppl] (Wien) 28: 375
63. Courriere P, Tremoulet M, Eche N, et al. (1985) Hormonal steroid receptors in intracranial tumours and their relevance in hormone therapy. Eur J Cancer Clin Oncol 21: 711
64. Courville CB (1941) On the classification of meningiomas. Bull Los Angeles Neurol Soc 6: 21
65. Crompton MR, Gautier-Smith PC (1970) The prediction of recurrence in meningiomas. J Neurol Neurosurg Psychiatry 33: 80
66. Cushing H (1922) The meningiomas (dural endotheliomas) their source and favoured seats of origin (Cavendish Lecture). Brain 45: 282
67. Cushing H, Eisenhardt L (1938) Meningiomas, their classification, regional behaviour, life history and surgical and results. Thomas, Springfield
68. Deen HG, Scheithauer BW, Ebersold MJ (1982) Clinical and pathological study of meningiomas of the first two decades of life. J Neurosurg 56: 317
69. Dell S, Ganti SR, Steinberger A, McMartry J III (1982) Cystic meningiomas: a clinocoradiological study. J Neurosurg 57: 8
70. Di Chiro G, Hatazawa J, Katz DA, Rizzoli HV, de Michele DJ (1987) Glucose utilization by intracranial meningiomas as an index of tumor aggressivity and probability of recurrence: A PET study. Radiology 164: 521
71. Dietemann JL, Heldt N, Burguet JL, Medjeck L, Maitrot D, Wackenheim A (1982) CT findings in malignant meningiomas. Neuroradiology 23: 207
72. Dilenge D, Calderon H (1976) Cathéterisme super-sélectif et embolisation des pedicules artériels de deux meningiomes de la fosse posterieure. Neurochirurgie 22: 711
73. Djindjian R, Merland JJ (1978) Superselective arteriography of the external carotid artery. Springer, Berlin Heidelberg New York
74. Doyon D (1980) A case of intratympanic meningioma. J Neuroradiol 7: 209

75. Drayer BP, Rosenbaum AE (1979) Brain edema defined by cranial computed tomography. J Comput Assist Tomogr 3: 317
76. Du Boulay GH (1984) The plain x-ray characteristics of particular diseases of the skull and brain. In: du Boulay GH (ed) A textbook of radiological diagnosis, vol 1, pp 49-53
77. Dyke CG (1941) The roentgen-ray diagnosis of diseases of skull and intracranial contents. In: Golden R (ed) Diagnostic roentgenology. Nelson, New York
78. El-Banhawy A, Walter W (1962) The incidence and significance of the early filling of veins in carotid angiography of supratentorial meningiomas. Acta Neurochir (Wien) 10: 247
79. Fabiani A, Torta R, Favero M, Brignolio F, Benech F, Mostert M (1983) Atypical and polymorphic angioblastic tumors of the central nervous system. Neurosurgery 13: 223
80. Fagioli L, Mavilla L, Nuzzo G, Calbucci F, Trevisan C (1981) Preoperative embolization of brain meningiomas. Acta Neurochir (Wien) 57: 307
81. Ferrante L, Matronardi L, Acqui M, Fortuna A (1987) Recurrent cystic meningiomas. J Neurosurg Sci 31: 177
82. Ferszt R, Bradac GB (1988) Edema surrounding meningiomas: Radiological and histological considerations. In: Cervós-Navarro J, Ferszt R (eds) Stroke and microcirculation. Raven, New York
83. Ferszt R, Neu S, Cervós-Navarro J, Sperner J (1978) The spreading of focal brain edema induced by ultraviolet irradiation. Acta Neuropathol (Berl) 42: 223
84. Ferszt R, Hahm H, Cervos-Navarro J (1980) Measurement of the specific gravity of the brain as a tool in brain edema research. Adv Neurol 28: 15 "Brain Edema", Cervos-Navarro J, Ferszt R (eds). Raven Press, New York 1980
85. Ferszt R, Aruffo C, Iglesias J (1988) Immunohistochemische Befunde bei Hirntumoren. Zentralbl Pathol (in press)
86. Fine M, Brazis P, Palacios E, Neri G (1980) Computed tomography of sphenoid wing meningiomas: Tumor location related to distal edema. Surg Neurol 13: 385
87. Fletcher WA, Imes RK, Hoyt WF (1986) Chiasmal gliomas: appearance and longterm changes demonstrated by computerized tomography. J Neurosurg 65: 154
88. Fohanno D, Bitar A (1986) Sphenoidal ridge meningeoma. Adv Tech Stand Neurosurg 14: 137
89. Fohanno D, Metzger J, Margent P, Pertuiset B (1971) Les signes de thrombose totale ou partielle du sinus longitudinal superieur dans les meningiomes parasagittaux. Neurochirurgie 17: 25
90. Fornari M, Savoiardo M, Morello G, Solero CL (1981) Meningiomas of the lateral ventricles. Neuroradiological and surgical considerations in 18 cases. J Neurosurg 54: 64
91. Fukui M, Kitamura K, Ohgami S, Takaki T, et al. (1977) Radiosensitivity of meningiomas-analysis of five cases of highly vascular meningiomas treated by pre-operative irradiation. Acta Neurochir (Wien) 36: 47
92. Gabibov GA, Blinkov SM, Tcherekayev VA (1988) The management of optic nerve meningiomas and gliomas. J Neurosurg 68: 889
93. Gado MH, Phelps ME, Coleman RE (1975) An extravascular component of contrast enhancement in cranial computed tomography. I. The tissue blood ratio of contrast enhancement. Radiology 117: 589
94. Gado MH, Phelps ME, Coleman RE (1975) An extravascular component of contrast enhancement in cranial computed tomography. II. Contrast enhancement and the blood tissue barrier. Radiology 117: 595
95. Gautier-Smith PC (1970) Parasagittal and falx meningiomas. Butterworth, London
96. Geoffray A, Lèe YY, Jing B, Wallace S (1984) Extracranial meningiomas of the head and neck. AJNR 5: 599
97. Girard PF, Trillet M, Confavreux C, et al. (1977) Méningiomatose multiple et familiale. Un syndrome voisine de la neurofibromatose de Recklinghausen. Rev Neurol (Paris) 133: 359
98. Giuffre R (1984) Successful radical removal of an intracranial meningioma in 1835 by Professor Pecchioli of Siena. J Neurosurg 60: 47
99. Go KG, Wilmink JT, Molemaar WM (1988) Peritumoral brain edema associated with meningiomas. Neurosurgery 23: 175
100. Godel V, Samuel Y, Shanon E, et al. (1981) Maxillary meningioma appearing as exophthalmus. Arch Otolaryngol 107: 626
101. Goldberg R, Byrd S, Winter J, et al. (1980) Varied appearance of trigeminal neuroma on CT. AJR 134: 57
102. Graif M, Bydder GM, Steiner RE, Niendorf P, Thomas DGT, Young IR (1985) Contrast enhanced MR imaging of malignant brain tumors. AJNR 6: 855
103. Granich MS, Pilch BZ, Goodman ML (1983) Meningiomas presenting in the paranasal sinuses and temporal bone. Head Neck Surg 5: 319
104. Gregorus FK, Hepler RS, Stern WE (1975) Loss and recovery of vision with suprasellar meningiomas. J Neurosurg 42: 69
105. Grunberg SM, Daniels AM, Muensch H, et al. (1987) Correlation of meningioma hormone receptor status with hormone sensitivity in a tumor stem-cell assay. J Neurosurg 66: 405
106. Guarnaschelli JJ, Dzenitis AJ, Ogden LL (1985) Ectopic subgaleal meningioma and familial Neurofibromatosis. Surg Neurol 23: 371
107. Guidetti B, Delfini R, Gagliardi FM, Vagnozzi R (1985) Meningiomas of the lateral ventricles. Clinical, neuroradiological and surgical considerations in 19 cases. Surg Neurol 24: 364
108. Guidetti B, Ciappetta P, Domenicucci M (1988) Tentorial meningiomas: surgical experience with 61 cases and long-term results. J Neurosurg 69: 183
109. Guzowski J, Paprella M, Rao KN, Hoshiro J (1976) Meningiomas of the temporal bone. Laringoscope 86: 1141
110. Hadani MA, Rappaport ZH, Findlor G, Tadmor R, Sahar A (1985) Recurrent cystic meningioma. Neurochirurgia (Stuttg) 28: 202
111. Hahm H, Ferszt R, Müller J, Cervos-Navarro J (1980) Topography of diffuse brain edema. Adv Neurol 28: 299 "Brain Edema", Cervos-Navarro J, Ferszt R (eds). Raven Press, New York 1980
112. Hallgrimsson J, Bjornsson A, Gudmundsson G (1970) Meningioma of the neck. Case report. J Neurosurg 32: 695
113. Halliday WC, Yeger H, Dune GF, Phillips MJ (1985) Intermediate filaments in meningiomas. J Neuropathol Exp Neurol 44: 617
114. Hekster RE, Matricali B, Luyendjik W (1974) Presurgical transfemoral catheter embolization to reduce operative blood loss. J Neurosurg 41: 396
115. Heppner F (1955) Meningiomas of the third ventricle in children. Review of the literature and report of 2 cases

with uneventful recovery after surgery. Acta Neurol Psychiatr Belg 30: 472
116. Hieshima GB, Everhart FR, Mehringer CM, et al. (1980) Preoperative embolization of meningiomas. Surg Neurol 14: 119
117. Hitchcock E, Morris CS (1987) Immunocytochemistry of intracranial meningiomas. J Neurooncology 5: 357
118. Hiyama H, Kobayashi N, Ono Y, Kakinoki Y, Ebihara R, et al. (1987) Correlation between MR signal intensity and histologic findings in neurinomas and meningiomas of the brain. Acta Radiol [Suppl] (Stockh) 369: 176
119. Hoessly GF, Olivecrona N (1955) Report on 280 cases of verified parasagittal meningiomas. J Neurosurg 12: 614
120. Holden J, Dolman CL, Churg A (1987) Immunohistochemistry of meningiomas including the angioblastic type. J Neuropathol Exp Neurol 46: 50
121. Holtas S, Nyman V, Cronquist S (1984) Computed tomography of malignant limphoma of the brain. Neuroradiology 26: 33
122. Hoye SJ, Hoar CS, Murray JE (1960) Extracranial meningioma presenting as a tumor of the neck. Am J Surg 100: 486
123. Iba-Zizen MT, Cabanis EA, Stoffels C, Vignaud J, Kujas A, Kujas M, van Effenterre R, Pasquet G (1984) Apport de l'IRM à la pathologie de la region sphénoidale. J Neuroradiol 11: 285
124. Inoue YK, Nishibe Y, Hollinshead AC, Takeuchi J, Uchida Y, Handa H (1987) Isolation of Inoue-Melnick virus from human meningioma-derived cell cultures and detection of antibody in patients with meningioma. J Med Virol 21: 201
125. Iwaki T, Takeshita I, Fukui M, Kitomura K (1987) Cell kinetics of malignant evolution of meningothelial meningioma. Acta Neuropathol (Berl) 74: 243
126. Jääskeläinen J, Haltia M, Servo A (1986) Atypical and anaplastic meningiomas: Radiology, surgery, radiotherapy and outcome. Surg Neurol 25: 233
127. Jääskeläinen J, Laasonen E, Karkkainen J, Troupp H (1986) Hormone treatment of meningiomas: Lack of response to medroxyprogesterone acetate (MPA). A pilot study of five cases. Acta Neurochir (Wien) 80: 35
128. Jacobs DH, McFarlane MJ, Holmes FF (1987) Female patients with meningioma of the sphenoid Ridge and additional primary neoplasms of the breast and genital tract. Cancer 60: 3080
129. Jagadha V, Deck JHN (1987) Massive cerebral edema associated with meningioma. J Can Sci Neurol 14: 55
130. Jay JR, McLanghlin DT, Riley KR, Maituza RL (1985) Modulation of meningioma cell growth by sex steroid hormones in vitro. J Neurosurg 62: 757
131. Jellinger K, Slowik F (1975) Histological subtypes and prognostic problems in meningiomas. J Neurol 208: 279
132. Kakizoe S, Kajiro M, Hikita N (1987) Primary cutaneous meningioma. Report of a case. Acta Pathol Jpn 37: 511
133. Kalm H (1950) Ein malignes Tentorium meningeom mit Metastasierung in die Medulla oblongata und in die subarachnoidale Liquorräume. Dtsch Z Nervenheilkd 613: 131
134. Kapila A, Chakeres DW, Blanco E (1984) The Meckel cave: Computed tomographic study. Radiology 152: 425
135. Karasick JL, Mullan SF (1974) A survey of metastatic meningiomas. J Neurosurg 39: 206
136. Karp LA, Zimmerman LE, Borit A, Spencer W (1974) Primary intraorbital meningiomas. Arch Ophthalmol 91: 24
137. Katayama Y, Tsubokava T, Yoshida K (1985) Cystic meningiomas in infancy. Surg Neurol 25: 43
138. Kazner E, Wende S, Grumme T, et al. (1982) Computed tomography in intracranial tumors. Springer, Berlin Heidelberg New York
139. Kendall BE, Lee BCP (1977) Cranial chordomas. Br J Radiol 50: 687
140. Kendall BE, Moseley I (1977) Therapeutic embolization of the external carotid arterial tree. J Neurol Neurosurg Psychiatry 40: 937
141. Kendall BE, Symon L (1977) Investigation of patients presenting with cerebellopontine angle syndromes. Neuroradiology 13: 65
142. Kendall B, Pullicino P (1979) Comparison of consistency of meningiomas and CT appearances. Neuroradiology 18: 173
143. Kendall B, Reider-Grosswasser I, Valentine A (1983) Diagnosis of masses presenting within the ventricles and computed tomography. Neuroradiology 25: 11
144. Kennedy F (1911) Retrobulbar neuritis as an exact diagnostic sign of certain tumours and abscesses of the frontal lobes. Am J Med Sci 142: 355
145. Kepes JJ (1982) Meningiomas. Biology, pathology and differential diagnosis. Masson, New York
146. Kepes JJ (1986) The histopathology of meningiomas. A reflection of origins and expected behavior? J Neuropathol Exp Neurol 45: 95
147. Kernohan JW, Sayre GP (1952) Tumors of the central nervous system. AFIP, Washington
148. Kieffer SA, Larson DA, Gold LHA, Prentice WB, Stadlan EM, Seifert S (1973) Rapid circulation in intracranial meningiomas. Radiology 106: 575
149. Kim KS, Rogers LF, Lee C (1983) The dural lucent line; characteristics signs of hyperostosing meningioma en plaque. AJNR 141: 1217
150. Kim KS, Rogers LF, Goldblatt D (1987) CT features of hyperostosing meningioma en plaque. AJNR 8: 853
151. Klatzo L (1967) Neuropathologic aspects of brain edema. J Neuropathol Exp Neurol 26: 1
152. Klatzo I, Chui E, Fujiwara K, Spatz M (1980) Resolution of vasogenic brain edema. Adv Neurol 28: 359-373
153. Kleinschmidt-de Masters BK, Avakian JJ (1985) Wallenberg syndrome caused by CSF metastasis from malignant intraventricular meningioma. Clin Neuropathol 4: 214
154. Kochi N, Tani E, Morimura T, Itagaki T (1983) Immunohistochemical study of fibronectin in human glioma and meningioma. Acta Neuropathol (Berl) 59: 119
155. Kolluri VRS, Reddy DR, Reddy PK, Nardu MRC, Rao SBP, Sumathe C (1987) Meningiomas in childhood. Childs Nerv Syst 3: 271
156. Kotwica Z, Jagodzinski Z, Polis L (1985) Meningiomas of the lateral ventricle. Neurochirurgia (Stuttg) 28: 199
157. Kubota T, Hirano A, Sato K, Yamamoto S (1985) Fine structure of psammoma bodies at the outer aspect of blood vessels in meningioma. Acta Neuropathol (Berl) 66: 163
158. Kunert-Radek J, Stepien H, Radek A, Pawlikowki M (1987) Somatostatin suppression of meningioma cell proliferation in vitro. Acta Neurol Scand 75: 434
159. Lanksch WR (1982) The diagnosis of brain edema by computed tomography. In: Hartmann A, Brock M (eds) Treatment of cerebral edema. Springer, Berlin Heidelberg New York
160. Lanuza M, Poon TP, Belmonte A (1985) Mixed teratoma and meningioma in the temporoparietal region. Surg Neurol 23: 399

161. Lasjaunnias PL (1981) Craniofacial and upper cervical arteries. Williams and Wilkins, Baltimore
162. Lee Y, Lin S, Horner FA (1979) Third ventricular meningioma mimicking a colloid cyst in a child. AJR 132: 669
163. Leeds NE, Seaman WE (1962) Fibrous dysplasia of the skull and its differential diagnosis: a clinical and roentgenographic study of 46 cases. Radiology 78: 570
164. Leeds NE, Taveras JM (1969) Dynamic factors in diagnosis of supratentorial brain tumors by cerebral angiography. Saunders, Philadelphia, pp 76-85
165. Leibel AS, Wara WM, Sheline GE, et al. (1976) The treatment of meningiomas in childhood. Cancer 37: 2709
166. Lesoin F, Jomin M, Bouchez B, Durot MS, Clarisse J, Arnott G, Pellerin P, Francois P (1985) Management of cavernous sinus meningiomas. Neurochirurgia (Stuttg) 28: 195
167. Lesoin F, Jomin M, Dupard T, Rousseaux M, Viand C, Krovisic I, Lozes C, Delhandsheer JM (1985) Les méningiomas kystiques. 3 observations. Neurochirurgie 31: 421
168. Ljunggren B (1982) The case of General Wood. J Neurosurg 56: 471
169. Llyod GA (1982) Primary orbital meningioma: a review of 41 patients investigated radiologically. Clin Radiol 33: 181
170. Lombardi G (1967) Radiology in neuro-ophthalmology. Williams and Wilkins, Baltimore
171. Long DM (1973) Vascular ultrastructure in human meningiomas and schwannomas. J Neurosurg 38: 409
172. Lopez MJ, Olivares JL, Ramos F, Redondo JA, Ramon y Cayal S, Banzo J, Legido A (1988) Giant meningioma in a 5 month-old infant. Childs Nerv Syst 4: 112
173. Louis A (1774) Mémoire sur les tumeurs fongueuses de la dura-mère. Mem Acad R Chir (Paris) 5: 1
174. Ludwin SK, Conley FK (1975) Malignant meningioma metastasizing through the cerebrospinal pathways. J Neurol Neurosurg Psychiatry 38: 136
175. Ludwin SK, Rubinstein LJ, Russell DS (1975) Papillary meningioma, a malignant variant of meningioma. Cancer 36: 1363
176. Lusins JO, Nakagawa H (1981) Multiple meningiomas evaluated by computed tomography. Neurosurgery 9: 137
177. Magdelenat H, Pertuiset BF, Poisson M, et al. (1982) Progestin and oestrogen receptors in meningiomas. Biochemical characterization, clinical and pathological correlations in 42 cases. Acta Neurochir (Wien) 64: 199
178. Magliocco C, Santucci N, Tenenbaum P, Kropp F (1978) Meningiomi del recesso laterale del IV° ventricolo. Riv Neurobiol 24: 274
179. Manelfe C, Guiraud B, David J, Eymeri J, Tremoulet M, Espagno J, Rascol A, Geraud J (1973) Embolisation par cathétérisme des méningiomes intracraniens. Rev Neurol (Paris) 128: 339
180. Manelfe C, Djindjian R, Picard L (1975) Embolisation par cathétérisme fémoral des tumeurs irriguées par l'artère carotide externe. A propos de 40 cas. Acta Radiol [Suppl] (Stockh) 347: 175
181. Manelfe C, Lasjaunias P, Ruscalleda J (1986) Preoperative embolization of intracranial meningiomas. AJNR 7: 963
182. Mani RL, Hedgcock MW, Mass SI, et al. (1978) Radiographic diagnosis of meningiomas of the lateral ventricle. Review of 22 cases. J Neurosurg 49: 249
183. Maniglia AJ (1978) Intra- and extra-cranial meningiomas involving the temporal bone. Laryngoscope [Suppl] 88: 12
184. Markwalder TM, Markwalder RV, Markwalder HM (1979) Meningioma of the anterior part of the third ventricle. J Neurosurg 50: 233
185. Markwalder TM, Seiler RW, Zava DT (1985) Antiestrogenic therapy of meningiomas. A pilot study. Surg Neurol 24: 245
186. Markwalder TM, Gerber HA, Waelti E, Schaffner T, Markwalder RV (1988) Hormonotherapy of meningiomas with medroxyprogesterone acetate. Immunohistochemical demonstration of the effects of medroxyprogesterone acetate on growth fractions of meningioma cells using the monoclonal antibody Ki-67. Surg Neurol 30: 97
187. Marmarou A, Takagi H, Shulman K (1980) Biomechanics of brain edema and effects on local cerebral blood flow. Adv Neurol 28: 345-358
188. Martuza RL, Miller DC, MacLaughlin DT (1985) Estrogen and progestin binding by cytosolic and nuclear fractions of human meningiomas. J Neurosurg 62: 750
189. Mayberg MR, Symon L (1986) Meningiomas of the clivus and apical petrous bone. Report of 35 cases. J Neurosurg 65: 160
190. McCarty CS, Taylor WF (1979) Intracranial meningiomas: Experiences at the Mayo Clinic. Neurol Med Chir (Tokyo) 19: 569
191. Melamed S, Sahar A, Beller AJ (1979) The recurrence of intracranial meningiomas. Neurochirurgia (Stuttg) 22: 47
192. Mendiratta SS, Rosenblum JA, Strobos RJ (1967) Congenital meningioma. Neurology (Minneap) 17: 914
193. Mennig H (1970) Geschwülste der Augenhöhle und ihre operative Behandlung. Thieme, Stuttgart
194. Meyer JE, Lepke LA, Lindfors KK, et al. (1983) Chordomas: their CT appearance in the cervical, thoracic and lumbar spine. Radiology 153: 693
195. Michel RG, Woodard BH (1979) Extracranial meningioma. Ann Otol 88: 407
196. Mikhael MA (1977) Diminished density surrounding a meningioma verified to be an overlying cystic astrocytoma. J Comput Assist Tomogr 1: 349
197. Mikhael MA, Ciric IS, Wolff AP (1985) Differentiation of cerebello pontine angle neuromas and meningiomas with MRI imaging. J Comput Assist Tomogr 9: 852
198. Miller DC, Ojemann RG, Proppe KN, McGinnis BD, Grillo HC (1985) Benign metastasizing meningiomas. J Neurosurg 62: 763
199. Miller E, Crockard HA (1987) Transoral transclival removal of anteriorly placed meningiomas at the foramen magnum. Neurosurgery 20: 966
200. Mirimanoff RO, Dosoretz DE, Linggood RM, Ojemann RG, Martuza RL (1985) Meningioma: Analysis of recurrence and progression following neurosurgical resection. J Neurosurg 62: 18
201. Moller A, Hatam A, Olivecrona H (1978) The differential diagnosis of pontine angle meningioma and acoustic neuroma with computed tomography. Neuroradiology 17: 21
202. Monajati A, Heggeness L (1982) Patterns of edema in tumours versus infarcts: visualization of white matter pathways. AJNR 3: 251
203. Moss SD, Rockswold GL, Chow SN, Yock D, Berger MS (1988) Radiation-induced meningiomas in pediatric patients. Neurosurgery 22: 758
204. Nager GT (1964) Meningiomas involving the temporal bone. Thomas, Springfield

205. Nakamura M, Inoue HK, Ono N, Kunimine H, Tamada J (1987) Analysis of hemangiopericytic meningiomas by immunohito-chemistry, electron microscopy and cell culture. J Neuropath Exp Neurol 46: 58
206. Nauta HJM, Tucker WS, Horsey WS, Bilbao JM, Gonsalves C (1979) Xanthochromic cysts associated with meningiomas. J Neurol Neurosurg Psychiatry 42: 529
207. New PFJ, Aronow S, Hesselink JR (1980) National Cancer Institute study. Evaluation of computed tomography in the diagnosis of intracranial neoplasms-meningiomas. Radiology 136: 665
208. New PFJ, Hesselink JR, O'Carroll CP, Kleinman GM (1982) Malignant meningiomas: CT and histologic criteria, including a new CT sign. AJNR 3: 267
209. Nijensohn DE, Aranjo JC, MacCarthy CS (1975) Meningioma of Meckel's cave. J Neurosurg 43: 197
210. Oberson R, Tribolet N, Campiche R, Probst A (1974) Embolisation de l'artère méningée moyenne cathétérisée par voie fémorale pour l'hémostase pré-opératoire d'un méningiome de la convexité. Schweiz Med Wochenschr 104: 388
211. Olivecrona H (1934) Die parasagittalen Meningiome. Thieme, Leipzig
212. Olson JJ, Beck DW, Schlechte JA, et al. (1986) Hormonal manipulation of meningiomas in vitro. J Neurosurg 65: 99
213. Olson JJ, Beck DW, MacJindre JW, et al. (1988) Androgen receptors in meningiomas. Cancer 61: 952
214. Ono M, Ono M, Rhoton AL Jr, Barry M (1984) Microsurgical anatomy of the region of the tentorial incisura. J Neurosurg 60: 365
215. Osborn AG (1980) Craniofacial venous plexus: angiographic study. AJNR 1: 541
216. Parisi C, Tropea R, Giuffrida S, Lombardo M, Giuffrè F (1986) Cystic meningiomas. J Neurosurg 64: 35
217. Parkinson D (1965) A surgical approach to the cavernous portion of the carotid artery. J Neurosurg 23: 474
218. Pech A, Cannoni M, Zanaret M, Triglia JM (1981) ENT manifestations of extracranial meningioma. J Fr Otorhinolaryngol 30: 87
219. Peña CE (1977) Meningioma and intracranial hemangiopericytoma. A comparative electron microscopy study. Acta Neuropathol (Berl) 39: 69
220. Penn RD (1980) Cerebral edema and neurological function; CT evoked responses and clinical examination. Adv Neurol 28: 383-394
221. Philippon J, Foucin JF, Grob R, et al. (1984) Cerebral edema associated with meningiomas: Possible role of secretory - excretory phenomenon. Neurosurgery 14: 295
222. Piatt J Jr, Campbell GA, Oakes WJ (1986) Papillary meningioma involving the oculomotor nerve in infant. J Neurosurg 64: 809
223. Pullicino P, Kendall BE, Jakubowski J (1980) Difficulties in diagnosis of intracranial meningiomas by computed tomography. J Neurology Neurosurg Psychiatry 43: 1022
224. Pykett JL, Newhouse JH, Buonanno FS, Brady TJ, Goldman MR, Kistler JP, Pohost GM (1982) Principles of nuclear magnetic resonance imaging. Radiology 143: 157
225. Ramos F Jr, Ba Zeze V, Velut S, Jan M (1987) Les méningiomes kystiques. Intérêt d'une classification radiochirurgicale. J Neuroradiol 14: 271
226. Reit KG, Fujiwara K, di Chiro G, et al. (1980) Serial measurements of CT attenuation and specific gravity in experimental cerebral oedema. Radiology 135: 343
227. Reubi JC, Maurer R, Klyn JGM, et al. (1986) High incidence of somatostatin receptors in human meningiomas: biochemical characterization. J Clin Endocrinol Metab 63: 433
228. Reulen HJ, Graham R, Spatz M, Klatzo I (1977) Role of pressure gradients and bulk flow in the dynamics of vasogenic brain edema. J Neurosurg 46: 24
229. Reulen HJ, Tsayumu M, Tack A, et al. (1978) Clearance of edema fluid into CSF. A mechanism for resolution of vasogenic brain edema. J Neurosurg 48: 754
230. Richter HP, Schachenmayr W (1983) Preoperative embolization of intracranial meningiomas. Neurosurgery 13: 261
231. Rodriguez-Carbajal J, Palacios E (1974) Intraventricular meningiomas of the fourth ventricle. AJR 31: 120
232. Rosalki SB, McGee LE (1962) Meningioma presenting as nasopharyngeal tumour. Report of two cases. J Laryngol 76: 133
233. Rosario R, Adelman L, Prager JR, Stein MB (1979) Meningioma of the pineal region and third ventricle. J Neurosurg 50: 489
234. Rose WS, Makhija MC, Sattenspiel S (1980) Meningioma presenting as a tumor in the neck. AJR 134: 1070
235. Rubenstein AB, Shalit MN, Cohen ML, Zandbank U, Reichental E (1984) Radiation-induced cerebral meningioma: A recognizable entity. J Neurosurg 61: 966
236. Russell DS, Rubinstein LJ (1989) Pathology of tumours of the nervous system. Arnold, London
237. Russell EJ, George AE, Kricheff II, Budzilovich G (1980) Atypical computed tomographic features of intracranial meningioma. Radiology 135: 673
238. Rutka JT, Muller PJ, Chui M (1985) Preoperative gelfoam embolization of supratentorial meningiomas. Can J Surg 21: 441
239. Rutka JT, Giblin JR, Dougherty DV, et al. (1986) An ultrastructural and immunocysto chemical analysis of leptomeningeal and meningeoma cultures. J Neuropathol Exp Neurol 45: 285
240. Rutka JT, Apodoca G, Stern R, Rosenblum M (1988) The extracellular matrix of the central and peripheral nervous system: Structure and function. J Neurosurg 69: 155
241. Sadar ES, Conomy JP, Benjamin SP, Levine HL (1979) Meningiomas of the paranasal sinuses, benign and malignant. Neurosurgery 4: 227
242. Salama N, Stafford N (1982) Meningiomas presenting in the middle ear. Laryngoscope 92: 92
243. Salamon G, Guerinel G, Combalbert A, et al. (1969) Etude artériographique des meningiomes intracrâniens. Correlations radio-anatomiques. Ann Radiol (Paris) 12: 661
244. Sasaki S, Ferszt R, Cervos-Navarro J (1977) Transendothelial vesicular transport of protein in brain induced by ultraviolet irradiation. Acta Neuropathol (Berl) 40: 207
245. Saunders ML, Young HF, Becker DP, Greenbeg RP, Newton PG, Corales RL, Ham WT, Porlishock JT (1980) The use of the laser in neurological surgery. Surg Neurol 14: 1
246. Schnegg JF, Gomez F, Le Marchand-Beraud T, de Tribolet N (1981) Presence of sex steroid hormone receptors in meningioma tissue. Surg Neurol 15: 415
247. Schoenberg BS, Christine BW, Whisnant JP (1975) Nervous system neoplasms and primary malignancies of other sites: The unique association between meningiomas and breast cancer. Neurology (Minneap) 25: 705
248. Schörner W, Felix R, Claussen C, Fiegler W, Kazner F, Speck U, Niendorf HP (1984) Kernspintomographische

Diagnostik von Hirntumoren mit dem Kontrastmittel Gadolinium-DTPA. ROFO 141: 511
249. Schwechheimer K, Kartenbeck J, Moll R, Franke WW (1984) Vimentin filament-desmosome cytoskeleton of diverse types of human meningiomas. A distinctive diagnostic feature. Lab Invest 51: 584
250. Scotti G, Yu CY, Colombo N, Norman D, Dillon W, Newton H (1987) Magnetic resonance imaging of cavernous sinus involvement by pituitary adenomas. In: Calabrò A, Leonardi M (eds) Computer aided neuroradiology. CIC, Rome
251. Sekhar LN, Jannetta PJ (1984) Cerebello-pontine angle meningiomas. Microsurgical excision and follow up results. J Neurosurg 60: 500
252. Sekhar LN, Jannetta PJ, Maroon JC (1984) Tentorial meningiomas. Surgical management and results. Neurosurgery 14: 268
253. Servo A, Jääskeläinen J, Wahlström T, Haltis M (1985) Diagnosis of intracranial haemangiopericytomas with angiography and CT scanning. Neuroradiology 27: 38
254. Shaungshoti S, Panyathanya R (1973) Ectopic meningiomas. Arch Otolaryngol 98: 102
255. Sheehy JP, Crockard A (1983) Multiple meningiomas: A long-term review. J Neurosurg 59: 1
256. Sigel ZM, Messina AV (1976) Computed tomography: the anatomic basis of the zone of diminished density surrounding meningiomas. AJR 127: 139
257. Simpson D (1957) The recurrence of intracranial meningiomas after surgical treatment. J Neurol Neurosurg Psychiatry 20: 22
258. Skullerud K, Löken AC (1974) The prognosis of meningiomas. Acta Neuropathol (Berl) 29: 337
259. Smith HP, Challa VR, Moody DM, Kelly DL Jr (1981) Biological features of meningiomas that determine the production of cerebral edema. Neurosurgery 8: 428
260. Soffer D, Pittaluga S, Feiner M, Beller AJ (1983) Intracranial meningiomas following low-dose irradiation to the head. J Neurosurg 59: 1048
261. Som PM, Sacher M, Strenger SW, Biller HF, Malis LI (1987) Benign metastasizing meningiomas. AJNR 8: 127
262. Spagnoli MV, Goldberg HI, Grossmen RI, Bilaniuk LT, Gomori JM, Hackeny DE, Zimmerman RA (1986) Intracranial meningiomas: High-field MR imaging. Radiology 61: 369
263. Stattin S (1986) Significance of some angiographic signs of intracranial meningiomas. Acta Radiol [Diagn] (Stockh) 5: 530
264. Stevens JM, Ruiz JS, Kendall BE (1983) Observations on peritumoral oedema in meningioma. II. Mechanism of oedema production. Neuroradiology 25: 125
265. Stevens JM, Ruiz JS, Kendall BE (1983) Observations on peritumoral oedema in meningioma. I. Distribution, spread and resolution of vasogenic oedema seen on computed tomography. Neuroradiology 25: 71
266. Stevens JM, Kendall BE, Love S (1984) Radiological features of subpendymoma with emphasis on computed tomography. Neuroradiology 26: 223
267. Suyama T, Tamaki N, Fujiwara K, Hamano S, Kimura M, Matsumoto S (1987) Peritumoral and intratumoral hemorrhage after gelatin sponge embolization of malignant meningioma: Case report. Neurosurgery 21: 944
268. Symon L (1977) Olfactory grove and suprasellar meningiomas. Adv Tech Stand Neurosurg 4: 67
269. Takahashi M, Lombardi G, Passerini A, Ohno S (1973) Primary intraorbital meningiomas: A roentgenologic study. Neuroradiology 5: 95
270. Takase M, Watanabe O (1988) Radiosensitive hemangiopericytoma of the falx. Case report. J Neurosurg 68: 640
271. Tampieri D, Pokrupa P, Melanson D, Ethier R (1987) Primary ectopic meningioma of the neck: MR features. J Comput Assist Tomogr 11: 1054
272. Tani E, Ikeda K, Yamagata S, Nishiura M, Higashi N (1974) Specialized junctional complexes in human meningioma. Acta Neuropathol (Berl) 28: 305
273. Taptas JN (1982) The so called cavernous sinus: A review of the controversy and its implications for neurosurgeon. Neurosurgery 11: 712
274. Taveras JM, Wood EH (1969) Diagnostic neuroradiology. Williams and Wilkins, Baltimore
275. Teasdale E, Patterson J, McLelland D, Macpherson P (1984) Subselective preoperative embolization for meningiomas: A radiological and pathological assessment. J Neurosurg 60: 506
276. Telenius R (1966) Angiographic appearance of angioblastic meningiomas. Acta Radiol [Diagn] (Stockh) 5: 554
277. Theron J, Clay C, Djindjian R (1975) Etude angiographique et embolisation d'une fistule artério-veineuse durale paracaverneuse d'une type anatomique particulier. Ann Radiol (Paris) 18: 729
278. Tilzer LL, Plap PU, Evans JP, Stone D, Alward K (1982) Steroid receptor proteins in human meningiomas. Cancer 49: 633
279. Tobler WD, Tew JM (1987) The role of the carbon dioxide lase in skull base tumours. Neurosurgery 2: 397
280. Tognetti F, Donati R, Bollini C (1987) Metastatic spread of benign intracranial meningioma. J Neurosurg Sci 31: 23
281. Treisch J, Schörner W, Laniado M, Felix R (1987) Charakteristika intrakranieller Meningeome in der magnetischen Resonanztomographie. ROFO 146: 207
282. Valavanis A, Schubiger O, Hayek J, Pouliadis G (1981) CT of meningiomas on the posterior surface of the petrous bone. Neuroradiology 22: 111
283. Valavanis A, Schubiger O, Naidich TP (1987) Clinical imaging of the cerebello-pontine angle. Springer, Berlin Heidelberg New York
284. Vidovszky T, Benoist G (1979) Comparative study of trigeminal neurinomas and parasellar meningiomas. Acta Neurochir [Suppl] (Wien) 28: 397
285. Wang AM, Power TC, Rumbaugh CL (1985) Lateral ventricular meningioma. Comput Tomogr 9: 355
286. Wara WM, Sheline GE, Newman H, Townsed JJ, Boldrey EB (1975) Radiation therapy of meningiomas. AJR 123: 453
287. Weinberger JM, Birt BD, Lewis AJ, Nedzelski JM (1985) Primary meningioma of the nasopharynx. Case report and review of ectopic meningioma. J Otolaryngol 14: 317
288. Wende S, Bohe J, Schubert R, Schulz V (1983) Lung metastasis of a meningioma. Neuroradiology 24: 287
289. Wharen RE, Anderson RE, Scheithauer B, Sundt TM (1984) The Nd:YAG lase in neurosurgery. I. Laboratory investigations: dose-related biological response of neural tissue. J Neurosurg 60: 531
290. Wharen RE, Anderson RE, Sundt TM (1984) The Nd: YAG laser in neurosurgery. II. Clinical studies: and adjunctive measure for hemostasis in resection of arteriovenous malformations. J Neurosurg 60: 540
291. Whittle IR, Foo MS, Besser M, et al. (1984) Progesterone and oestrogen receptors in meningiomas: biochemical

and clinico-pathological considerations. Aust NZ J Surg 54: 325
292. Wickbom I (1953) Angiographic determination of tumor pathology. Acta Radiol (Stockh) 40: 529
293. Wilner D (1982) Radiology of bone tumors and allied disorders, vol 1. Saunders, Philadelphia
294. Wolf BS, Huang YP, Newman CM (1963) The superficial sylvian venous drainage system. AJR 89: 398
295. Wolff M, Rankow RM (1971) Meningioma of the parotid gland: An insight into the pathogenesis of extracranial meningioma. Hum Pathol 2: 453
296. Wolters B, Kleinsasser O (1985) Intranasale extradurale Meningiome. Laryngol Rhinol Otol 64: 198
297. Wood MW, White RJ, Kernohan JW (1957) One hundred intracranial meningiomas found incidentally at necropsy. J Neuropathol Exp Neurol 16: 337
298. Worthington C, Caron JL, Melanson D, Leblanc R (1985) Meningioma cysts. Neurology (NY) 35: 1720
299. Wu JK, Kadson DL, Whitemore EL (1985) Metastatic meningioma to cervical vertebra. Case report. Neurosurgery 17: 75
300. Yagishita A, Hassonn J, Vincentelli F, Jiddane M, Salamon G (1985) Neuroradiological study of hemangiopericytomas. Neuroradiology 27: 420
301. Yamashima T (1985) Meningiothelial rosettes in the canine subrachnoid space. Acta Neuropathol (Berl) 66: 223
302. Yamashita J, Handa H, Iwaki K, Abe M (1980) Recurrence of intracranial meningiomas with special reference to radiotherapy. Surg Neurol 14: 33
303. Yasargil MG, Mortara RW, Curic M (1980) Meningiomas of the basal posterior cranial fossa. Adv Tech Stand Neurosurg 7: 3
304. Yasuoka S, Okazoki H, Danbe JR, McCarty CS (1978) Foramen magnum tumours: Analysis of 57 cases of benign extramedullary tumours. J Neurosurg 49: 828
305. Yeakley JW, Kulkarni MV, McArdle CB, Haar FL, Tang RA (1988) High-resolution MR imaging of juxtasellar meningiomas with CT and angiographic correlation. AJNR 9: 279
306. Zava DT, Markwalder TM, Markwalder RV (1984) Biological expression of steroid hormone receptors in primary meningioma cells in monolayer culture. Clin Neuropharmacol 7: 382
307. Zimmerman RD, Fleming CA, Sant-Louis LA, Lee BCP, Manning JJ, Deck MDF (1985) Magnetic resonance imaging of meningiomas. AJNR 6: 149
308. Zink PM, Trappe AE (1989) Intraossäre Meningiome. Ein Bericht über zwei Fälle. Nervenarzt 60: 52
309. Zülch KJ (1979) Histological typing of tumours of the central nervous system. WHO, Geneva
309a. Zülch KJ (1956) Biologie und Pathologie der Hirngeschwülste. In: Olivecrona H, Tönnis W (eds) "Handbuch der Neurochirurgie". Springer, Berlin Heidelberg

MIX
Papier aus verantwortungsvollen Quellen
Paper from responsible sources
FSC® C105338

If you have any concerns about our products,
you can contact us on
ProductSafety@springernature.com

In case Publisher is established outside the EU,
the EU authorized representative is:
Springer Nature Customer Service Center GmbH
Europaplatz 3, 69115 Heidelberg, Germany

Printed by Libri Plureos GmbH
in Hamburg, Germany